Exercise Therapy in the Management of Musculoskeletal Disorders

Exercise Therapy in the Management of Musculoskeletal Disorders

Edited by

Fiona Wilson

John Gormley

Juliette Hussey

Discipline of Physiotherapy
School of Medicine
Trinity College, Dublin
Ireland

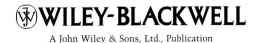

A John Wiley & Sons, Ltd., Publication

Library of Congress Cataloging-in-Publication Data
Exercise therapy in the management of musculoskeletal disorders / edited by Fiona Wilson, John Gormley, Juliette Hussey.
      p. ; cm.
   Includes bibliographical references and index.
   ISBN 978-1-4051-6938-7 (pbk. : alk. paper)   1. Musculoskeletal system–Diseases–Exercise therapy.
I. Wilson, Fiona, 1966-   II. Gormley, John.   III. Hussey, Juliette.
   [DNLM: 1. Musculoskeletal Diseases–therapy.   2. Exercise Therapy. WE 140]
   RC925.5.E94   2011
   616.7'0642–dc22
                                                              2010041337

A catalogue record for this book is available from the British Library.

This book is published in the following electronic formats: ePDF 9781444340143; ePub 9781444340150

Set in 9.5/11.5pt Sabon by Toppan Best-set Premedia Limited
Printed and bound in Malaysia by Vivar Printing Sdn Bhd

1 2011

Contents

Contributors

Leanne Bisset PhD, MPhty (Sports and Musculoskeletal), BPhty
Research Fellow, Physiotherapy Department, Royal Brisbane & Women's Hospital, Herston, Queensland; School of Physiotherapy and Exercise Science, Griffith University, Gold Coast, Queensland, Australia

Thomas J. Gill IV, MD
Chief, Sports Medicine Service, Massachusetts General Hospital; Associate Professor of Orthopedic Surgery, Harvard Medical School; Medical Director, Boston Red Sox Baseball Club, Boston, Massachusetts, USA

John Gormley BSc (Hons), DPhil
Senior Lecturer, Discipline of Physiotherapy, School of Medicine, Trinity College Dublin, Ireland

Juliette Hussey MA, MSc, PhD, Dip Phys, Dip Advanced Physiotherapy Studies
Senior Lecturer and Head of Discipline, Discipline of Physiotherapy, School of Medicine, Trinity College Dublin, Ireland

Mandy Johnson PhD, MPhil, Grad Dip Phys, MCSP
Senior Academy Physiotherapist, Manchester United Football Club, Sir Matt Busby Way, Old Trafford, Manchester, UK

Ruth Magee MPHty, BA (Hons), BSc, MISCP, MCSP
Physiotherapist in private practice, Enniskerry Physiotherapy Clinic, Enniskerry Medical Centre, Enniskerry, County Wicklow, Ireland

Nicholas J. Mahony BA, MB, MSc, FFSEM, MICGP
Lecturer, Department of Anatomy, School of Medicine, Trinity College Dublin, Ireland

Alison H. McGregor PhD, MSc, MCSP
Reader in Biodynamics, Human Performance Group, Biosurgery & Surgical Technology, Division of Surgery, Oncology, Reproductive Biology & Anaesthetics (SORA), Faculty of Medicine, Imperial College London, Charing Cross Hospital, London, UK

Grace O'Malley BSc, MSc, MISCP
Senior Paediatric Physiotherapist, The Children's University Hospital, Dublin, Ireland

Kirsty Peacock BSc, MSc (Sports Med), MISCP
Formerly Physiotherapist to Munster Rugby and Irish Rowing Team; Currently Physiotherapist in Private Practice, Munster Sports Physiotherapy, Limerick, Ireland

Michael M. Reinold PT, DPT, ATC, CSCS
Rehabilitation Coordinator/Assistant Athletic Trainer, Boston Red Sox Baseball Club; Coordinator of Rehabilitation Research and Education, Department of Orthopedic Surgery, Division of Sports Medicine, Massachusetts General Hospital, Boston, Massachusetts, USA

Kyle J. Rodenhi MS, PT
Physical Therapist, Massachusetts General Hospital Sports Physical Therapy, Boston, MA, USA

Dr Kevin Sims MPhty St, PhD, FACP
Clinical Supervisor/Casual Lecturer, University of Queensland; Physiotherapist, Cricket Australia, Centre of Excellence, Australia

Michelle Smith PhD, MPhty (Sports Phty), BMR (Phty), BPhysEd
Lecturer, Division of Physiotherapy, School of Health and Rehabilitation Sciences, The University of Queensland, Queensland, Australia

Professor Bill Vicenzino PhD, MSc, Grad Dip Sports Phty, BPhty
Chair in Sports Physiotherapy and Head of Division of Physiotherapy, School of Health and Rehabilitation Sciences, The University of Queensland, Queensland, Australia

Anne S. Viser PT, DPT, ATC
Physical Therapist, Massachusetts General Hospital Sports Physical Therapy, Boston, Massachusetts, USA

Fiona Wilson BSc, MSc (Sports Med), MA, MISCP
Lecturer/Chartered Physiotherapist, Discipline of Physiotherapy, School of Medicine, Trinity College Dublin, Ireland

Preface

In recent years, the balance of evidence has led to exercise as the treatment of choice in musculoskeletal dysfunction. This has seen a shift in focus in both undergraduate and postgraduate training towards exercise therapy with an accompanying demand for appropriate texts. This book addresses this need and covers the fundamentals of using exercise as a treatment modality in the broad range of pathologies including osteoarthritis, inflammatory arthropathies and osteoporosis. It is anticipated that this book will provide a good progression from the fundamental principles described in this text and would specifically relate these principles to specific areas and pathologies.

The specific aims of this book are to:

- Provide the student with a comprehensive overview of the role of exercise therapy in the management of musculoskeletal disorders

- Evaluate the evidence for use of exercise therapy as a treatment modality
- Educate the student in the potential of exercise as a treatment modality
- Provide practical ideas for use of exercise therapy in the management of musculoskeletal disorders in different areas of the body and for differing pathologies
- Promote the use of exercise among physiotherapists.

This book is primarily aimed at undergraduate physiotherapy students and postgraduate physiotherapists and other clinicians who are starting to design rehabilitation programmes for patients. An emphasis of the book is the relevance of evidence but there is also a practical bias with ideas of rehabilitation programmes and specific exercises.

To
Olly and Daisy,
Sean,
Robert and Gavin

The Principles of the Use of Exercise in Musculoskeletal Disorders

1

Introduction

1

John Gormley

Historical perspectives

In many countries physiotherapy or physical therapy is the one of the largest health care professions after medicine and nursing. One of the major modalities of treatment at a physiotherapist's disposal is exercise. Examining the history of the profession demonstrates that exercise is a fundamental component of treatment. Indeed many would argue that exercise is the most important treatment available to physiotherapists. The use of exercise in both the prevention and treatment of disease and disorders pre-dates the formation of the physiotherapy profession. This chapter examines the history of exercise and its role in disease management.

History of exercise

The use of exercise to promote health was recognised in China in approximately 2500BC, when Hua T'o, a Chinese surgeon, promoted exercise based on the movement of animals (MacAuley, 1994). The ancient Greeks encouraged physical wellbeing and the greatest exponent of exercise was Galen. In his work, De Sanitate Tuenda dealt with the beneficial effects of exercise. In explaining how exercise worked, the amount of exercise and the types of exercise, he used numerous case studies to illustrate his ideas (Bakewell, 1997). What is clear is that not only was the importance of exercise recognised by the Greeks, but also the need for a prescription, encompassing not only the type of exercise, but also the dose or amount necessary for wellbeing. Galen believed that exercise in a moderate form was beneficial but that excess was dangerous as it worked by balancing the effects of eating and drinking, and therefore it was important to avoid excess of either.

In the seventeenth century, the Italian mathematician Giovanni Borelli (1608–1679) first described the body as a machine and used mathematics to describe the functioning of the body. This was the first attempt to apply scientific principles to human movement and Borelli would be regarded as the father of biomechanics. As the body was described as a machine with moving parts, it could be concluded that it needed movement for optimum effectiveness (Bakewell, 1997). In 1740, a French doctor, Nicolas Andry (1658–1742) wrote a book entitled *L'Orthopedie*, in which he described the need for

Exercise Therapy in the Management of Musculoskeletal Disorders, First Edition. Edited by Fiona Wilson, John Gormley and Juliette Hussey.
© 2011 Blackwell Publishing Ltd

correct posture to prevent and treat deformities of the spine and also the need for active exercise rather than passive movement.

The idea that exercise was beneficial for the human body was hampered in the eighteenth century by a number of renowned British physicians including John Hunter (1728–1793), who promoted rest for the treatment of 'disablements' (Buckwalter, 1995). One of the greatest exponents of the use of rest was the Liverpool physician Hugh Owen Thomas (1834–1878), who is regarded as the father of British orthopaedics and during his career invented the Thomas splint for a fractured femur. He advocated that healing was enhanced by rest and that early mobilisation only caused adhesions. It is interesting that this philosophy is contrary to modern-day treatments for musculoskeletal disorders.

Contrary views to this pervading opinion were put forward by Julius Wolff (1836–1902) and Just Lucas-Championniere (1843–1913). Wolff proposed Wolff's Law: that mechanical stress altered bone and that bone was laid down at sites of stress and reabsorbed at sites where there was little stress. Lucas-Championniere, a French physician, argued that rest was detrimental to the musculoskeletal system and that fractures (especially those near joints) were best treated by early mobilisation and by massage. Although Wolff and Lucas-Championniere's theories have been subsequently proved to be correct, it was not until the mid 1950s that early exercise and mobilisation in the treatment of fractures started to become accepted.

Exercise and physiotherapy

The major changes in the use of exercise came about in the twentieth century, with an increase in knowledge and with the formation of the physiotherapy profession. The origins of the physiotherapy profession can be traced back to 1894 as the Society of Trained Masseuses, which became a legal and professional organisation in 1900 as the Incorporated Society of Trained Masseuses. In 1920, exercise was incorporated as part of the profession when the Incorporated Society of Trained Masseuses amalgamated with the Institute of Massage and Remedial Gymnastics. In 1944 the society was renamed the Chartered Society of Physiotherapists. Treatment at this time primarily consisted of exercise, electrotherapy and massage. Gymnasiums were a common sight in physiotherapy schools and exercise was a major component of the physiotherapy curriculum, which required students to undertake physical education classes.

Physiotherapists at this time, however, were not autonomous professionals as they had their treatments prescribed by doctors. In 1977, physiotherapists gained professional autonomy, therefore allowing them to treat patients as they felt appropriate. The fact that up to 1977 physiotherapists were unable to carry out treatment as they thought appropriate was not conducive to either innovation or to research. Despite physiotherapists using exercise on a daily basis, most of the advances in exercise therapy came from the fields of exercise physiology, biomechanics and medicine. This research led to a greater understanding of how the body works and how exercise can benefit all the major systems in the body.

The changes in 1977 and the movement of physiotherapy education into universities provided an opportunity for increased innovation and research in exercise therapy. Furthermore, in 1986 the Remedial Gymnasts Board was disbanded and remedial gymnasts became members of the physiotherapy profession. It is therefore surprising that interest in exercise as a treatment appeared to decrease in the 1990s. The reasons for this are unclear but are probably multifaceted, spanning changes in undergraduate curricula, increased specialisation and new technology. In recent years there has been a renewed interest in exercise and its beneficial effects not only among physiotherapists but also in health care in general.

The benefits of exercise

Exercise has beneficial effects on the cardiovascular system and the musculoskeletal system and indeed other body systems, but it is in the cardiovascular and musculoskeletal systems that the effects are most obvious. Aerobic exercise leads to a decreased demand on the heart at any particular workload with decreased blood pressure and decreased heart rate, increased stroke volume and consequently at a given heart rate, an increased cardiac output. Muscles become more efficient in extracting oxygen from the circulating blood through an increase in the number and size of mitochondria. In bone, there is an increase in the density of weight-bearing bones and therefore is recommended for the prevention of osteoporosis in at-risk groups, e.g. post-menopausal women. Exercise also has beneficial effects on the density of bone in non-weight-bearing bones. Upper limb athletes, e.g. tennis players, have greater bone density in their dominant arm compared with their non-dominant arm (Kontulainen *et al.*, 1999).

Strength training in itself will not necessarily lead to the changes in blood pressure, heart rate and stroke volume as seen with aerobic exercise. At the level of muscle there will be an increase in the size of fast twitch muscle fibres, which accounts for the hypertrophy of muscles and also neuromuscular adaptations, leading to a more efficient muscle contraction. Strength training increases the strength of ligaments and tendons and can lead to increased bone density. The increase in bone density seen in resistance training is greater compared with the changes seen in aerobic training. Cumulatively exercise has effects throughout the body.

Exercise is an active treatment which needs the co-operation and assent of the individual to be treated. Exercise programmes and exercise prescriptions therefore rely on the participation of the individual, and will not be successful if an individual is not compliant with their prescription. The lack of compliance or adherence to exercise programmes is one of the greatest reasons for poor results. Individuals often want a 'quick fix', i.e. a painkiller or a manipulation, so exercise may not be popular with many patients. It is therefore important that physiotherapists explain and educate people about their condition and their exercise programme in order to achieve high levels of adherence.

This chapter reviewed how the use of exercise has developed over the centuries. The following chapter examines the practical application of exercise in the management of musculoskeletal disorders.

References

Bakewell, S. (1997) Medical gymnastics and the Cyriax collection. *Medical History*, 41(4), 487–495.

Buckwalter, J.A. (1995) Activity vs. rest in the treatment of bone, soft tissue and joint injuries. *Iowa Orthopaedic Journal*, 15, 29–42.

Kontulainen, S., Kannus, P., Haapasalo, H., Heinonen, A., Sievänen H., Oja, P. and Vuori, I. (1999) Changes in bone mineral content with decreased training in competitive young adult tennis players and controls: a prospective 4-yr follow-up. *Medicine and Science in Sports and Exercise*, 31(5), 646–652.

MacAuley, D. (1994) A history of physical activity, health and medicine. *Journal of the Royal Society Medicine*, 87(1), 32–35.

2 The Role of Exercise in Managing Musculoskeletal Disorders

Fiona Wilson

SECTION 1: INTRODUCTION AND BACKGROUND

Chapter 1 reviewed how the use of exercise has developed over the centuries. This chapter will examine the practical application of exercise in the management of musculoskeletal disorders. The intention is not to be too condition- or joint-specific as these areas will be examined in detail later in the book. The aims of this chapter are to:

- Review current evidence and emerging bias towards exercise as a modality of choice over the past 10 years
- Discuss different areas of exercise: aerobic training; strength training; range of movement and flexibility exercise; proprioceptive and balance training
- Examine modalities and techniques employed when prescribing exercise.

Evidence for the role of exercise in managing musculoskeletal disorders

A search of the literature was conducted using the keywords musculoskeletal ± disorder, disease, injury, dysfunction and exercise. The search engines that were employed were: Medline, PubMed, Cinahl, Science Direct, PEDro, *Cochrane Database of Systematic Reviews* and Google Scholar. A number of trials have focused on the efficacy of therapeutic exercise in specific areas of disorder such as low back pain and whiplash. Other trials are less specific and have examined the influence of exercise on pain or disability associated with musculoskeletal disorders.

A small number of trials have examined the role of exercise on long-term musculoskeletal health in a large cohort. These trials are both prospective and longitudinal in design. Bruce *et al.* (2005) studied the long-term impact of running and other aerobic

Exercise Therapy in the Management of Musculoskeletal Disorders, First Edition. Edited by Fiona Wilson, John Gormley and Juliette Hussey.
© 2011 Blackwell Publishing Ltd

exercises on musculoskeletal pain in a cohort of healthy ageing male and female seniors. The prospective study was carried out over 14 years. The cohort of 866 individuals was stratified into runners and community-based controls. Pain was the primary outcome measure and was assessed in annual surveys. The subjects were further stratified into 'ever-runners' and 'never-runners' to include runners who had stopped running. It was found that runners had a lower body mass index (BMI) and less arthritis than community controls, and although they reported slightly more fractures, this result was not significant. Likewise, the ever-runners had lower BMI and less arthritis than controls. Exercise was associated with significantly lower pain scores in both the runners and ever-runners when compared with controls. The authors concluded that consistent exercise patterns over the long term in physically active seniors are associated with about 25% less musculoskeletal pain than reported by sedentary controls.

Berk *et al.* (2006) concluded that exercise can have a beneficial effect on postponement of disability due to musculoskeletal disease, even if introduced at a later stage in life. A prospective cohort of 549 patients was studied annually for 16 years using a Health Assessment Disability Index as the outcome measure. All patients were given a rating to describe their levels of general activity at baseline and at the end of the study. While active exercisers performed well at the end of the study in comparison with the cohort that had remained sedentary, it was found that participants who were initially inactive but increased their activity levels as the study progressed achieved excellent end-of-study values, which were similar to the values in those who were active throughout. The authors concluded that exercise has benefits for the musculoskeletal system even if introduced later in life. The implications for the clinician of the above studies relate to the importance of education for all patients and that exercise can be introduced at any time for any patient to provide benefit to the musculoskeletal system. The studies also clearly point to the fact that lack of activity is a risk factor for musculoskeletal disease.

Establishment of risk factors for any disorder or disease is one of the first lines of long-term management for any clinician. A small number of studies have specifically addressed exercise/activity and its relationship to the onset of musculoskeletal disorders. Heesch *et al.* (2006) examined this relation-

ship between levels of physical activity and stiff or painful joints in a 3-year prospective study. In a cohort of 8770 women (mid-age and older) it was found that both mid-age and older women who were active at low, moderate or high levels had significantly lower odds of reporting stiff or painful joints than their sedentary counterparts. This was particularly noted in the older age group and the authors suggested that this study was the first to show a dose–response relationship between physical activity and arthritis symptoms. While the previous study focused on older women, Pihl *et al.* (2002) examined whether the physically active lifestyle of physical education teachers reduced their risk of musculoskeletal disorders when compared with sedentary controls. The researchers established that the lifestyle of physical education teachers led them to have significantly lower adjusted risk of all musculoskeletal disorders as well as improved body composition in comparison with the control group.

The evidence reviewed above and that which will follow in the book, on balance, supports therapeutic exercise in the management of musculoskeletal disorders. However, it is pertinent to examine the role of exercise or activity in itself as a risk factor for musculoskeletal disease. There are two main areas where exercise or activity has been established as increasing the risk of developing musculoskeletal disorders, that is, in sport and in certain occupations. Increasing evidence from the past decade has strengthened the relationship between occupational activities and the risk of developing and accelerating osteoarthritis (Conaghan, 2002). McLindon *et al.* (1999) established that the number of hours of heavy physical activity was linked to the risk of radiographic knee osteoarthritis with the risk increasing in obese people. However, the injuries were associated with heavy lifting and high levels of squatting and kneeling. Kujala *et al.* (1994) demonstrated an increased risk of developing osteoarthritis in the lower limbs in former male elite athletes in a retrospective study of 2049 subjects. However, the evidence is still biased towards moderate levels of activity having beneficial effects on the musculoskeletal system for both management and prevention of musculoskeletal disorders. Studies which highlight exercise as a risk factor for disorders consistently identify high levels of loading as being the causative element, and clinicians who prescribe exercise must be aware of this.

In conclusion, exercise has been shown in a number of high-quality trials to have benefits both in the management and prevention of musculoskeletal disorders. While there is some evidence that exercise may have harmful effects on the musculoskeletal system in the form of disease or injury, this is almost exclusively associated with abnormal or high levels of loading.

SECTION 2: PRACTICAL APPLICATION OF EXERCISE

Components of fitness

The components of fitness may be described as the following: aerobic or cardio-respiratory fitness; muscle strength and endurance; flexibility or range of motion (ROM); and body composition (American College of Sports Medicine (ACSM), 2000). However, a frequent inclusion in recent years is balance, co-ordination and proprioception (Shankar, 1999). Body composition depends on many factors including genetics, activity levels and diet, and for the purposes of this text will be addressed primarily in Chapter 15, which deals with obesity. Therefore, the components of fitness which will be referred to throughout this text may be summarised as:

- Aerobic or cardio-respiratory fitness
- Muscle strength and endurance
- Flexibility or ROM
- Balance, co-ordination and proprioception.

Exercise prescription

Prescription of exercise requires a clear understanding of the components of fitness and knowledge of appropriate levels of intensity, frequency and duration of each element that will be suitable for each patient. Beyond prescribing specific exercise, the health benefits of general exercise should be considered, particularly at initial assessment. In 2007, the ACSM revised its guidelines for levels of physical activity that are required to see health benefits. For healthy adults under age 65, it is now recommended that they (ACSM, 2008):

Do moderately intense cardio 30 minutes a day, 5 days a week
Or
Do vigorously intense cardio 20 minutes a day, 3 days a week
And
Do 8–10 strength-training exercises, 8–12 repetitions of each exercise twice a week.

The clinician who is prescribing exercise must consider the two main principles of training, which are overload and specificity. When considering the components of fitness, these principles can be most effectively applied to aerobic fitness, muscle strength, and endurance and flexibility. The principle of overload states that for an organ or tissue to improve its function, it must be exposed to loading at a level to which it is not accustomed (ACSM, 2000). The principle of specificity states that training effects form an exercise modality are specific to the exercise performed and the muscles involved. This is seen when high-repetition, low-load exercise produces an increase in muscular endurance but little increase in strength. Conversely, high-load and low-repetition exercise will increase strength but will have little effect on endurance (ACSM, 2000).

Components of an exercise session

Designing an exercise programme requires consideration of the distinct phases of a session, which are defined in sequence as:

- Warm-up
- Endurance phase
- Recreational activities
- Cool-down.

Traditional clinical treatment sessions would frequently introduce exercise to include one or more components at the end of a modality, such as manipulation. However, best practice is to structure a programme and to ensure that all components are covered. It is common to focus on one area such as strength training and neglect to include other areas in the patient's treatment plan, which demonstrates a lack of consideration for the patient's general health. Focusing on one area such as strength training does not consider the overall benefits of all components of fitness to the musculoskeletal system, as outlined in the previous chapter. A programme that is designed into the phases listed above is more likely to cover all components of fitness in a more structured way.

Warm-up

The warm-up facilitates a transition for the body to move from a state of rest to exercise. It allows the heart rate to achieve a steady increase to exercising levels, facilitates increased blood flow to muscles and may increase soft tissue extensibility and thus enhance performance and reduce injury. The warm-up should consist of around 10 minutes of low-intensity exercise which facilitates activity in large joints such as the hips, knees and shoulders and uses large muscle groups. A good example of such exercise would be deep knee bends with arm swinging or step-ups.

Stretches should follow this activity with specific joint and muscle groups targeted individually for the patient. Consideration should also be given to the level of loading which specific muscle groups will experience during the activity which will follow. A generic stretching programme should be avoided as this may fail to target important areas for individual patients and may lead to lengthy stretching programmes that interrupt the flow of the warm-up. Stretching and flexibility are discussed later in this chapter.

The final stage of the warm-up will allow the heart rate to reach the target exercise levels and thus will include more high-level aerobic activity, which may start to replicate that used during the endurance phase.

Endurance phase

The endurance phase develops cardio-respiratory fitness and should comprise about 10–60 minutes of continuous or intermittent aerobic activity. This should be set at a level that is appropriate for the patients and is based on previous assessment of levels of fitness. Activities which use large muscle groups should be employed for optimal effect. The duration of this phase should be inversely related to the intensity of the activity. Resistance training and specific exercise in a rehabilitation programme may be included in this phase (ACSM, 2000).

Recreational activities

Inclusion of games, skills or challenges following the endurance phase may make the programme more interesting and encourage the patient to adhere to the programme. This may be particularly important in the rehabilitation of an athlete or an individual with an occupational injury.

Cool-down

The purpose of the cool-down is to facilitate a graduated return to the pre-exercise state. It allows heart rate and blood pressure to return to normal and enhances lactate removal. The format should be very similar to the warm-up and should include exercise of diminishing intensity. In practical terms, it presents an opportunity for the clinician to further assess the patient's response to the programme.

Prescription of aerobic exercise

The benefits of aerobic exercise for the musculoskeletal system were outlined in the previous chapter. The aim of prescription of aerobic exercise is to generate an improvement in maximal oxygen consumption (VO_{2max}). The VO_{2max} of an individual defines their aerobic capacity and is a measure of their maximal oxygen uptake. Endurance training has the effect of making the cardio-respiratory system more efficient when the training is performed regularly, and consequent improvements will be seen in the VO_{2max}. As the VO_{2max} and heart rate of an individual are related in a linear fashion, measurement of heart rate during exercise is a good reflection of the individual's VO_{2max} or aerobic capacity. It must be remembered that changes not only take place in the cardiac and pulmonary systems but also at a localised muscular level. Changes in VO_{2max} are directly related to the intensity, frequency and duration of the prescribed exercise and these elements should be given primary consideration in exercise prescription.

Type of exercise

There are many factors to consider when prescribing aerobic exercise for the patient with a

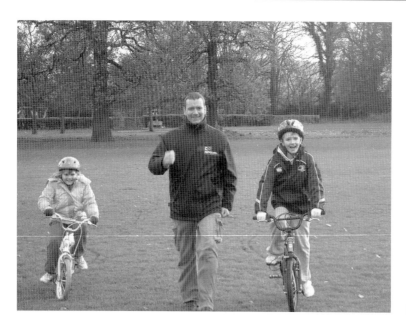

Figure 2.1 Power walking.

musculoskeletal disorder. The usual recommendation is to prescribe exercise which uses as many large muscle groups as possible in a repeated, aerobic pattern – clear examples are running and swimming. However, prescribing exercise in a patient with a musculoskeletal disorder can present a challenge as their condition may limit their function. The clinician needs to have a good understanding of the limitations of the disorder and prescribe a mode of exercise accordingly. One of the most challenging aspects of designing an aerobic exercise programme is to plan one to which the patient will adhere in the long term. Short-term adherence is frequently managed by asking the patient to attend for supervision on a regular basis, however, long-term benefits to the patient's health will only be seen when the mode of exercise is maintained. Therefore it is important that very careful consideration is given to the mode of exercise that is selected. Most ambulant patients with a musculoskeletal disorder, provided it is not severe and in the lower limbs, will be able to commence a walking programme. The benefits of walking are that patients are familiar with the exercise and that they are often easily able to fit it into their lifestyle as no equipment is needed. However, there is a risk that walking would be performed at a level which is too low and therefore insufficient to challenge the cardiovascular system, particularly as it may be performed with minimal movement of the trunk and upper limbs. Some simple and safe adaptations

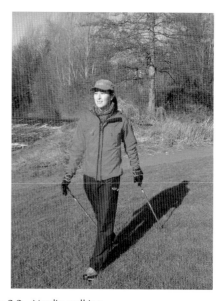

Figure 2.2 Nordic walking.

can make the exercise more challenging such as adding in definite arm movements with weights in the hands, as seen in power walking (Fig. 2.1), which encourages the recruitment of more muscle groups and enhances the aerobic effect. Nordic walking uses poles in the hands, which not only encourages greater use of the trunk and upper limbs but also enhances stability for those who may be challenged by balance (Fig. 2.2).

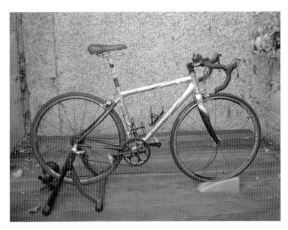

Figure 2.3 Bicycle on 'rollers'.

Swimming is an excellent exercise as it does not load the joints and recruits most of the major muscle groups. However, many adults are poor swimmers or may not have easy access to a pool as public leisure centres become scarcer. However, if it is enjoyed by the patient, a good swimming programme can be very beneficial. Hydrotherapy which involves exercise in heated water has been shown to present numerous benefits in patients with musculoskeletal disease. Many hospital physiotherapy departments would have such a pool and this should be considered if it is available. However, this is frequently only offered as a short course of treatment and consideration needs to be given to a mode of exercise which will be used in the long term.

Cycling is a good source of challenge to the cardio-respiratory system and has the advantage that it may be used as a mode of transport for some patients and therefore can be a lifestyle change. Exercise of the trunk and upper limbs is minimal but it may be suitable for patients who have a lower limb disorder. An exercise bike can be used by those who are nervous of cycling in traffic; patients can purchase cycling 'rollers' from any bicycle shop to convert a normal bike into one that is stationary (Fig. 2.3).

Prescription of exercise when rehabilitating an athlete requires specific consideration. The aim should be to return the athlete to their sport as quickly as possible. Loss of aerobic fitness during rehabilitation of an injury will prevent a rapid return to a competitive environment, which is the primary concern for most athletes. The type of aerobic exercise should be as close to their sport as possible, with adaptations if necessary. For example, a runner with

a lower limb injury may commence aqua jogging using a flotation vest, which will ensure that similar muscle groups and kinematics will be employed during rehabilitation. It should also be remembered that an athlete will have a much higher starting point in terms of fitness and may need to be prescribed higher intensity exercise as their goal is to maintain fitness rather than achieve it.

Exercise intensity

There are a number of different methods of setting the exercise intensity but the mode which may be most practical and simple for the musculoskeletal clinician involves prescribing as a percentage of maximum heart rate (HR_{max}). The ACSM (2008) recommends between 55/65% up to 90% of HR_{max} to achieve benefit. While those individuals whose are very unfit at the start of the programme would require prescription at the lower end of intensity, those who are fit would be working at the upper end of intensity. For the average individual, prescription at 70–80% of HR_{max} would be suitable to see improvement. Best practice requires establishment of the patient's HR_{max} by means of a progressive physiological or 'step' test. However, the equation which estimates the HR_{max} (below) may be used when this is not available, i.e.

$$\text{Estimated } HR_{max} = 220 - \text{age}.$$

Exercise duration

The duration of exercise is governed by the intensity as high intensity exercise will require shorter duration periods than low intensity to achieve the same benefits. The ACSM guidelines outlined earlier in the chapter should be reviewed to establish minimum requirements for each patient. In general, for the average individual who is exercising at 70–80% of HR_{max}, a duration of 20–30 minutes excluding warm-up and cool-down will be sufficient to benefit the patient. As mentioned previously, this should be adapted accordingly for the very unfit or conversely, the very fit patient.

Exercise frequency

Exercise frequency for the musculoskeletal patient may be governed by clinical visits which may be limited to once or twice per week. However, optimal benefits will be achieved with three to five sessions per week. This demands adherence by the patient that may be achieved in a number of ways, the most successful of which requires that the patient is supervised in a clinic or gym. However, this is both costly and not practical, particularly as long-term benefits are only achieved by maintenance of the programme following discharge. Training diaries may be useful as are classes at a local gym, and the aim should be to educate the patient regarding the importance of maintaining the exercise frequency. Of course, for the Olympic athlete who is already doing two aerobic training sessions daily, this should be replicated in rehabilitation to maintain fitness. The patient who is starting from a very low fitness level may achieve benefits by starting at two sessions per week. Although the frequency must be adjusted for each patient, the ultimate goal for the average individual should be to at least meet the minimum requirements as recommended by the ACSM and outlined earlier in the chapter.

Progression of the programme

The rate of progression of the programme will depend on the patient and their goals, which will have been established at the original assessment. As this text is concerned with rehabilitation of musculoskeletal injury, it will also depend on the rate of resolution of the injury. The intensity, duration and frequency of exercise may be low (40–50% HR_{max}), short (15 minutes) and limited to three times per week for the patient who is commencing the programme. The ultimate aim would be that this patient will have progressed to moderately intense exercise for 30 minutes, five times a week, or vigorously intense exercise for 20 minutes, three times a week. The programme should be commenced with caution, and assessment should always be ongoing and the patient's response to the programme should be constantly monitored. As the patient finds that the programme becomes less challenging, which may be demonstrated when the established exercise intensity is no longer enough to reach heart rate goals, then intensity, frequency and duration may be increased gradually and with caution. Maintenance of improvement should be considered at discharge and a programme should be planned

which the patient may adapt to their lifestyle to facilitate long-term benefits.

Prescription of muscle strength and endurance exercise

Strength is regarded as the maximum force that a muscle can exert and endurance refers to the ability to maintain the force over time. Both are required for normal function of muscles and different muscles have different functions. Some muscles have a greater proportion of slow twitch or type I fibres and thus demonstrate greater endurance, such muscles are associated with functions such as postural control. Other muscles have a greater proportion of fast twitch or type II fibres and are associated with rapid generation of force. Resistance training improves the capacity of a muscle to generate and/or maintain force. When prescribing resistance training, the overload principle should be applied. This may be achieved by increasing the load, the number of repetitions or the number of weight-training sessions above levels normally experienced. Muscle strength is developed by using low repetitions, typically 8–12 repetitions, with a resistance or weight which is close to the maximum that may be lifted or moved. To improve muscle endurance, high repetitions with low load are employed.

Types of resistance

Huber and Wells (2006) define the modes of resistance exercise as *isometric* (constant length), *isotonic* (constant tension), *isokinetic* (constant velocity) and *plyometric* (increased length). The most commonly used resistance exercise is isotonic muscle work in the form of free or machine-based weights. Resistance may be manual, given by the clinician, or mechanical, in the form of resistance from machine, free, pulley or elastic-based weights.

Isometric exercise

Isometric resistance may be given by the therapist, gravity or by a constant weight. Isometric exercise

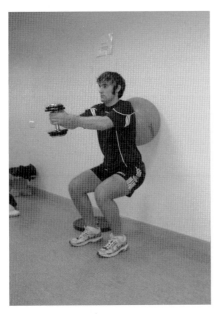

Figure 2.4 Isometric activity of a number of muscle groups.

is beneficial when low loading and low levels of balance and control are required. It is also useful in rehabilitation of musculoskeletal injury when range of joint motion is limited or when there is a desire to strengthen a muscle in a particular point in a movement arc. There is a lack of consensus regarding time of contraction, but 10 seconds is a good minimum starting point. Isometric exercise may be selected to work a small group of muscles. Multiple muscle groups may be exercised isometrically by using a more complex activity such as a squat while holding a medicine ball (Fig. 2.4).

Isotonic exercise

Isotonic exercise may be facilitated using machine, elastic resistance, pulleys, hydraulic or free weights with or without gravity assistance or resistance. One of the advantages of this method is that it is frequently measurable in that the weight can be fixed at a specific resistance (measured in kilograms). This enhances prescription and measurement of progression. Machines and pulleys frequently help isolate activity to a joint or limb by fixing the rest of the patient's body. The disadvantage of this is that incorrect technique and 'trick movements' may be easily applied, decreasing the

efficacy of the exercise as the patient compensates for muscle weakness by activating other muscle groups. Free weights using hand-held weights, bars and discs such as Olympic weights, elastic resistance and gym balls among others are perhaps the most effective but most challenging mode of muscle strengthening. Free weights require good control and good technique that should be taught by the therapist prescribing the exercise. Trick movements are common when free weights are employed particularly as a patient tries to employ gravity or momentum to aid movement of a weight. Figure 2.5a demonstrates poor technique in a squat exercise; the weight is too heavy and the patient cannot maintain good position of the lower limbs as they return to a standing position. In Figure 2.5b, the weight is lighter and the patient is encouraged to keep the hips and knees in the midline to facilitate the correct exercise.

Plyometric exercise

Plyometric exercise prescription is based on the physiological principle that a maximum contraction follows a maximum stretch during an eccentric action. A concentric action follows an eccentric action to produce an optimum concentric action (Huber and Wells, 2006). A typical example is a high jump followed by a deep squat. Such exercise is most suitable in the rehabilitation of athletes where it will replicate their sport and thus apply the principle of specificity well.

Open versus closed kinetic chain exercise

It is pertinent at this point to make a short note regarding the benefits of open versus closed kinetic chain exercise. The kinetic chain refers to the limb which is linked by a series of joints. In a closed kinetic chain, the end of the chain is in contact with or 'planted' on a surface so the foot or the hand will be resisted by the surface, for example, when performing a standing squat. In an open kinetic chain, it is not fixed and can move freely as seen when sitting on a stool and swinging the lower leg forwards. The type of muscle activity which is observed is quite different in the two types of exercise. One of the advantages of the closed kinetic

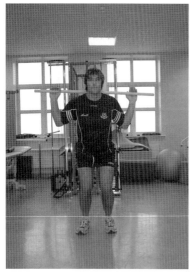
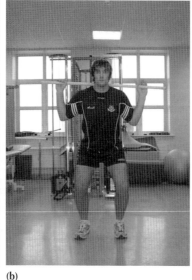

(a)   **(b)**

Figure 2.5 (a) Poor technique in a squat exercise, note the position of the lower limbs. (b) Correct technique in a squat exercise.

chain is that multiple muscle groups are recruited and that there are increased proprioceptive demands on the joints.

Intensity, frequency and volume of exercise

The intensity of exercise is measured by establishing the 1RM, which is the maximum weight that an individual can lift or move once through the full ROM. Strength gains will be established when the weight is set at 60–70% of the 1RM and repetitions of up to 15 performed twice a week (see ACSM guidelines above). To improve endurance, lighter weights and higher repetitions are prescribed. When rehabilitating a musculoskeletal injury, it may not be possible to establish the 1RM; in this instance a conservative estimate with careful monitoring may be the most appropriate approach. There are many theories regarding muscle strengthening and the reader is encouraged to explore this further to develop a more comprehensive understanding.

Strength and endurance training is frequently at the core of a programme to rehabilitate a patient with a musculoskeletal disorder. The later chapters of this book will describe the joint-specific approaches to this modality with supporting evidence. As many patients have multiple pathologies, other factors must be considered in the prescription of strengthening exercise, in particular its effect on

blood pressure. Increases in blood pressure during high resistance exercise, particularly isometric exercise, are much greater than that during continuous aerobic exercise. Thus prescription of resistance exercise for the patient with both musculoskeletal and cardiovascular disease must be considered carefully.

Prescription of range of motion or flexibility exercise

The area that appears to inspire the greatest controversy in inclusion in fitness programmes is that of prescription of stretching exercises, which are also known as flexibility or ROM exercises. The area of greatest debate is around the benefits of stretching programmes in reducing risk of musculoskeletal injury. There is a wealth of research in the area and the reader is encouraged to analyse this in a critical manner. Many of the studies lack robust methodology and there still appears to be no clear consensus (Thacker *et al.*, 2004; Fradkin *et al.*, 2006; Small *et al.*, 2008) although many experienced clinicians and patients alike (particularly athletes) present anecdotal evidence of its efficacy. Some of this research is presented in the later chapters dealing with specific joints. For the purposes of this chapter, a simplistic view is taken in that a healthy and functioning joint will move through its full ROM and rest in a neutral position, allowing those around it to do likewise. When there is limitation of ROM, which may be due to many factors including muscle shortness or imbalance, the normal function of the whole kinetic chain is compromised. Thus a fitness programme should aim to achieve optimal ROM of joints and extensibility of soft tissues to enhance function with an argument that it may also reduce risk of injury.

A number of different types of exercise increase ROM: passive, active and active-assisted.

Passive exercise

Passive ROM exercise is the most simple and must be performed by a clinician on a patient. Such a movement will be performed during routine assessment of a patient with a musculoskeletal disorder to establish joint integrity and limitations of movement. It is useful when active movement is painful, as in the case of muscular injury, but of course it is labour intensive. Passive ROM exercise will frequently be a starting point with little stretching taking place, however, to progress the joint ROM, the joint should be stretched at the end of range except in cases where further damage or instability may occur.

Active range of motion

Active ROM exercise involves the patient actively taking the joint through the full ROM. Stretches may then be added on to increase the ROM by pushing the movement beyond its original end point. Such exercises can be easily included in an aerobic programme. The sedentary patient who is starting a programme may have limited ROM in a number of joints as a result of inactivity and may benefit from inclusion of very simple ROM exercises, which often are well placed in the warm-up section of a programme.

Active-assisted range of motion exercise

Some patients may be unable to achieve full ROM actively but with limited help may reach target levels. Use of the other limb or props such as sticks

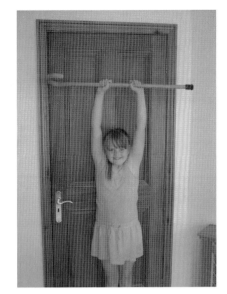

Figure 2.6 Active-assisted exercise using a stick to increase range of motion in the shoulder.

or pulleys may help the patient move the joint further (Fig. 2.6).

Types of stretching

Stretching exercises should complement ROM exercise and good practice demands that stretching is preceded by active or passive ROM exercise to assess the integrity and limitations of a joint. The addition of stretching exercise allows increases in the ROM. There are a number of different types of stretches, which are frequently described as *static*, *proprioceptive neuromuscular facilitation* (PNF) and *ballistic*.

Static stretching

A static stretch involves moving a joint to its end point or slowly stretching a muscle until mild discomfort is experienced. The position is held for an extended period of time. There is no consensus regarding the optimal time to hold the stretch and anywhere between 10 and 30 seconds has been suggested. However, most clinicians would suggest that a stretch time of at least 20 seconds and preferably 30 seconds or more is required to observe a relaxation in the muscle as the stretch response of the muscle spindle subsides, which allows further

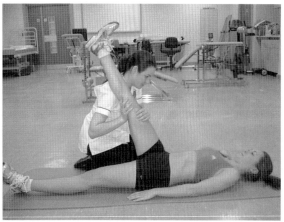
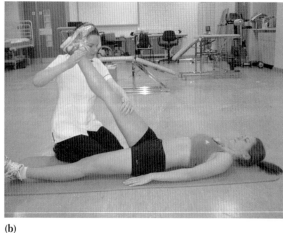

(a)   **(b)**

Figure 2.7   (a) A therapist resists isometric contraction of the hip extensors prior to a stretch. (b) A therapist assists in a stretch of the hip extensors.

movement or stretch. The stretch can be performed by a therapist, who assists in achieving optimum length of the muscle or joint ROM, or a patient may apply overpressure themselves to facilitate the same action. This is probably the safest type of stretch.

PNF

PNF stretching involves activating either the agonist or antagonist muscles immediately before a stretch is performed. This is based on the theory of reciprocal inhibition in which the maximum activation of one muscle inhibits activation of its antagonist, thus allowing optimal relaxation and stretching. This type of stretching often includes the 'hold-relax' technique, where a therapist stretches a muscle to resistance, resists an isometric contraction of a muscle for around 10 seconds, following which the therapist asks the patients to relax and stretches the muscle further. In Figure 2.7a the therapist resists an isometric contraction of the hip extensors and follows this with a stretch (Fig. 2.7b).

Ballistic stretching

Ballistic stretching involves bouncing movements with the aid of momentum to increase ROM, for example kicking a straight leg in the air to increase hip ROM and lengthen hamstrings. It is less popular as it has been suggested that the rapid movement involved may activate the muscle spindle and thus reduce the potential to increase ROM. This type of stretching may not be suitable for many patients with musculoskeletal disorders but is popular with athletes (following a static stretch) as it replicates movements performed during sporting activity.

Frequency, intensity and duration

Compared with the other areas of fitness, there is limited consensus regarding optimal dosage required to achieve good ROM and flexibility. A good rule to follow would be to include stretches in the warm-up of any aerobic or strengthening programme and to pay regular attention to those muscle groups or joints where limitations have been noted. The ACSM (2000) suggests:

Type: A general stretching routine that exercises major muscle and/or tendon groups using static or PNF techniques
Frequency: A minimum of 2–3 days per week
Intensity: To a position of mild discomfort
Duration: 10–30 seconds for static, 6-second contraction followed by 10–30 seconds of assisted stretch for PNF
Repetitions: three to four for each stretch.

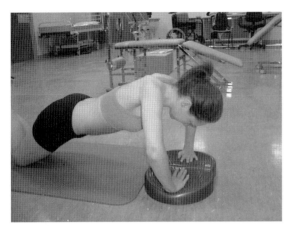

Figure 2.8 Press-up exercise on an unstable surface.

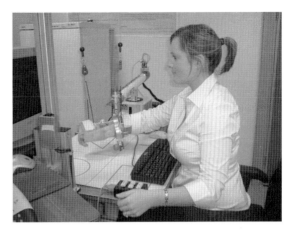

Figure 2.9 Use of a virtual reality device to simulate normal movement.

Prescription of proprioception, co-ordination and balance exercise

The concepts of balance, co-ordination and proprioception are important to consider when assessing and rehabilitating normal function in the patient. Balance may be defined as either static, which is the ability to maintain a position, or dynamic, which is the ability to move smoothly between positions. Co-ordination is the ability to produce a smooth, ordered movement and proprioception is the ability to identify joint position in space. Thus these concepts are all functions of the nervous system and are necessary to achieve normal movement. There is emerging evidence that musculoskeletal injury can compromise these functions, particularly proprioception, and so it is important to include exercises to address deficits in rehabilitation. These concepts will be discussed in the joint-specific chapters but the reader is encouraged to investigate further to glean knowledge of examining these disorders in patients.

There is limited literature regarding prescription of exercise in these areas, particularly when considering frequency, intensity and duration. However, it would be pertinent to ensure that the balance, co-ordination and proprioceptive systems are challenged throughout the rehabilitation programme while doing other exercises and are accordingly done daily if possible. The simplest way is to introduce unstable surfaces on which the patient performs their normal exercise as seen in Figure 2.8, which illustrates a patient with a shoulder injury performing a press-up on a wobble board to introduce a balance and proprioceptive component to rehabilitation.

Introduction of exercise which moves out of the simple planes of movement will make the exercise challenging and stimulating to the systems discussed above. Increasing balance demands by making the base smaller or standing on one foot introduces further challenge. The revolution in computer games, which have now become interactive, means that programmes have been introduced which simulate real movement without risk of injury, stimulating use of all systems above. Their use in rehabilitation is likely to increase, particularly with the use of imagination by those working in rehabilitation (Fig. 2.9).

References

American College of Sports Medicine (2000) *ACSM'S Guidelines for Exercise Testing and Prescription*, 6th edn. Lippincott Williams & Wilkins, Maryland, USA.

American College of Sports Medicine (2008) Available at: www.acsm.org/physicalactivity (accessed June 2008).

Berk, D.R., Hubert, H.B. and Fries, J.F. (2006) Associations of changes in exercise level with subsequent disability among seniors: A 16-year longitudinal study. *Journals of Gerontology – Series A Biological Sciences and Medical Sciences*, 61, 97–102.

Bruce, B., Fries, J.F. and Lubeck, D.P. (2005) Aerobic exercise and its impact on musculoskeletal pain in older adults: a

14 year prospective, longitudinal study. *Arthritis Research and Therapy*, 7, R1263–R1270.

Conaghan, P. (2002) Update on osteoarthritis part 1: current concepts and the relation to exercise. *British Journal of Sports Medicine*, 36, 330–333.

Fradkin, A.J., Gabbe, B.J. and Cameron P.A. (2006) Does warming up prevent injury in sport? The evidence from randomised controlled trials? *Journal of Science and Medicine in Sport*, 9, 214–220.

Heesch, K.C., Miller, Y.D. and Brown, W.J. (2006) Relationship between physical activity and stiff or painful joints in mid-aged women and older women: a 3-year prospective study. *Arthritis Research and Therapy*, 9, R34.

Huber, F.E. and Wells, C.L. (2006) *Therapeutic Exercise, Treatment Planning for Progression.* Saunders/Elsevier, Missouri.

Kujala, U.M., Kaprio, J. and Sarno, S. (1994) Osteoarthritis of weight bearing joints of lower limbs in former elite male athletes. *British Medical Journal*, 308, 231–234.

McLindon, T.E., Wilson, P.W.F., Aliabadi, P., Weissman, B. and Felson, D.T. (1999) Level of physical activity and the risk of radiographic and symptomatic knee osteoarthritis in the elderly: the Framingham study. *American Journal of Medicine.* 106, 151–157.

Pihl, E., Matsin, T. and Jurimae, T. (2002) Physical activity, musculoskeletal disorders and cardiovascular risk factors in male physical education teachers. *Journal of Sports Medicine and Physical Fitness*, 42, 466–471.

Shankar, K. (1999) *Exercise Prescription.* Hanley & Belfus, Philadelphia, Pennsylvania.

Small, K., McNaughton, L. and Matthews, M. (2008) A systematic review into the efficacy of static stretching as part of a warm – up for the prevention of exercise related injury. *Research in Sports Medicine*, 16, 213–231.

Thacker, S.B., Gilchrist, J., Stroup, D.F. and Kimsey, C.D. (2004) The impact of stretching on sports injury risk: A systematic review of the literature. *Medicine and Science in Sports and Exercise*, 36, 371–378.

Measurement and Assessment in the Management of Musculoskeletal Disorders

Alison H. McGregor

Introduction

There are numerous diseases and conditions that can affect the musculoskeletal system and its consequent function. These range from diseases of the joints to osteoporosis, back pain, spinal disorders, childhood musculoskeletal disorders, and injury or trauma to the musculoskeletal system. Since musculoskeletal disorders are believed to be one of the most common causes of severe long-term pain and physical disability and affect hundreds of millions of people, it is important to understand the impact of these disorders on function to be able to determine effective treatment pathways and preventative strategies. However, before one can understand musculoskeletal dysfunction one needs to understand normal function and its assessment.

What is normal function?

Function can be defined as the special work performed by an organ or structure in its normal state (Roper, 1987). In the context of the musculoskeletal system this is the ability of the body to move and interact within its environment. An understanding of movement, particularly human movement is important to therapists, doctors, biomechanists, orthotists as well as many other health professionals. It is equally important that this understanding or description of motion can be communicated between specialists in a consistent and meaningful manner.

The study of human movement is often referred to as kinesiology and can take place at a segmental local level or at a whole body level. In understanding movement it is important to appreciate the systems involved in creating this movement, many of which involve simple mechanical and physical principles. When considering movement, several systems are working together in harmony to produce normal function including muscles, bones, and ligaments.

The concept of integrated systems was introduced by Panjabi (1992) in describing the function of the spine. He proposed that to move and function normally, the spine requires a series of systems working together, namely: a control system (the central nervous system), a system of active elements (the muscles), and a system of passive elements (the vertebrae and discs). It was further proposed that a dysfunction of any part of one of these systems

Exercise Therapy in the Management of Musculoskeletal Disorders, First Edition. Edited by Fiona Wilson, John Gormley and Juliette Hussey.
© 2011 Blackwell Publishing Ltd

could lead to: (1) an immediate response from the other systems to compensate; (2) a long-term adaptation response of one or more systems; or (3) an injury to one or more components of any system. In the first, function would be impaired, in the second, although apparently normal, the stabilising system would be altered and in the third dysfunction/back pain would present. Although our understanding at present of the control system is limited, there has been extensive research to understand the mechanics of movement from the perspective of the passive and active systems.

Many factors can influence the working of the systems described above, including environmental influences such as gravitational fields (Davey *et al.*, 2004) and objects within that environment, for example workplace surroundings (Davis and Marras, 2003) and physiological factors, namely the effects of fatigue, training, etc. (Fulton *et al.*, 2002; Holt *et al.*, 2003), and psychosocial factors (Pincus *et al.*, 2002; Marras, 2005). Of particular interest is the relationship of mechanical influences induced by our environment and lifestyle on the health and functioning of our locomotor system, an area worthy and in need of further exploration (Brinkman *et al.*, 2002). What is relevance of this statement?

In simplistic terms the body can be considered as consisting of a skeleton that provides a rigid framework which acts as a series of struts and levers. These struts and levers in turn can be moved by the actions of muscles, and can also be used to protect and support vulnerable soft tissues and organs. This framework of bones or struts is connected through joints and it is at these joints that growth is permitted, and force in the form of compression (a force that squeezes things together), tension (a force that pulls apart two connected structures), shear (a force that causes two adjacent layers or surfaces to slide relative to each other) and torsion (a force that causes to structures to twist on each other) loads are transmitted and movement occurs. These forces and movements in turn are generated by the action of muscles. As well as moving joints, muscles can also be used to stabilise joints. These roles are often occurring at the same time as the muscle and act not only to allow the motion but also to convey the functional load that this motion creates and keep the joint stable.

For a joint to be stable it must be in equilibrium, which means that after any slight displacement it will return to its original position and if it was unstable it would buckle and fail. To understand stability, one must consider gravity and its effects. Gravity is the attractive force the earth has on the mass of an object, and our weight, for instance, is the combined effect of this mass and gravity. This weight can then be thought of as a force that acts through a single point, which in mechanical terms is called the centre of mass or centre of gravity. This point in the upright human is approximately around the umbilicus. When a body is in an unsupported state, gravity will act to create a force that will accelerate and move this body so it is no longer in equilibrium. If, however, it has a supported or stable base it would not move. Simplistically for a body to be stable, the centre of gravity/mass must lie within the base of support of that body to stop it from toppling over. So in considering motion of the body one also has to think about what is happening to keep the body in a stable state to allow this motion to occur.

The skeletal framework is often subdivided into the axial or central skeleton, which comprises the head, neck and trunk, and the appendicular skeleton, which comprises of the upper (arm, forearm and hand) and lower limb (thigh, leg and foot). Motion is considered within each system. However, all these systems need to link together and like all structures or buildings these need to be based on stable foundations. This means that in assessing a body region, one cannot neglect the rest of the body. For humans, the axial or central skeleton as its name suggests could be considered as 'mission control' in terms of stability. If it is not stable then the rest of the body's function will be compromised. Unfortunately for humans, the spine in mechanical terms is considered 'inherently unstable', and research on cadaveric spines devoid of musculature has shown that the spine in the neutral position with the pelvis fixed will buckle under loads of around 20 N (Panjabi *et al.*, 1989). This load would be considerably less if the pelvis had not been fixed. Thus for the spine, its base of support, i.e. the pelvis and its muscular system, are of importance for stability to be achieved, and without such stability the appendicular system may lack optimal functionality. Therefore care should be taken when using the term 'core stability' as this involves not only the muscles acting on the spine, of which there are numerous, but also on the muscles that achieve a stable base of support for the spine, namely the muscles acting on the pelvis i.e. gluteals, oblique abdominal and lower abdominals.

Biomechanics of movement

Winter (1990) defines the biomechanics of human movement as the interdiscipline that describes, analyses and assesses human movement. Movement is often defined in terms of either kinematics or kinetics or both. Kinematics is the term used in the description of a movement and as such, includes the pattern and speed of movement, and the coordination and displacement of the different body segments relative to some form of spatial reference system. Kinetics, by contrast, is the study of the forces associated with motion and these include both internal forces, i.e. those resulting from muscle activity etc., and external forces, i.e. those generated from external loads or bodies. For example, considering a person who is walking, a kinematic assessment would include the phases of gait and a description of the motion occurring, for example, at the knee; a kinetic assessment however, would be a description of the forces generated at the knee during the phases of gait. These forces can rarely be directly measured and kinetic analysis frequently requires some form of mathematical link segment modelling. This type of modelling, however, relies on appropriately measured kinematic and anthropometric data. Anthropometric measures include dimensions, weight, shape, centre of gravity, and other properties of the body segments according to race, age and sex, and a number of databases describing these are available (Dempster, 1955; Chandler *et al.*, 1975; Pheasant, 1996).

Thus the kinematic assessment of motion is an important factor in understanding the biomechanics of movement. In the clinical environment, motion is assessed at a very primary level by the human eye. Although one gains an appreciation of what is occurring, it is a subjective measure and one that places huge overload on the observer, particularly if it is a complex and fast movement. Furthermore, what is seen then needs to be described and recorded. However, if measurements of the movement are performed quantitatively the task of documentation is easier, objective and more likely to be repeatable. Using quantitative techniques of

analysis, databases of normal and abnormal can be developed permitting more detailed analyses with time. The choice of measurement and analysis technique is, however, dependent on the situation/task to be assessed, the person, the facilities and equipment available.

A description of movement, whether quantitative or qualitative, requires use of standard reference terminology. Clinicians tend to use the anatomical position as the reference position when describing motion and then make use of the following directional terms:

Superior – towards the head
Inferior – away from the head
Anterior – the front of the body
Posterior – the back of the body
Medial – towards the midline of the body
Lateral – away from the midline of the body
Proximal – close to the centre of the body
Distal – away from the centre of the body

A limitation of this method is that it only describes the position of one body segment relative to another and it does not give information on where in space is the body segment. To be able to achieve this necessitates a spatial reference system. This reference system can either be relative or absolute; a relative system requires that all coordinates are reported relative to an anatomical co-ordinate system while an absolute system reports the co-ordinates to an external spatial reference system.

Movement from the anatomical position are then described using anatomical reference planes which divide the body into equal parts, lie at right angles to each other and intersect at the centre of gravity of the body (Fig. 3.1). These planes are as follows.

- The frontal plane – which is also referred to as the coronal or z axis, is a vertical plane that divides the body equally into front and back halves.
- The sagittal plane – which is also referred to as the antero-posterior plane or x axis, is a vertical plane that divides the body equally into left and right halves.
- The transverse plane – which is also referred to as the horizontal plane or y axis, is a horizontal plane that divides the body into equal upper and lower halves.

Further to the planes of motion are three axis of rotation which each lie perpendicular to the plane

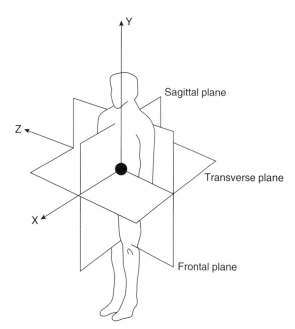

Figure 3.1   Anatomical frames of reference and co-ordinate systems.

of motion. So the transverse (also referred to as antero-posterior) axis of motion lies perpendicular to the sagittal plane; the sagittal axis is perpendicular to the frontal plane and the frontal (also referred to as longitudinal) axis is perpendicular to the transverse plane.

Using these definitions, movements in the sagittal plane about a frontal axis include flexion, extension, dorsiflexion and plantar flexion; movements in the frontal plane about a sagittal axis include abduction, adduction, ulnar deviation, radial deviation and lateral flexion of the trunk; and movements in the transverse plane about a frontal axis include medial and lateral rotation, supination and pronation.

However, many of these descriptions are simplifications of what is occurring at the joint or body segment since motion in the body usually arises as a result of both linear and angular motion. Linear motion can be simplistically thought of as motion occurring along a line where all the parts of the body move in the same direction at the same speed, e.g. a block sliding across a surface. Angular motion on the other hand is motion involving rotation around a central point. Frequently, human motion is simplified to angular motion occurring about a fixed centre of joint rotation. A more precise assess-

ment would involve a description of the translations (linear movements) and rotations the segment makes around each axis of motion relative to a fixed point in space. Descriptions of both linear and angular motion include the magnitude or degree of motion occurring, and its respective velocities and accelerations.

Furthermore, motion can be considered to be either static or dynamic. Static motion is where a body is in a constant state of motion that is at rest with no movement or moving with a constant velocity, while dynamic motion is where motion is occurring and creating accelerations or decelerations. Sometimes a complex dynamic motion is broken into phases or 'snap shot' moments of time and this is usually referred to as quasi-static motion.

With all the tools to describe motion one needs to consider how to assess it. There are many factors that influence the choice of methodology when it comes to assessing motion, including logistics such as time, facilities, equipment available, costs as well as the depth and repeatability of the assessment required, which in turn depends upon how this information is to be used and what level of precision, accuracy and repeatability is required.

Observed analysis

Traditionally in medical fields, there is a reliance on qualitative description of motion. This often takes the form of direct observations of the movement that is occurring and forms the primary level of assessment. Although quick, cheap and effective, it places a huge overload on the skills of even the most experienced clinicians due to the complexity of joint movements in most functional tasks. It also lacks robustness as different observers will focus on different aspects of the movement and describe them in different ways.

The use of video footage of movement is often used to overcome these problems as it facilitates the reviewing and freezing of the images. However, any assessment remains descriptive and limited objective measures can be made. Software is increasingly available to perform measures from video footage or digital photographs, but the terms or frames of reference need to be consistent when the images are obtained and any information derived is limited to

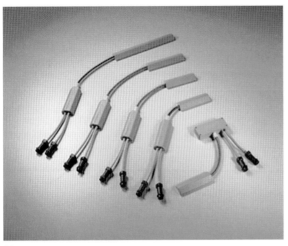
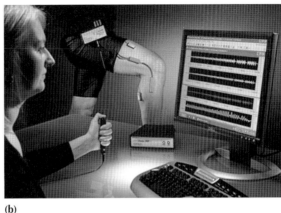

(a)   (b)

Figure 3.2   (**a**) Range of electrogoniometer sizes. (**b**) An example of electrogoniometer usage at the knee joint. Reproduced with kind permission from Biometric Ltd, UK.

the plane of motion in which the image has been obtained. Bearing in mind these considerations, such analysis is feasible to do and can provide valuable information if resources are limited.

Kinematic assessment methods and measurement tools

To take an assessment up the next level, some form of measurement needs to be made. This can be done with measurement tools that can essentially be divided into goniometers, imaging tools such as X-rays, and optical motion analysis system. Each tool will be considered in turn.

Goniometers

Routinely, many therapists use a simple hand-held goniometer consisting principally of a protractor with arms, which permits measurement of joint angles relative to an assumed centre of joint rotation. Used in its simplest form, it is cheap but in many ways clumsy, and it is difficult to obtain repeatable measures of a joint angle. It is also further limited to simple end-range measurements.

Engineering technology has expanded on this with a variety of electrogoniometers in existence,

each utilising different technologies. The most simple is the single axis potentiometer, which has a potentiometer at the junction of the two goniometer arms. Movement of the arms changes the resistance output of the potentiometer and this is calculated into an angular change. This approach relies on accurate identification of the joint's centre of rotation. In the late 1980s flexible goniometers using strain gauge technology were developed. These are lightweight and easy to use, without the need to locate the joint's centre of rotation. They are able to measure motion in real time, permitting assessments of not only range but also joint velocity and acceleration. Further developments have meant that they are now able to measure single and multi-axis motion and come in a variety of sizes and dimensions for use in the different regions of the body (Fig. 3.2). Although they are primarily limited to measuring local movement of a body system rather than whole body movement, they are capable of robust repeatable measures (Goodson *et al.*, 2007).

Using similar principles, electromagnetic systems have been developed to measure changes in angle. These devices consist of an electromagnetic source and a number of sensors that move in the resultant magnetic field (Fig. 3.3). Movement changes the electromagnetic field between the sensor and source and these changes are translated into measurements of movement. These systems are robust and permit

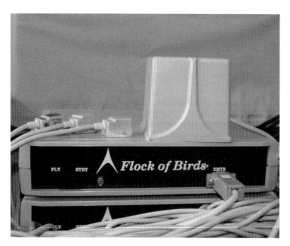

Figure 3.3 The Flock of Birds™, an electromagnetic motion tracking system. Reproduced with kind permission from Ascension Technology, Vermont, USA.

the assessment of rotations and translations in each orthogonal axis. Thus, detailed measurement can be made of segmental kinematics, as well as simple joint range measures (McGregor *et al.*, 1995; Bull and McGregor, 2000). However, such systems tend to be more expensive, and require more programming and associated software. A further limitation is that the electromagnetic field can be distorted by ferrous materials and thus location and usage has to be considered carefully. Finally, these systems are limited to regional or local motion systems as they permit only a relatively small number of motion tracking sensors to be used. As with the electrogoniometers above they also rely on secure fixation to the skin at valid and appropriate skeletal landmarks.

Increasingly, accelerometer technology is being used to assess motion. As the name suggests these devices measure acceleration and consist of force transducers. In simple terms, a small mass is attached to a beam which is attached to the body; as the body moves, the beam is deflected and this deflection is used to measure the acceleration of the mass, with strain gauges being used to measure the deflection. These devices can be uniaxial or biaxial and with advances in electronics are now available in compact form and can store large volumes of recorded data. One problem with accelerometers is that they respond to the field of gravity and thus the output represents the vector sum of the kinematic acceleration and the acceleration of gravity (Ladin, 1995). Attempts have been made to com-

pensate for this and such devices are increasingly being used to assess gait and motion (Moe-Nilssen, 1998; Moe-Nilssen and Helbostad, 2004).

Care must also be taken with investigating the accuracy, precision, validity and repeatability of motion systems, since there is no such thing as the perfect measurement. When determining the accuracy of a piece of equipment one needs to see how well the system measures each motion component with respect to a gold or known standard. Precision on the other hand is how close together a group of measurements are to each other. This means that your instrument might be very precise but inaccurate, a common feature in many measurement tools. Reliability is the variability of the measurements obtained by one person (intra-operator) measuring the same parameter repeatedly, and one can also assess reliability between two different people measuring the same parameter (inter-operator). Validity, by contrast, is a measure of how representative your measurement is of the actual motion occurring, and this often requires comparison with some form of imaging measurement.

Imaging

Often considered the 'gold standard' method of kinematic assessment, imaging has frequently been used to assess range of motion in joints. The simplest systems used are those utilising two-dimensional X-ray images taken at the limits of joint range from which measures can be obtained (Dvorak *et al.*, 1993; Frobin *et al.*, 2002). Many researchers have attempted to overcome the two-dimensional nature of these measures by using stereo-radiography techniques (Pearcy, 1985). Such imaging is limited particularly with respect to normative studies due to ionising radiation exposure. This problem and that of the static nature of the measurements has been overcome in part through the development of videofluoroscopy techniques, which at lower levels of radiation exposure permit dynamic two dimensional X-rays. Such techniques have been adapted for many body regions (Baltzopoulos, 1995; Breen *et al.*, 2006). Computed tomography permits the extension of such imaging to three dimensions (Shapeero *et al.*, 1988; Sun *et al.*, 2000) but this modality is associated with increased exposure to ionising radiation, thus limiting its widespread usage. It was hoped that the development of cine magnetic resonance imaging

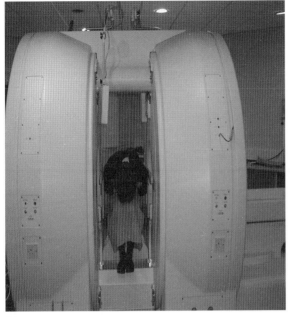
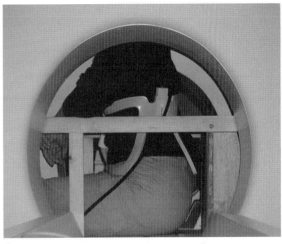

(a)   (b)

Figure 3.4   The interventional magnetic resonance imaging (MRI) scanner being used to assess lumbar intersegmental motion.

(MRI) (Brossmann *et al.*, 1995) and dynamic interventional open MRI techniques (Fig. 3.4) (McGregor *et al.* 2001; Johal *et al.* 2005) would overcome these problems. A well as limited availability and cost there are many other problems associated with dynamic interventional MRI, including slow image acquisition and poor image quality, leading to a focus on end-range measures of motion (McGregor *et al.*, 2001, 2002; Hill *et al.*, 2005a).

Optical motion analysis systems

Optical motion analysis in many ways is an expansion of video recording techniques. A camera is able to record a two-dimensional image of a three-dimensional object, and in movement analysis, often it is the three-dimensional image that is of interest if one is to make a detailed analysis of the movement occurring. This is achieved using multiple cameras and techniques such as photogrammetric reconstruction. For more details of this methodology, see Ladin (1995). Inherent in these techniques is the need to digitise the images obtained, which is facilitated by the use of active markers such as light emitting diodes (LEDs) that emit infrared light, or by passive markers such as light reflecting devices. This allows the identification of bony landmarks and the estimation of the centre of rotation of a joint, etc. To be able to capture all markers during a movement task usually requires three to six cameras, thereby increasing the complexity of the analysis; and yet despite this, the movement of some markers has to be interpolated. Such systems are growing in number and availability. They are however, expensive, require detailed calibration, are not always portable and are time consuming to set up and use correctly. Like all dynamic motion analysis systems they produce vast quantities of data and it is wise to consider how one will analyse these prior to commencing measurement. Most research to date using optical motion systems has focused on gait analysis.

How can kinematic assessments be used?

There are many uses for kinematic assessment and the method used is often governed by the intended use of the information. For therapists these uses are many. Traditionally, measures of joint range have been used as outcome measures or markers of treatment progression. Such measures not only let the therapist know that their intervention is working but also provide feedback to the patient on the progression of their condition. These have often relied on visual observation; however, if the intention was to research a treatment package and its effect on a disease process, greater accuracy would be required and in such situations it may be wise to opt for an electrogoniometric technique.

For more complex and fast movement patterns, particularly gait or dynamic activities such as running, it is often difficult to observe the movements that are occurring. Using appropriate motion analysis techniques one can either focus on the region of interest or perform a more detailed analysis of the global movement. This permits comparisons between subjects or allows one to perform serial measurements which can provide information on alterations to movement patterns as a result of injury or as a result of coaching or therapy intervention. For instance, Holt *et al.* (2003) were able to identify patterns of movement of the spine in competitive rowers during rowing and relate these to the force generated at the handle of a rowing ergometer. This provided a model to investigate the implications of fatigue, ergometer type (Steer *et al.*, 2006), level of experience (McGregor *et al.*, 2004), and level of intensity (McGregor *et al.*, 2005). The information obtained in real time provided biofeedback to coaches and athletes that led to changes in training and coaching. Performance was therefore enhanced as the athletes were more biomechanically efficient for the same physiological workload (McGregor *et al.*, 2007). Through kinetic modelling this information could also be used to understand the loading that occurs at specific regions of the body during the motion which will provide insight into injury mechanisms. Such techniques can be applied to a variety of activities and sports and are also used in the animation and robotic industry.

Assessment of muscles

An alternative way of looking at a movement or injury is to look at the functioning of the muscles. Usually there is a complex interaction of different muscles occurring to generate movement, and the intention here is not to explore this in detail but to give indication of approaches that could be used to look at this more closely.

One method of exploring muscle function is based on monitoring the electrical signal associated with the contraction of the muscle, namely the electromyogram or EMG. This signal gives an indication of voluntary muscular activity and it is known to increase as the tension in the muscle increases. The signal can be detected by using either surface electrodes or needles electrodes. Surface electrodes are less invasive but still only record from the motor units underlying that area. The signal can be influenced by cross-talk from underlying muscles and closely associated muscles and surface electrodes cannot assess deep muscle groups. Needle electrodes permit the analysis of activity in deeper muscles, but are invasive and often uncomfortable and isolate activity to that of the motor units in contact with the electrode. Furthermore EMG only permits an assessment of the activity that is occurring and not of the force being produced, thus limiting its usefulness. A detailed account of EMG is beyond the scope of this chapter but a number of texts and other publications are available on this technique.

Often more applicable to the therapist is the strength characteristic of a muscle. It is rarely possible to isolate this assessment to a particular muscle non-invasively and consequently muscles are assessed in groups, such as the quadriceps/knee extensors. Simple grading systems, such as the Oxford grading scale, a five-point scale with 0 representing no contraction and 5 normal contraction, have been derived. Although such a scale is suitable for neurological rehabilitation it has less scope in musculoskeletal conditions, in which more people would be expected to have normal contraction. As a result, a variety of tools ranging from simple weight lifting to fixed weight systems and, ultimately, isokinetic systems are used to measure strength (Fig. 3.5). Weight lifting and fixed weight systems do not accommodate the force length–tension curve of a muscle and as a consequence only assess the maximal weight lifted by the weakest component of joint range. Consequently, isokinetic systems have been developed that control the speed of movement of the joint rather than maintain a constant resistance and thus permit maximal torque to be assessed throughout joint range. Such meas-

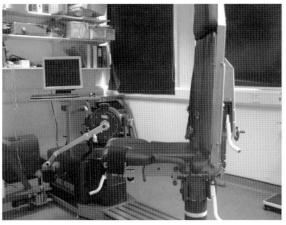
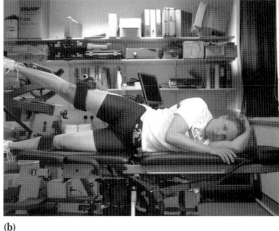

(a)   (b)

Figure 3.5 Cybex isokinetic dynamometer. (**a**) Set-up for testing knee function. (**b**) In use for testing hip abduction and adduction.

ures can be applied to both concentric and eccentric work of the muscles. These systems also allow static or isometric assessment. Such systems were once very popular in the field of performance and rehabilitation but have fallen out of fashion and are currently used primarily in the research field. They can, however, provide useful information on joint symmetry and information on performance at different velocities which give indicators of explosive strength and power. A key issue with these systems is the poor levels of repeatability (Hupli *et al.*, 1997; Hill *et al.*, 2005b; Laheru *et al.*, 2007). However, despite this they can still be used to provide important information on relative strength ratios, weaknesses and fatigue (Parkin *et al.*, 2001; McGregor *et al.*, 2004).

References

Baltzopoulos, V. (1995) A videofluoroscopy method for optical distortion correction and measurement of knee-joint kinematics. *Clinical Biomechanics*, 10, 85–92.

Breen, A.C., Muggleton, J.M. and Mellor, F.E. (2006) An objective spinal motion imaging assessment (OSMIA): reliability, accuracy and exposure data. *Biomedical Central Musculoskeletal Disorders*, 7, 1.

Brinkman, P., Frobin, W. and Leivseth, G. (2002) *Musculoskeletal Biomechanics*. Thieme, Stuttgart.

Brossmann, J., Muhle, C., Bull, C.C., Zeiples, J., Melchert, U.H., Brinkmann, G., Schronder, C. and Heller, M. (1995) Cine MR imaging before and after realignment surgery for patellar maltracking – comparison with axial radiographs. *Skeletal Radiology*, 24, 191–196.

Bull, A.M.J. and McGregor, A.H. (2000) Measuring spinal motion in rowers: use of an electromagnetic device. *Clinical Biomechanics*, 15, 772–776.

Chandler, R.F., Clauser, C.E., McConville, J.T., Reynolds, H.M. and Young, J.W. (1975) *Investigation of inertial properties of the human body*. Wright-Patterson Air Force Base, Ohio.

Davey, N.J., Rawlinson, S.R., Nowicky, A.V., McGregor, A.H., Dunois, K., Strutton, P.H. and Schroter, R.C. (2004) Human corticospinal excitability in microgravity and hypergravity during parabolic flight. *Aviation, Space & Environmental Medicine*, 75, 359–363.

Davis, K.G. and Marras, W.S. (2003) Partitioning the contributing role of biomechanical, psychosocial, and individual risk factors in the development of spine loads. *Spine Journal*, 3, 331–338.

Dempster, W.T. (1955) WADC Technical Report: Space requirements of the seated operator – geometrical, kinematic, and mechanical aspects of the body with special reference to the limb, pp. S5–S159. University of Michigan, Michigan.

Dvorak, J., Panjabi, M.M., Grob, D., Novotny, G.E. and Antinnes, J.A. (1993) Clinical validation of functional flexion/extension radiographs of the cervical spine. *Spine*, 18, 120–127.

Frobin, W., Leivseth, G., Biggemann, M. and Brinckmann, P. (2002) Sagittal plane segmental motion of the cervical spine. A new precision measurement protocol and normal motion data of healthy adults. *Clinical Biomechanics*, 17, 21–31.

Fulton, R.C., Strutton, P.H., McGregor, A.H. and Davey, N.J. (2002) Fatigue-induced change in corticospinal drive to back muscles in elite rowers. *Experimental Physiology*, 87, 593–600.

Goodson, A., McGregor, A.H., Douglas, J. and Taylor, P. (2007) Direct, quantitative clinical assessment of hand function: usefulness and reproducibility. *Manual Therapy*, 12, 144–152.

Hill, A.M., McGregor, A.H., Wragg, P., Brinckmann, P. and Burton, A.K. (2005a) The assessment of cervical spine kinematics: a comparison of iMR and conventional radiographic techniques. *Journal of Back and Musculoskeletal Rehabilitation*, 18, 29–35.

Hill, A.M., Pramanik, S. and McGregor, A.H. (2005b) Isokinetic dynamometry in assessment of external and internal axial rotation strength of the shoulder: Comparison of two positions. *Isokinetics & Exercise Science*, 13, 187–195.

Holt, P.J.E., Bull, A.M.J., Cashman, P.M.M. and McGregor, A.H. (2003) Rowing technique: The influence of fatigue on anteroposterior movements and force production. *International Journal of Sports Medicine*, 24, 597–602.

Hupli, M., Sainio, P., Hurri, H. and Alaranta, H. (1997) Comparison of trunk strength measurements between two different isokinetic devices used at clinical settings. *Journal of Spinal Disorders*, 10, 391–397.

Johal, P., Williams, A., Wragg, P., Hunt, D. and Gedroyc, W. (2005) Tibio-femoral movement in the living knee. A study of weight bearing and non-weight bearing knee kinematics using 'interventional' MRI. *Journal of Biomechanics*, 38, 269–276.

Ladin, Z. (1995) Three dimensional instrumentation. In: *Three-dimensional Analysis of Human Movement*. Allard, P., Stokes, I.A.F. and Blanchi, J.P. (eds). Human Kinetics, Illinois.

Laheru, D., Kerr, J.C. and McGregor, A.H. (2007) Assessing hip abduction and adduction strength: can greater segmental fixation enhance the reproducibility? *Archives of Physical Medicine and Rehabilitation*, 88, 1147–1153.

Marras, W.S. (2005) The future of research in understanding and controlling work-related low back disorders. *Ergonomics*, 48, 464–77.

McGregor, A.H., McCarthy, I.D. and Hughes, S.P.F. (1995) Motion characteristics of the lumbar spine in the normal population: *Spine*, 20, 2421–2428.

McGregor, A.H., Anderton, L., Gedroyc, W., Johnson, J. and Hughes, S.P. (2001) The assessment of spinal kinematics using interventional magnetic resonance imaging. *Clinical Orthopaedics and Related Research*, 392, 341–348.

McGregor, A.H., Anderton, L., Gedroyc, W., Johnson, J. and Hughes, S.P. (2002) The use of interventional open MRI to assess the kinematics of the lumbar spine in patients with spondylolisthesis. *Spine*, 17, 1582–1586.

McGregor, A.H., Bull, A.M.J. and Byng-Maddick, R. (2004a) A comparison of rowing technique at different stroke rates – a description of sequencing, force production and kinematics. *International Journal of Sports Medicine*, 25, 465–470.

McGregor, A.H., Patankar, Z. and Bull, A.M.J (2005) Spinal kinematics in elite oarswomen during a routine physiological 'step test'. *Medicine and Science in Sport and Exercise*, 37, 1014–1020.

McGregor, A.H., Patankar, Z. and Bull, A.M.J. (2007) Changes in the spinal kinematics of oarswomen during step testing. *Journal of Sports Science and Medicine*, 6, 29–35.

Moe-Nilssen, R. (1998) A new method for evaluating motor control in gait under real-life environmental conditions. Part 2. *Gait Analysis*, 13, 328–335.

Moe-Nilssen, R. and Helbostad, J.L. (2004) Estimation of gait cycle characteristics by trunk accelerometry. *Journal of Biomechanics*, 37, 121–126.

Panjabi, M., Kuniyoshi, A., Duranceau, J. and Oxland, T. (1989) Spinal stability and intersegmental muscle forces – a biomechanical model. *Spine*, 14, 194–199.

Panjabi, M.M. (1992) The stabilizing system of the spine. Part II. Neutral zone and instability hypothesis. *Journal of Spinal Disorders*, 5, 390–396.

Parkin, S., Nowicky, A.V., Rutherford, O.M. and McGregor, A.H. (2001) Do sweep stroke oarsmen have asymmetries in the strength of their back and leg muscles? *Journal of Sport Science*, 19, 521–526.

Pearcy, M.J. (1985) Stereo radiography of lumbar spine motion. *Acta Orthopaedica Scandinavia Supplementum*, 212, 1–45.

Pheasant, S. (1996) *Bodyspace: Anthropometry, Ergonomics and the Design of Work*, 2nd edn. Routledge, London.

Pincus, T., Burton, A.K., Vogel, S. and Field, A.P. (2002) A systematic review of psychological factors as predictors of chronicity/disability in prospective cohorts of low back pain. *Spine*, 27, 109–120.

Roper, N. (1987) *Pocket Medical Dictionary*, 14th edn. Churchill Livingstone, Edinburgh.

Shapeero, L.G., Dye, S.F., Lipton, M.J., Gould, R.G., Galvin, E.G. and Genant H.K. (1988) Functional dynamics of the knee joint by ultrafast, cine-CT. *Investigative Radiology*, 23, 118–123.

Steer, R.R., McGregor, A.H. and Bull, A.M.J. (2006) Repeatability of kinematic measures of rowing performance and their use to compare two different rowing ergometers. *Journal of Sports Science and Medicine*, 552–559.

Sun, J.S., Shih, T.T., Ko, C.M., Chang, C.H., Hang, Y.S. and Hou, S.M. (2000) In vivo kinematic study of normal wrist motion: an ultrafast computed tomographic study. *Clinical Biomechanics*, 15, 212–216.

Winter, D.A. (1990) *Biomechanics and Motor Control of Human Movement*, 2nd edn. John Wiley & Sons, USA. Available at: www.boneandjointdecade.org (accessed September 2008).

Regional Application of Exercise

2

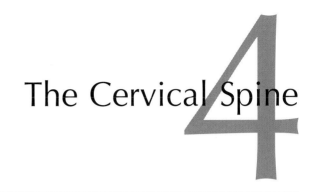

The Cervical Spine

Kirsty Peacock

SECTION 1: INTRODUCTION AND BACKGROUND

Cervical spine dysfunction is widely prevalent and forms a large percentage of the therapist's caseload both in the public and private sectors. After back pain, neck pain is the most frequent musculoskeletal cause of consultation in primary care worldwide (Binder, 2007). It has been estimated that 67% of people in Western populations will have neck pain at some point in their lives (Cote *et al.*, 1998; Vernon and Humphries, 2007) and that 300 per 100 000 inhabitants will experience whiplash-associated disorder (WAD; Holm *et al.*, 2008). Bourghouts *et al.* (1999) estimated the total cost of neck pain in the Netherlands in 1996 to be €686 million, with about 1.4 million workdays lost. In an epidemiological study of professional rugby players, the incidence of injuries to the cervical and lumbar spine was approximately 11 injuries per 1000 match-playing hours and 4 per 1000 training hours (Fuller *et al.*, 2007).

Acute neck pain can be caused by sudden application of external forces, such as an acceleration/deceleration mechanism, or internal forces, such as over-reaching, or by repetitive micro-trauma caused by consistent poor posture or repetitive strain situations. The natural history of acute neck pain is thought to involve no more than several days to a few weeks for significant recovery (Vernon and Humphries, 2007). The prognosis of chronic neck pain is more vague. Many people can be affected for up to 2 years' post-injury. Caroll *et al.* (2008) report that 50–85% of people who have suffered neck pain do not experience complete resolution of their symptoms. Brison *et al.* (2000) reported that 44% of those involved in a rear-end collision complained of neck stiffness at 6 months after the incident. Chronic neck pain produces a high level of morbidity by affecting the activities of daily living and quality of life (Webb *et al.*, 2003; Wolsko *et al.*, 2003). As is the case with low back pain, cervical pain is being recognised as a 'multifaceted phenomenon incorporating physical impairment, psychological distress and social interruption' (Harvey and Cooper, 2005). For an in-depth classification of subgroups of neck pain the reader is referred to Guzman *et al.* (2008).

This section will first outline the common cervical spine pathologies seen by physiotherapists and discuss the impairments in the neuro-musculoskeletal system caused by these pathologies. The evidence supporting the use of exercise in the management of the impairments will then be presented. In Section 2, the concepts discussed in Section 1 will be practically applied in the clinical setting.

Exercise Therapy in the Management of Musculoskeletal Disorders, First Edition. Edited by Fiona Wilson, John Gormley and Juliette Hussey.
© 2011 Blackwell Publishing Ltd

Cervical spine dysfunction and neuromuscular impairment

Most neck pain is 'non-specific', with symptoms having a postural or mechanical basis (Binder, 2007). However a number of conditions have been identified in the research:

- Spondylosis
- WAD
- Cervical postural syndromes
- Disc dysfunction
- Acute torticollis
- Acute nerve root pain
- Cervicogenic headache/dizziness
- Brachial plexus injury/'stingers'.

Several approaches have been put forward for the treatment of these conditions; however, recently there has been greater emphasis on therapeutic exercise in the management of neck pain, regardless of pathology. This is due to an increasing amount of research concluding that the pattern of neuromuscular dysfunction is very similar regardless of the underlying cause (Falla *et al.*, 2004; Jull *et al.*, 2004a).

When discussing exercise and the cervical spine it is essential to have a thorough understanding of the relevant *functional anatomy* and the concept of *stability dysfunction/uncontrolled movement*. The reader should refer to Panjabi *et al.* (1998) and Comerford *et al.* (2008) for further clarification of these areas.

Efficacy of exercise for cervical dysfunction

Systematic reviews have concluded that exercise is of benefit to individuals with mechanical neck pain or WADs (Sarig-Bahat, 2003; Kay *et al.*, 2005; Hurwitz *et al.*, 2008).

Aerobic exercise

There is very little evidence in the literature to support the use of aerobic exercise in the management of neck pain. In a study examining the effect of exercises such as stepping and dynamic exercises of the trunk and extremities in women with neck pain, Takala *et al.* (1994) found no significant difference in neck pain between the exercise and control groups. However, the general concept that cardiovascular exercise has a hypoalgesic effect can be applied to patients with neck pain.

Muscle strength and endurance training

The overall impression from the recent substantial evidence for exercise and neck pain is that stability dysfunction and functional control should be addressed early on with low load-specific exercises. Once an individual is able to control their area of uncontrolled movement through range and function, general strengthening exercises can be prescribed.

The needs of each individual must be addressed and rehabilitation tailored appropriately. If the patient is an elite athlete, end-stage rehabilitation must be aggressive to return them to their original condition. Failure to do this could result in treatment failure and the patient 'breaking down'.

The research on low load-specific muscle re-education has demonstrated the following pertinent findings:

- Isometric function of the cranio-cervical flexors can be improved with deep flexor exercises with a resultant decrease in pain (O'Leary *et al.*, 2007).
- Manipulative therapy combined with exercise therapy can reduce the symptoms of cervical headache and the effects are maintained for at least 12 months (Jull *et al.*, 2002).
- Patients with neck pain show a reduced ability to maintain an upright posture. An exercise programme aimed at strengthening the cranio-cervical flexors showed an increased ability to maintain an upright posture (Falla *et al.*, 2007).

The research for high load resistance training has demonstrated the following mixed results:

- Patients with chronic neck pain can benefit from a 6-week neck-strengthening programme including low load and high load resistance training. Patients completing the programme had a significant improvement in disability, pain and isometric neck muscle strength in different directions (Chiu *et al.*, 2004).

■ A long-term Finnish study by Ylinen *et al.* (2003) demonstrated that both strength and endurance training for 12 months are effective methods for decreasing pain and disability in women with chronic neck pain. Stretching and aerobic exercise alone proved to be a much less effective form of training than strength training. The improvements were maintained at 3-year follow-up assessments and the results indicated that exercise may not need to be performed regularly for the remainder of the participants' lives (Ylinen *et al.*, 2007).

■ Studies by Bronfort *et al.* (2004), Highland *et al.* (1992), and Jordan *et al.* (1998) have suggested that there is a reduction in pain and improvement in function with high load-resistance training. Viljanen *et al.* (2003) found that a programme of dynamic muscle training and relaxation was no better than ordinary activity for women office workers. A combination of isometric exercise, postural correction and use of a neck support pillow has been shown to be effective in the management of chronic neck pain. Isometric exercise in isolation has no effect (Helewa *et al.*, 2007).

■ A systematic review by Sarig-Bahat (2003) concluded that there is strong evidence supporting the use of dynamic-resisted exercises but that they are no more effective than endurance training, body awareness and passive physiotherapy. Kay *et al.* (2005) concluded that there is strong evidence of benefit favouring a multimodal care approach of exercise combined with mobilisations or manipulation for mechanical neck pain. From a best evidence synthesis of the literature from 1980 to 2006 Hurwitz *et al.* (2008) conclude that for WAD, educational videos, mobilisation and exercise appear to be the most effective form of management.

To summarise, there is some indication that both low load training and high load strength training may be beneficial in the management of neck pain.

Range of movement and flexibility exercises

Active range of motion exercises consist of any exercises that include active movement without resistance. A systematic review by Sarig-Bahat (2003) found strong evidence to support the effectiveness of early active mobilising exercises in acute whiplash patients based on the findings of McKinney (1989a), Rosenfeld *et al.* (2000) and Soderlund *et al.* (2000).

Sensorimotor and proprioceptive exercise

Rehabilitation exercises to improve sensorimotor deficits aim to restore co-ordinated movement or cervicocephalic kinaesthesia using visual training techniques. Systematic studies have demonstrated that a programme of eye fixation/proprioception exercises included in a complete rehabilitation programme is associated with strong to moderate evidence for reducing pain and improving function in mechanical neck pain and whiplash, with or without headache (Sarig-Bahat, 2003; Kay *et al.*, 2005). Joint positioning can be improved with home exercises of eye, head and arm co-ordination (Humphreys and Irgens, 2002). A comparative study of conventional proprioceptive training and cranio-cervical flexion training found that both regimens were effective in retraining joint position sense, implying that either programme can improve sensorimotor function in patients with neck pain (Jull *et al.*, 2007b).

SECTION 2: PRACTICAL USE OF EXERCISE

Aerobic exercise

When prescribing aerobic exercise for individuals with neck pain, it is important to consider the following points:

■ *Posture.* If a patient presents with symptoms related to a poking chin posture, with uncontrolled movement into upper cervical extension, he/she should be advised to avoid activities such as breaststroke, as this may aggravate the condition. Rowing or cycling may have a similar effect.

■ *Overhead movement.* If it has been noted that a patient has uncontrolled movement into

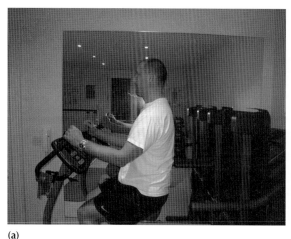
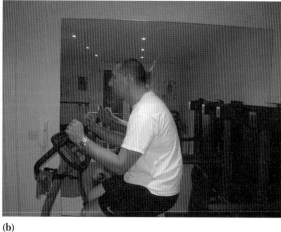

(a)   (b)

Figure 4.1   Suitable aerobic exercise for patients with neck pain, using a mirror to correct posture: (**a**) poor posture; (**b**) corrected posture.

extension, either at the upper or mid-cervical spine and this is related to the symptoms they experience, it is best to avoid any cardiovascular exercise that involves upper body work over 90° shoulder abduction/elevation, until the patient has learnt to control cervical spine movement into extension.

■ *Impact.* If patients have a shear or area of 'give', high-impact exercise such as aerobics or running may have a detrimental effect.

A static bike work-out, using a large mirror for visual feedback, may be the best form of aerobic exercise, as it is low impact and the patient can control neutral head position (Fig. 4.1). Walking has also been recommended (Soderlund *et al.*, 2000).

Endurance and strength training

Endurance training

Comerford and Mottram (2007) take the following four-point approach to rehabilitation.

(1) Teach the patient to control movement in the direction of symptom provocation, i.e. control the 'give' and move the restriction

This strategy is the key to controlling symptoms, as it helps to unload the tissues under stress. For

example, a patient presents with central low cervical spine pain. She reports that reading aggravates her pain. On assessment, the patient has stiffness into flexion at the mid-cervical spine but to compensate she moves into excess flexion at the low cervical spine (Figs 4.2a and 4.2b). On analysis, reading aggravates this patient's symptoms because she is looking down while reading and she has uncontrolled range of movement into lower cervical flexion, which put the soft tissues and cervical joints under stress. To control the symptoms, the therapist must instruct the patient to try to stabilise the lower cervical spine while moving into flexion from the mid-cervical spine (Fig. 4.2c). This can be done by explaining to the patient that you want her to move from higher up in the cervical spine, like a 'nodding' movement while keeping the lower neck still. This is not a 'normal movement', but the aim of the exercise is to teach the patient how to control the uncontrolled movement into flexion. The therapist can give auditory, visual and manual feedback to help the patient achieve this. Instruct the patient to move through only that much range as the restriction allows or as far as the 'give' is dynamically controlled. Scapula control is very important and patients need to be made aware of correct scapula positioning during the exercise (Mottram, 2003). The exercise should not reproduce the patients' symptoms. This is the first exercise that should be taught to the patient, as she can use it immediately to help her to control her symptoms. It needs to be repeated slowly, 15–20 repetitions, two to three

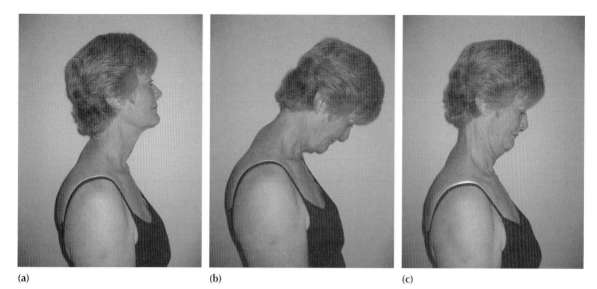

(a)   (b)   (c)

Figure 4.2 (**a**) Static posture. (**b**) Patient demonstrating lower cervical 'give' into flexion. Note how the mid-cervical spine remains in lordosis. (c) Controlling the 'give' and moving the restriction.

times per day. The patient should perform these exercises until the movement starts to feel familiar and it is easy to do. Start with the patient sitting against the wall, then progress to sitting away from the wall, standing, leaning forwards over the bed and then leaning back over the bed with their arms supporting them. Exercises can be progressed by asking the patient to repeat the exercises on an unstable surface such as a Swiss ball or Sit-Fit™.

The key is to control the excess movement from one or occasionally two areas. On observing the patient's movement patterns you may need to control:

- A 'give' into *flexion* in the *upper cervical spine*, by positioning the upper cervical spine in neutral and moving the lower cervical spine from extension to flexion and back again. The low cervical spine is moved by tilting the head forward from the base of the neck. The exercise should be repeated slowly for 15–20 repetitions, two to three times a day.
- A 'give' into *extension* in the *upper cervical spine*, by positioning the upper cervical spine in neutral, maintaining this neutral position and moving the low cervical spine through range from flexion to extension. Instruct the patient to perform a backward head tilt. Extension should occur at the low cervical

spine. The exercise should be repeated for 15–20 repetitions, two to three times a day.
- A 'translation' into *extension* in the *mid-cervical spine*, by positioning the upper and mid cervical spine in neutral, maintaining this neutral position and moving through range from flexion to extension. Extension should occur at the low cervical spine. Repeat the exercise but instruct the patient to extend from the upper cervical spine by performing a chin lift. Repeat the exercise for 15–20 repetitions, two to three times per day.
- *'Chin poke'*, or *lateral flexion* during *rotation*, by positioning the cervical spine and scapula in neutral and rotating the head through the available range without the substitution strategies. The patient should rotate through the whole cervical spine. Repeat for 15–20 repetitions, two to three times per day.
- *'Chin poke'* or *rotation* into *side flexion*, by positioning the cervical spine and scapula in neutral and side bending the head through the available range without the substitution strategies. The patient should side bend through the whole cervical spine. Repeat for 15–20 repetitions, two to three times per day.
- A 'give' into *side flexion* at the *lower cervical spine*, by positioning the cervical spine and scapula in neutral and tilting the head through

the available range of upper cervical side bending. Instruct the patient to tilt the head at the base of the skull. The patient should be sitting or standing, keeping the occiput against the wall. Repeat 15–20 for repetitions, two to three times per day.

- A 'give' into *side flexion* at the *upper cervical spine*, by positioning the cervical spine and scapula in neutral, tilting the head through the available range of lower cervical side bending by tilting the head at the base of the neck. The patient should be sitting or standing, keeping the occiput against the wall. Repeat 15–20 for repetitions, two to three times per day.

It is important that the symptoms experienced by the patient are related to the site of 'give'. A patient may present with a combination of these dysfunctions but the clinician must decide which dysfunction is most relevant to the patient's symptoms. It may be necessary to use manual therapy for articular or myofascial restriction in combination with the above movement for re-education.

(2) Teach the patient to control translation in a neutral joint position

This exercise is for the local stability muscles and aims to regain normal muscle stiffness in order to control translation. These exercises are low load and aim to stimulate the anterior and posterior local stabilisers in neutral. Several tests must be completed to assess the function of these local stabilisers and the rehabilitation of these muscles then uses the test positions.

(a) *Testing deep flexors of the cervical spine*

The cranio-cervical flexion test (Fig. 4.3) (Comerford and Mottram, 2007, adapted from the work by Jull *et al.*, 2004b, cited in Boyling *et al.*, 2004) assesses the deep neck flexors, i.e. rectus capitis anterior and lateralis ± longus capitis and deep multifidus.

(1) Position the patient in supine with the cervical spine, temporomandibular joints and scapulae in a neutral position.
(2) Place a small rolled-up towel under the top of the back of the head to support the cervical spine in neutral.
(3) Place the pressure biofeedback under the cervical lordosis, folded and clipped.

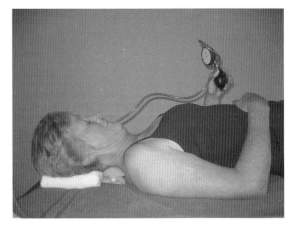

Figure 4.3 Cranio-cervical flexion test.

(4) Inflate the pressure biofeedback to a base pressure of 20 mmHg.

Instruct the patient to slide their head up the towel using a nodding action until the pressure increases from 20 mmHg to 22 mmHg; then ask the patient to hold for 5 seconds. Relax back to 20 mmHg, then increase the pressure to 24 mmHg using the same action and hold for 5 seconds. Then relax back to 20 mmHg and then increase the pressure from 20 mmHg to 26 mmHg and hold again for 5 seconds. This test should be repeated twice without substitution or fatigue. The patient must achieve cranio-cervical flexion during the test. Substitution strategies may include loss of neutral position and palpable or visible contraction of the sternomastoid, scalenes or hyoids (Falla *et al.*, 2003).

Rehabilitation of the deep flexors: If the patient does not have ideal recruitment, i.e. cannot sustain the holds or uses substitution strategies, the deep flexors must be retrained. The pressure that can be achieved using the biofeedback device, without substitution, and cranio-cervical flexion noted. Ask the patient to hold this pressure for 10 seconds and repeat 10 times. As the patient improves the ability to hold, the incremental pressures will become easier. There must be no co-contraction rigidity – this is manifested by dominance of the superficial global mobility muscles holding the head rigid. Once the patient has learnt the correct movement with the biofeedback, this exercise should start in sitting and progress to standing. To progress rehabilitation, the anterior stabilisers need to be functionally loaded, by positioning the patient in supine

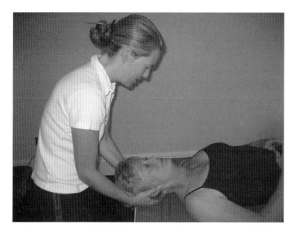

Figure 4.4 Test for deep extensor function.

and having their head resting in neutral in the physiotherapist's hand. The patient is instructed to keep the head stationary as the physiotherapist removes the supporting hand. On testing the patient should be able to support their head in neutral for about 15 seconds for two repetitions without fatigue or substitution strategies. The superficial mobility muscles will be active but should not dominate. Abnormal substitution strategies include chin poke and low cervical flexion. For a home programme, patients should start this exercise in supported incline sitting about 10–15° from the vertical (e.g. against an ironing board) and just lifting their occiput clear without substitution strategies and holding for 10 × 10 seconds. The angle of supported sitting can then be increased to 45°. The exercise can thereafter be done in different postures and progressed again with the use of unstable surfaces.

(b) *Testing the deep extensors of the cervical spine*

For the deep suboccipital extensor test (Fig. 4.4; adapted from Kennedy, 1998):

(1) Position the patient in supine with the cervical spine and scapulae in neutral. Keeping the jaw relaxed will help to keep the temporomandibular joints in neutral.
(2) Support the patient's occiput with the fingertips.
(3) Instruct the patient to keep the head in neutral as the therapist attempts to gently move the head into upper cervical flexion (using a suboccipital distraction action). On testing the patient should be able to maintain this position

isometrically against this light resistance for 15 seconds for two repetitions without any give into upper cervical flexion, substitution or fatigue. There should be no movement.
(4) Substitution strategies include active upper cervical extension, movement such as the head pushing down, indicating scalene and co-contraction rigidity, or contraction of the sternocleidomastoid.

Rehabilitation of the deep extensors: If the patient does not have ideal recruitment, the deep suboccipital extensors must be retrained. The patient holds their head themselves with the index and middle fingers along the occiput. They slowly and gently try to move the head passively into upper cervical flexion with their hands, while simultaneously trying to resist this motion. The resistance should be against very light pressure. Instruct the patient to hold for 10 seconds and repeat for 10 repetitions. This can be performed in different postures. The patient should beware of aggravating symptoms, particularly if there is neural sensitivity relating to headaches or dural sensitivity. To progress rehabilitation, load the posterior stabilisers functionally, by positioning the patient in prone and neutral. The operator should hold the patient's head with the forehead resting on the operators' hand. Instruct the patient to keep the head stationary as the operator removes the supporting hand. The patient should be able to hold the position for 15 seconds for 2 repetitions without fatigue or substitution strategies. For a home programme the patient should sit at a table with neutral alignment and lean forward to take weight on their forearms. Train 10-second holds for 10 repetitions. Progress the exercise to 45° prone incline position and then to prone. The exercise can then be progressed to different postures. Use of unstable surfaces, such as a Swiss ball, could then be introduced.

(3) Teach the patient to actively control the full available range of movement

This involves the rehabilitation of the global muscle system. These muscles must control full passive inner range and any hypermobile outer range. The ability to control rotation is a particularly important role of these muscles. For stability control, the eccentric role of these muscles is more important than their concentric role. To rate these muscles, three factors must be considered:

■ Does the inner range shortening of the muscle = the passive range of movement of the joint?

■ For stability control, if muscle active = joint passive, can the muscle support the neck in this position?

■ If the muscle can support the neck in its inner range, can it eccentrically control the lowering through the range of motion, in a smooth manner, without the loss of trunk and scapular stability?

Exercises for the rehabilitation of the global mobility muscles must start in basic postures and progress to functional positions such as sitting at a desk, or made sport-specific for the athletic population.

Patients presenting with upper or mid-cervical extension and rotation stability dysfunction: Rehabilitation of the anterior global stabiliser muscles (longus colli, oblique fibres and longus capitis) is a priority for patients with upper or mid-cervical extension and rotational stability dysfunction, as these muscles eccentrically control extension.

Testing the anterior global stabiliser muscles in **mid-inner range**:

■ Position the patient in supine and neutral.

■ With the back of the subjects head resting in neutral on the operators hand, instruct the subject to lift their head forward through range into full flexion and rotation (chin towards the sternum and at least half range rotation). At this point the operator passively supports the head and assesses if there is any more range available. If the operator can see more passive range than the patient was able to achieve actively, the patient has failed the test. If no more range can be seen from the passive assessment, instruct the patient to hold that inner range position for 15 seconds and then lower the head back to neutral. This should be completed twice. The patient should be able to hold the head and lower down to neutral smoothly with no substitution strategies.

■ Substitution strategies may include chin poke due to dominant sternomastoid, and shoulder girdle elevation/protraction due to dominant scalenes. If the plane of the face stays horizontal as the head lifts forwards, a combination of sternomastoid and scalenes are dominant. If the hyoids are dominant the patient will not be able to talk normally. Other strategies are the head pushing down or sideways, or rotation of the shoulder girdle or trunk.

Rehabilitating the anterior global stability muscles in **mid-inner range**: Reproduce the movement, but only to the range that is controlled. Initially, train without rotation i.e. hold in midline. Once 10×10 second holds in full range have been achieved, progress onto holds in flexion and rotation. If control is very poor this exercise can be started in incline sitting and progressed into supine.

Testing the anterior global stability muscles in **outer range**:

(1) Position the patient in sitting tall and supported with a neutral spine, with the mouth closed and a neutral bite (jaw not clenched).

(2) Instruct the patient to flex the upper cervical spine and then independently extend the lower cervical spine. Maintaining the low cervical spine in extension slowly extend the upper cervical spine by allowing the chin to lift towards the ceiling (initially only quarter range) and return to neutral, leading with active upper cervical flexion. Make sure the chin does not protrude; and the occiput must not lift vertically. The chin must move down and inwards and the occiput must move up. If control is good at quarter range, progress to half and then three-quarters, and finally full range upper cervical extension.

Rehabilitating the anterior global stability muscles in the **outer range**: Reproduce the movement, but only in the range that is controlled. Initially hold for 10×10 seconds in the midline and progress to adding rotation. If control is poor, this exercise can be started in incline sitting. It is important to regain inner range control before training outer range to prevent aggravating the patient's symptoms.

Patients presenting with low cervical flexion and rotation stability dysfunction: Rehabilitation of the posterior low-cervical global stabiliser muscles (multifidus, spinalis, and semispinalis cervicus) is a priority for low cervical flexion and rotation stability dysfunction.

Testing the posterior low cervical stabilisers in inner range:

(1) Position the patient in prone resting on the elbows with the scapulae and thoracic spine in neutral and the head hanging in flexion.
(2) Instruct the subject to maintain the upper cervical spine in flexion or neutral and lift the head with independent extension and rotation of the low cervical spine through full range and then return eccentrically to the starting position.
(3) The patient should be able to hold for 15 seconds twice without fatigue or substitution.

Rehabilitating the posterior low stabilisers: Reproduce the movement, but only in the range that is controlled. Initially hold for 10 × 10 seconds in midline and progress to adding rotation. If control is poor this exercise can be started in sitting, leaning at 45°, and then progress to prone on elbows.

For patients presenting with upper or mid-range flexion and rotation/side bending stability dysfunction: Rehabilitation of inner range *suboccipital stabiliser* muscles is a priority for upper or mid-cervical flexion and rotation/side bending stability dysfunction.

Testing the suboccipital stabilisers in inner range:

(1) Position the patient prone, resting on their elbows, with the cervicothoracic junction at end-range extension and a neutral upper cervical spine.
(2) Instruct the patient to perform active upper cervical lateral flexion. There should be symmetrical full range upper cervical lateral flexion without substitution or fatigue. The patient should hold the position for 15 seconds for two repetitions without fatigue or substitution.

Rehabilitating the suboccipital stabilisers: Reproduce the movement, but only in the range that is controlled. Instruct the patient to try to hold for 10 × 10 seconds. If this is not possible, first try to unload the exercise by asking the patient to leaning forwards on their forearms; if this does not work reduce the hold time.

(4) Regaining extensibility of the global mobilisers

This will be covered briefly in exercises for range of motion.

Strength training

Once the patient has been able to correct the stability dysfunction, overload training can be started. It is important to include functional postures as soon as possible, as this helps to retrain the sensorimotor system. Exercises can be combined with scapular and lumbar spine stability work. It is essential that rehabilitation be taken to its end stage. Functional activities and sporting activities rely on the successful combination of basic stability and strength of the entire body, moving with different forces, at various speeds. Functional training is 'training that conditions the body consistent with its integrated movement and/or use' (Santana, 2000).

Thera-Band®, pulleys and bungees can provide resistance, however, head harnesses and free weights are useful with elite athletes such as professional rugby players. Swiss balls and 'sit-fits' are useful for isometric exercises. A strength training programme should include exercises for the shoulders, upper back and chest. Ylinen *et al.* (2003) suggest dumbbell shrugs, presses, curls, bent over rows, flys or pullovers, completing three sets of 20 repetitions. The following text includes examples of cervical spine resistance exercises for patients who have progressed from stability training. Sensorimotor exercises need to be added to complete the programme. It is assumed that the patient has warmed up (including self-resisted isometric cervical exercises and gentle cervical self stretches).

(1) *Isometric exercises using the sit-fit:* Flexion, extension, side flexion (left and right). Stand 2–3 foot lengths from the wall. Place the sit-fit against wall (Fig. 4.5a). Keeping the cervical spine in neutral, the patient should place their head on the sit-fit and lean into the wall. Hold for 20 seconds. To progress this exercise, move the feet further away from the wall, and to progress again, the patient could stand on one leg or add in arm movement with weights. This exercise can also be completed with a Swiss ball on the floor (Fig. 4.5b).
(2) *Concentric/eccentric exercises with Thera-Band™ (Fig. 4.6):* Flexion; flexion plus oblique

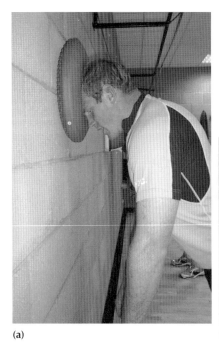

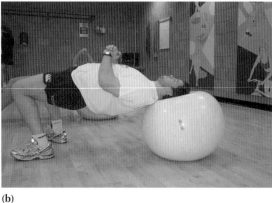

(a)   (b)

Figure 4.5   (**a**) Isometric flexion exercise with sit-fit. (**b**) Isometric extension exercise with a Swiss ball.

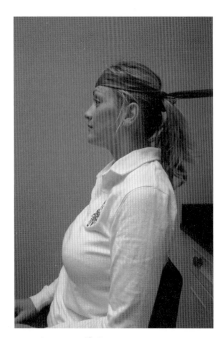

Figure 4.6   Thera-Band® flexion exercise.

right and left; extension; extension plus oblique right and left; side flexion.

These exercises can be completed in standing or sitting. Ensure that the patient can complete the movements without the dysfunction they originally presented with. The eccentric movement back into neutral must be slow and controlled. Ten repetitions × 2 sets in each direction should be completed.

Elite athletes such as professional rugby players may need more resistance, such as the 1-minute circuit exercises shown in Figure 4.7. It is important that these exercises are done under the supervision of the clinician, with no pain and only after successful progression of resistance exercises. These exercises could also be used as part of a prehabilitation session (Steele, 2007).

Range of movement/flexibility exercises

General sustained self-stretches for the cervical spine have been taught for many years and are well known. Holding time for the stretches range from

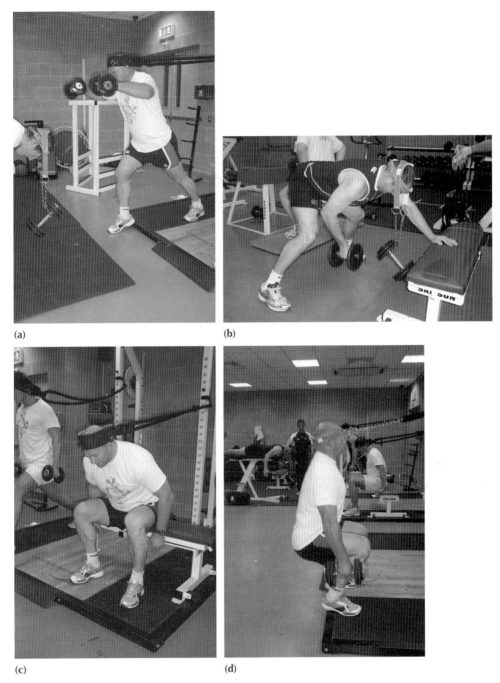

Figure 4.7   Resisted cervical exercises for elite rugby players (forward positions). (**a**) Flexion hold plus shoulder press. (**b**) Extension hold plus one arm fly. (**c**) Isometric flexion with trunk flexion. (**d**) Extension hold plus deep squat.

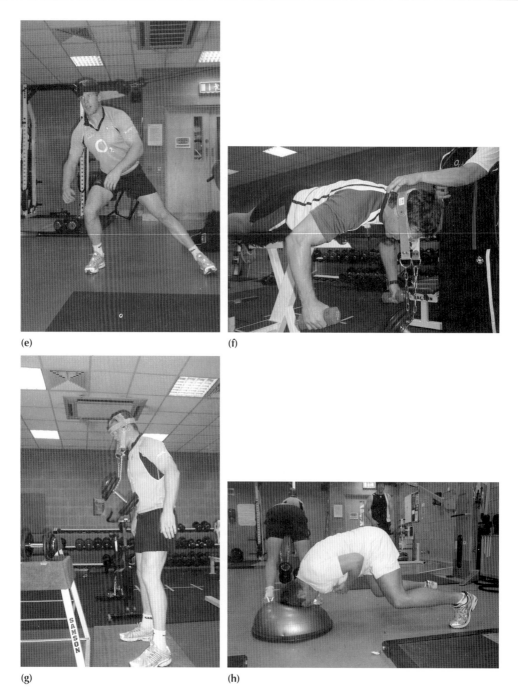

(e)

(f)

(g)

(h)

Figure 4.7   *(Continued)* (**e**) Lateral lunge plus side flexion hold. (**f**) Isometric extension plus bilateral fly. (**g**) Deep squat starting position. (**h**) Head bridge.

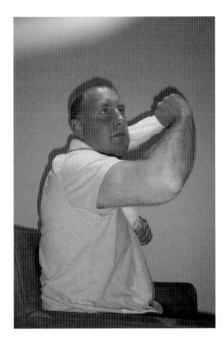

Figure 4.8 Self SNAG to improve rotation.

30 seconds to 2 minutes and these are repeated two to three times. A useful technique for increasing range of motion into extension, side flexion or rotation is a Mulligan (1999) sustained natural apophyseal glide (SNAG) with a towel (See Fig. 4.8).

The *ligamentum nuchae* becomes tight in subjects presenting with a loss of control into upper or mid-cervical extension, as the distance from the posterior occiput to the lower cervical spine is in a constantly shortened position. This can be a common problem in the athletic cycling population, due to the position of the hands on the handle-bars and the necessity to keep the head up. To assess the length of the ligamentum nuchae, the patient should be in prone resting position on their elbows, with the scapulae in neutral, the thoracic spine flexed and the head hanging so that the upper cervical and lower cervical spine is in flexion. The head should hang in full flexion with a midline groove between the paravertebral muscle bulk. If the ligamentum nuchae is tight, a prominent midline ligamentous ridge in the upper to mid-cervical spine can be seen and flexion is restricted. To stretch the ligamentum nuchae, use the position just described and let the head hang down for 30–120 seconds and repeated two to three times (Fig. 4.9).

The *scalenes* appear dominant in individuals with poor local stability function who present with pain related to low cervical flexion, upper cervical extension and rotation stability dysfunction. To assess whether the scalenes are overactive, position the patient in supine with the occiput on the bed. The therapist's hand supports the cervical lordosis as seen in Figure 4.9b and the other hand stabilises the first rib. The patient's head is then positioned to bias the particular scalene:

- Anterior scalene – half range rotation towards the stabilised rib and then 15° side bend away
- Middle scalene – no rotation and 15–20° side bend away
- Posterior scalene – one third rotation away and then 20–25° cervical side bend away.

To stretch the scalene, the patient actively repositions the test movement until either muscle resistance stops the movement or stability is lost. The physiotherapist then passively supports this position. The subject is asked to exhale and the stretch is held for 20–30 seconds and repeated three to five times (Fig. 4.9b).

The *levator scapulae* often appear overactive in patients presenting with cervical extension and rotation stability dysfunction. To test if the levator scapulae are overactive, position the patient in supine with the scapulae midway between elevation and depression, and the head forward in flexion to resistance. Rotate and side bend the head away until either muscle resistance stops or muscle tension causes a loss of proximal shoulder position. Ideally with the operator providing head fixation, there should be no further increase in neck range into side bend, when the muscle is unloaded by hitching the shoulder. The patient should be able to reproduce passive range without substitution or loss of proximal control. To stretch the levator scapulae, actively reproduce the test movement and passively support this position. Actively retract and depress the scapula and hold this stretch for 20–30 seconds, then repeat the stretch three to five times. The stretch should be felt mainly at the neck angle rather than the upper cervical spine (Fig. 4.9c).

Sensorimotor and proprioceptive rehabilitation

Treleaven (2008) regards the inclusion of rehabilitation of the sensorimotor system in cervical spine disorders to be as important as lower limb proprioception retraining following an ankle or knee injury.

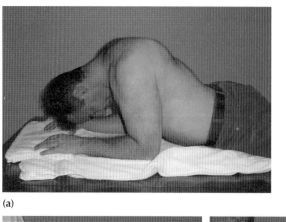

(a)

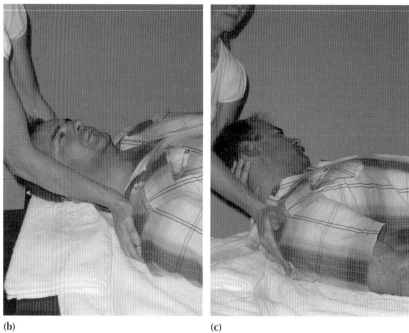

(b)   (c)

Figure 4.9 (a) Ligamentum nuchae stretch. (b) Scalene stretch. (c) Levator scapulae stretch.

Motor control

It has been demonstrated that individuals with neck pain have altered motor control. Clinical assessment and rehabilitation of the cervical sensorimotor system has three components (Whiplash and Neck Pain Research Unit, Sterling, 2005):

- Cervical joint position sense
- Standing balance
- Oculomotor function.

Cervical joint position sense (Whiplash and Neck Pain Research Unit, Sterling, 2005)

A small laser pointer can be mounted onto a headband. The patient is seated 90 cm away from the wall and asked to look straight ahead. This point is marked on the wall. The patient is then blindfolded and instructed to return to this point as accurately as possible following either left and right rotation or extension. The patient indicates verbally when they think they have returned to this position.

The final position can be marked and compared with the initial starting position, measured in centimetres. If the patient presents with dysfunctions in cervical joint position sense, they can commence relocation rehabilitation exercises immediately. The patient can practise relocating the head to predetermined positions in flexion, extension rotation and side flexion while blindfolded. Another useful exercise is the cranio-cervical flexion test as discussed above. The patient should practise targeting different pressures on the biofeedback device, with their eyes closed and then open their eyes to check on the pressure on the dial. Higher-level skills include following a moving target of a set speed and distance with the eyes open and replicating the same movement with the eyes closed. Speed and distance can be altered.

Alternative test for cervicohead repositioning accuracy (Comerford and Mottram, 2007): The patient is positioned in four-point kneeling. The head and neck are passively positioned in neutral alignment, and then the patient actively moves (turning side to side, looking up/down) and attempts to return to the neutral position. This is performed twice and rated with the following scale:

Good: the patient accurately and confidently returns to the neutral position both times without making adjustments.

Average: The patient returns to neutral position with reasonable accuracy but lacks the confidence – may need to make several adjusting movements or is 'not quite sure'.

Poor: The patient cannot return to the neutral position and is often very unsure of the correct position.

Standing balance (Sterling, 2005)

Clinical examination of standing balance involves progressively challenging the postural control system by altering foot position, visual input and the supporting surface. Each test should be assessed for 30 seconds and sway or rigidity noted. The progression can be as follows:

- Comfortable → narrow stance
- Firm → soft surface (e.g. 10 cm dense foam)
- Eyes open → eyes closed
- Double leg → single leg.

Exercises to improve standing balance are based on the tests and can be integrated with functional activities.

Oculomotor function (Sterling, 2005)

- *Eye follow* – the patient keeps the head still and follows a moving target with the eyes; from side to side, up and down, progressing to an H pattern (Fig. 4.10). The trunk is then rotated (up to 45° neck torsion) or to a point just short of pain. Again the head is kept still, and the test of following a moving target with the eyes is repeated (rotating the trunk biases the cervical receptors compared with the vestibular receptors). Keeping the head still, the patient follows saccadic movements at randomised eye positions. The starting position, speed and focus point can be altered accordingly. The therapist should monitor the patient's ability to follow the target. Jerky eye movements, dizziness, unsteadiness or nausea are noted. Exercises to improve eye follow function are based on the results of the tests described above.
- *Gaze stability* – ask the patient to keep the eyes focused on a point while moving the head

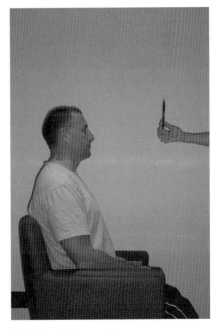

Figure 4.10 Eye follow exercise.

actively or passively in all directions. The therapist should note any reproduction in symptoms, such as inability to focus or dizziness. Progress to asking the patient to close their eyes, move their head and then open their eyes again to check that the eyes have maintained a stable gaze on the target. This tests imaginary gaze. To improve gaze stability, start with exercises in supine looking at the ceiling, and progress to exercises in sitting or standing. To progress this exercise, peripheral vision can be restricted by using a pair of swimming goggles that have been blackened out except for a small area in the centre of each eye.

■ *Eye/head co-ordination*:

(1) Rotate the eyes and head to the same side left and right.
(2) The eyes move first to a target. The patient then turns the head ensuring the eyes are kept focus on the target.

(3) The eyes move first and then the head to look between two targets placed either horizontally or vertically, maintaining focus between the two points.
(4) The eyes and head are rotated to the opposite side, left and right.

Exercises to improve eye follow are based on the tests which assess ability to follow a moving target (see above) (Sterling, 2005).

In conclusion, current literature supports the use of exercise in the management of mechanical neck pain, whiplash and cervicogenic headache. When designing a therapeutic exercise programme for individuals with neck pain, it is essential that all relevant components are included. Specific functional stability work is essential and is the key to symptom relief and strength training that prepares the body for function, return to work or sport. Sensorimotor training can be started the day the patient presents to the clinician and is an essential part of rehabilitation.

SECTION 3: CASE STUDIES AND STUDENT QUESTIONS

Case study 1

A 45-year-old right-handed painter presents with central neck pain and mild dizziness, following a rear-end collision 2 weeks ago. He returned to work but found that this aggravated the problem and he has had to take sick leave. On examination the patient has a head-forward-hinge posture, with the hinge at the mid-cervical spine.

Movements: flexion – no immediate pain but the lower cervical spine is relatively flexible into flexion compared to the upper cervical spine; extension – pain at half range over crease at the mid-cervical spine, where there is an area of relative flexibility into extension and low cervical extension is restricted. Right rotation is painful on the right and asymmetrical, with an increase in relative flexibility at the mid-cervical spine. Left rotation causes a mild pulling sensation. On palpation, ↓ C 4/5 is painful (soft end-feel) and C5/6/7 is stiff, with a hard end-feel. PPIVMs (passive physiological intervertebral movements) reveal that C4/5 is hypermobile into extension and rotation and hypomobile into flexion with

C5/6/7 stiff into extension. Cervical repositioning is assessed as being poor, with mild defects in standing balance and gaze stability.

Hypothesis: This patient has low cervical flexion give and a mid-cervical extension give.

Exercise programme

Treatment 1

(1) Control site and direction of movement. Teach the patient to control extension at the mid-cervical spine and move into extension from the low cervical spine. Position the patient in sitting with the upper and mid-cervical spine in neutral. Ask the patient to move through range from flexion to extension, maintaining neutral at the upper and mid-cervical spine. Use a mirror and your hands to guide the patient so that movement occurs at the lower cervical spine. Teach the patient rotation control in a similar manner. Check that the

Case study 1—cont'd

patient can do the exercises correctly without feedback. The patient needs to practise these exercises for 15–20 repetitions two to three times per day and then built to 1–2 minutes until it feels natural and familiar.

(2) Teach scapular stability exercises (Mottram, 2003).

(3) Hold a pen in front of the patient and ask him to move his head slowly into *small* ranges of flexion, left and right rotation and left and right side flexion, while keeping the gaze set on the pen. This should be repeated three times, two to three times per day.

(4) Ask the patient to try to balance on one leg for 30 seconds and repeat twice on each leg.

(5) He should aim for a 30-minute walk every day.

Treatment 2

(1) Teach the patient to control the uncontrolled hypermobility at C4/5. (a) Using the pressure biofeedback, teach the patient to recruit the deep flexors in neutral and hold for 10 seconds for 10 repetitions. Teach him to do this as a home exercise using the wall as feedback. (b) Teach the patient to recruit the deep suboccipital extensors and hold for 10 seconds for 10 repetitions. Once the patient can do this correctly, teach the home exercise using his own hands to give resistance.

(2) Progress exercise 1 from day 1. Ask the patient to repeat this exercise in standing and progress with the right upper limb in the functional position he uses for work.

(3) Teach scapula stability exercises holding a paintbrush.

(4) Progress the balance exercises to closed eyes.

(5) Progress the gaze stability exercises by asking the patient to close their eyes, move their head and then open their eyes to check the eyes have maintained a stable gaze on the target.

(6) Continue with walking.

Treatment 3

(1) Teach the patient to actively control the full available range of movement of extension and rotation, by aiming to rehabilitate the anterior stabilisers in inner and outer range.

(a) In incline sitting ask the patient to flex the neck as far as possible without substitution strategies. Hold 10×10 seconds in the midline. Progress the exercise to supine and then flexion and rotation holds. Once the patient has trained the anterior stabilisers in inner range, progress to outer range by instructing the patient to flex the upper cervical spine and then independently extend the lower cervical spine. This will help to unload the structures under strain due to the uncontrolled movement at the mid-cervical spine. Add in functional arm movements as able.

(2) Re-educate the posterior stabilisers by positioning the patient in prone, resting on the elbows with the head hanging in flexion. The patient should maintain the upper cervical spine in neutral and lift the head with independent extension and rotation of the low cervical spine. Hold for 10×10 seconds.

(3) Teach the patient to increase the extensibility of the right scalenes using the left hand for resistance and following the stretch procedure as discussed.

(4) Progress the balance exercises to wobble board work.

(5) Progress the gaze stability exercise, using the goggles to restrict peripheral vision.

Treatment 4

(1) Progress exercise 1 in treatment 3 by using Thera-Band® to resist extension and flexion.

(2) Progress into functional loading activities. For example, control cervical extension and maintain good scapulothoracic patterning, while elevating the arm through scaption with a 1 kg weight. Use different speeds and different angles. Another example is an exercise to replicate lifting a ladder. Start with a 65 cm Swiss ball and ask the patient to control the cervical extension as he picks up the ball from a chair and lifts it to a higher surface while looking up. Progress the exercise to lifting a box.

(3) Progress the gaze stability exercises into functional applications.

(4) Ask the patient to continue with walking or add in static bike cycling.

Case study 2

A 31-year-old front row rugby player presents to you after having sustained a 'stinger injury' during a tackle in a game last week. There are no residual symptoms and he has no neck pain. Cranioverterbral instability tests and vertebrobasilar insufficiency (VBI) tests are clear. This is the second stinger injury in 2 months. A magnetic resonance (MR) image shows mild spinal stenosis.

Management

The patient has been doing an exercise programme that includes:

(1) Exercises to improve a mild flexion give at the lower cervical spine
(2) Neural dynamic mobilisations for the median nerve
(3) Stretches for the anterior scalenes
(4) Stability exercises for the glenohumeral joint and thoracic spine, including rotator cuff exercises in functional positions
(5) Proprioceptive training for the cervical spine, thoracic spine and glenohumeral joint
(6) Tackle technique training with the coach.

The following is an example of an exercise programme for cervical strengthening. (To be completed 2–3 × week as part of the rehabilitation programme. Full exercise programme must include progressions of the exercises just described.)

Warm-up

- 10 minutes on a bike.
- Manual isometric holds 10 seconds, flexion, extension, left and right lateral flexion and left and right rotation.

- Cervical self-stretches all ranges × 5.
- Deep cervical flexor holds 10 × 10 seconds.
- Deep suboccipital extensor holds 10 × 10 seconds.
- Upper limb mobilisations for the median nerve (ULNT1).

Circuit – 1 minute per exercise with 30 seconds rest. Circuit to be completed twice.

(1) Flexion/extension/left side flexion/right side flexion holds with sit-fit against the wall.
(2) Extension hold plus deep squat.
(3) Flexion hold plus deep squat.
(4) Lateral lunge plus side flexion hold.
(5) Arm steps plus extension hold – using a weighted neck harness; position the patient in a press-up position directly in front of wall bars. Instruct the individual to walk up the wall bars with their hands. The cervical spine must be kept in neutral.
(6) Three-way front lunge – position the individual in standing about 1.2 m (4 ft) from wall bars with their back to the wall. Attach a head strap over the forehead and attach the strap to the wall bars with Thera-Band® or bungee. Instruct the individual to step into a running position, i.e. step standing with running arm position. The cervical spine must remain in neutral.
(7) Trunk roll-out – start in a supine position with the thoracic spine resting on a Swiss ball. Maintain cervical spine and trunk in neutral while rolling over the ball by flexing and extending the knees. The end position is when the ball reaches the occiput.

Warm down – relaxation drill in supine plus visualisation of correct tackling technique.

Case study 3

A 60-year-old medical secretary presents with insidious-onset neck pain. She has a 2-year history of mild, intermittent headache over the right temporal region associated with mild right neck ache. Her job involves a significant amount of reading

and she feels this may be aggravating her headaches. Her neck ache increases as the day goes on. X-rays show that she has a loss of disc height at C3, 4 and 5 cervical discs with associated degeneration. Her doctor has diagnosed cervical spond-

Case study 3—cont'd

ylosis and feels that the headache may be related to her neck. He has ruled out any other medical condition. On assessment she has a chin poke posture.

Movements: Flexion three-quarters range (resistance > pain) increase in relative flexibility of the lower cervical spine into flexion; extension half range (onset of pain = onset of resistance); left rotation/side flexion half range (resistance > pain), right rotation/side flexion half range (resistance = pain). On palpation ↓ C1/2 is stiff and painful, with unilateral right postero-anterior accessory movement being very sore early in range over C2/3. During the cranio-cervical flexion test the patient is unable to sustain target pressure levels of 24 mmHg for a period of 5 seconds without the chin poking out and the right sterno-cleidomastoid becoming significantly overactive. Cervical joint position sense and balance is assessed as being 'poor'. The patient has been attending physiotherapy for 3 weeks and has found that manual therapy for the upper cervical spine has helped, but has not resolved the problem. In addition her home programme has included static bike work, basic flexion control exercises, deep flexor and deep extensor exercises, anterior stabiliser exercises in inner range, cervical repositioning exercises and various oculomotor exercises.

Hypothesis: this woman has a low cervical flexion give, which is improving but has not yet completed mid-stage rehabilitation into function.

Management

Treatment 1

(1) Position the patient in sitting with a light Thera-Band™ around the head to provide resistance into extension. This exercise aims to improve eccentric control of cervical flexion. Instruct the patient to maintain the upper cervical spine in neutral, move the low cervical spine slowly through range from flexion to extension and back into flexion to do a backward head tilt. Make sure the patient extends through the low cervical spine. Progress this exercise to sitting on a Swiss ball.

(2) Position the patient in her working posture at a desk with a book. Complete deep flexor exercises 10 × 10 seconds in this position. Progress this exercise either by sitting on a Swiss ball or Sit-Fit™.

(3) With the patient in prone check that the patient is able to recruit the deep extensors. If she is able to do this progress the exercise to lying prone on a firm bed with the head overhanging the edge of the bed. Ask the patient to position the cervical spine in neutral, while recruiting the deep extensors. Hold for 10 × 10 seconds and try to increase the holding time.

(4) Once the patient has been training inner range anterior stabilisers and is able to hold in end-range flexion and rotation without substitution strategies, progress to outer-range anterior stabiliser exercises. Position the patient in sitting with a neutral spine. Maintain the low cervical spine in extension slowly, extend the upper cervical spine by allowing the chin to lift towards the ceiling a quarter range. Hold for 10 seconds × 10 at a quarter range. Then try to do this exercise at half range, three-quarters range and full range. Add in rotation and repeat the exercise. Then add in isometric resistance at different ranges.

(5) Complete the cervical repositioning exercises sitting on a Swiss ball. Add in scapular stability work. Add in functional postures. Progress to standing on a sit-fit.

(6) Check that as the deep flexors are improving (using the biofeedback), the right sternoclei-domastoid is becoming less dominant. If the sternocleidomastoid seems shortened get the patient to sit with the occiput and thorax against the wall. Instruct the patient to rotate her head half range towards the right and side flex away. Actively slide the occiput up the wall (upper cervical flexion) and hold for 20–30 seconds, repeating three to five times.

(7) If the suboccipitals still seem tight, instruct the patient to lie supine with the hands bringing the head into upper cervical flexion and then actively slide the occiput up tall. Hold the stretch for 20–30 seconds and repeat three to five times.

Student questions

(1) How would you describe the patient's posture in Figure 4.2a?
(2) Which muscles may be dominant or tight in this type of posture?
(3) What is the difference between a 'global mobiliser' muscle and a 'global stabiliser' muscle?
(4) If a patient presents with two areas of 'give' how would you decide which area is the clinical priority?
(5) Why do you need to be careful when prescribing suboccipital extensor stretches to patients with neural irritability?
(6) A patient presents to you with neck pain. (He also has chronic obstructive pulmonary disease). Which muscles are likely to be overactive and contributing to the neck dysfunction?
(7) How many repetitions of exercise would you recommend when using Thera-Band® for resistance?
(8) What advice would you give to your patient following completion of an exercise programme?
(9) Why is it important to vary the speed, range and starting positions of exercises?
(10) Give three exercises for the rehabilitation of the cervical sensorimotor system. How would you progress these exercises for the following appointment?

Acknowledgements

The authors are grateful to Sarah Mottram, MSc, MMACP, MCSP, Chartered Physiotherapist, Private Practitioner, The Movement Works, Ludlow, UK, and Kinetic Control Accredited Tutor, Kinetic Control, UK, and Mark Comerford, BPhty MAPA, Physiotherapist, Performance Rehab, Australia, and Kinetic Control Accredited Tutor, Kinetic Control, UK for inclusion of their exercise programme and discussion of their concepts in this chapter.

References

Binder, A. (2007) cervical spondylosis and neck pain. *British Medical Journal*, 334, 527–531.

Bourghouts, J.A. J., Koes, B. W., Vondeling, H. and Boulter, L.M. (1999) Cost of illness in neck pain in the Netherlands in 1996. *Pain*, 80, 629–636.

Boyling, J.D., Jull, G.A. and Twomey, L.T. (2004) *Grieve's Modern Manual Therapy – The Vertebral Column*, 3rd edn. Elsevier/Churchill Livingstone, Edinburgh.

Brison, R.J., Hartling, L. and Pickett, W. (2000) A prospective study of acceleration-extension injuries following rear end motor vehicle collisions. World congress on whiplash-associated disorders in Vancouver, British Columbia, Canada, February 1999. *Journal of Musculoskeletal Pain*, 8, 7–13.

Bronfort, G., Nilsson, N., Hass, M., Evans, R., Goldsmith, C.H., Assendelft, W.J.J. and Bouter, L.M. (2004) Non-invasive physical treatments for chronic/recurrent headaches. *Cochrane Database of Systemic Reviews*, 3, CD001878.

Caroll, L.J., Hogg-Johnson, S., van der Velde, G., Haldeman, S., Holm, L.W., Carragee, E.J., Hurwitz, E.L., Côté, P., Nordin, M., Peloso, P.M., Guzman, J., Cassidy, J.D. and Bone and Joint Decade 2000–2010 Task Force on Neck Pain and Its Associated Disorders. (2008) Course and prognostic factors for neck pain in the general population. *Spine*, 33(4 Suppl.), S75–S82.

Chiu, T., Lam, T. and Hedley, A. (2004) A randomised controlled trial on the efficacy of exercise for patients with chronic neck pain. *Spine*, 30, E1–7.

Comerford, M.J. and Mottram, S.L. (2007) *Diagnosis of Mechanical Dysfunction and Stability Retraining of the Neck and Shoulder Girdle*. Kinetic Control, UK.

Comerford, M.J., Mottram S.L. and Gibbons, S.G.T. (2008) *Understanding Movement & Function – Concepts Course*. Kinetic Control, UK.

Cote, P., Cassidy, J.D. and Carroll, L. (1998) The Saskatchewan Health and Back Pain Survey: the prevalence of neck pain and related disability. *Spine*, 23, 1689–1698

Falla, D., Campell, C.D., Fagan, A.E., Thompson, D.C. and Jull, G.A. (2003) Relationship between craniocervical flexion R.O.M. and pressure changes during the craniocervical flexion test. *Manual Therapy*, 8, 92–96.

Falla, D., Jull, G., Russell, T., Vicenzino, B. and Hodges, P. (2007) Effect of neck exercise on sitting posture in patients with chronic neck pain. *Physical Therapy*, 87, 408–417.

Falla, D., Jull, G.A. and Hodges, P.W. (2004) Neck pain patients demonstrate reduced E.M.G. activity of the deep cervical flexor muscles during performance of craniocervical flexion. *Spine*, 29, 2018–2014.

Fuller, C.W., Brooks, J.H. and Kemp, S.P. (2007) Spinal injuries in professional rugby union: a prospective cohort study. *Clinical Journal of Sports Medicine*, 17, 10–16.

Guzman, J., Haldeman, S. and Carroll, L.J. (2008) Clinical practice implications of the bone and joint decade 2000–2010 task force on neck pain and its associated disorders – from concepts and findings to recommendations. *European Spine Journal*, 17, S199–S213.

Harvey, H. and Cooper, C. (2005) Physiotherapy for neck and back pain. *British Medical Journal*, 330, 53–54.

Helewa, A., Goldsmith, C.H., Smythe, H.A., Lee, P., Obright, K. and Stitt, L. (2007) Effect of therapeutic exercise and sleeping neck support on patients with chronic neck pain: A randomised clinical trial. *Journal of Rheumatology*, 34, 1.

Highland T.R., Dreisinger, T.E., Vie, L.L. and Russell, G.S. (1992) Changes in isometric strength and range of motion of the isolated cervical spine after eight weeks of clinical rehabilitation. *Spine*, 17(6 Suppl.), S77–82.

Holm, L., Carroll, L.J., Cassidy, J.D., Hogg-Johnson, S., Cote, P., Guzman, J., Pelsoa, P., Nordin, M., Hurwitz, E., van der Velde, G., Carragee, E., Haldeman, S. and Bone and Joint Decade 2000–2010 Task Force on Neck Pain and Its Associated Disorders. (2008) The burden and determinants of neck pain in whiplash associated disorders after traffic collisions. *Spine*, 33(4 Suppl.), S52–S59.

Humphreys, B. and Irgens, P. (2002) The effect of a rehabilitation exercise programme on head repositioning accuracy and reported levels of pain in chronic neck pain subjects. *Journal of Whiplash and Related Disorders*, 1, 99–112.

Hurwitz, E., Carragee, E.J., van der Valde, G., Carroll, L.J., Nordin, M., Guzman, J., Peloso, P.M., Holm, L.W., Côté, P., Hogg-Johnson, S., Cassidy, J.D., Haldeman, S. and Bone and Joint Decade 2000–2010 Task Force on Neck Pain and Its Associated Disorders. (2008) Treatment of neck pain: Non invasive interventions. *Spine*, 33(4 Suppl.), S123–S152.

Jordan, A., Bendix, T., Neilson, H., Hansen, F., Host, D. and Winkel, A. (1998) Intensive training, physiotherapy, or manipulation for patients with chronic neck pain. *Spine*, 23, 311–319.

Jull, G., Trott, P., Potter, H., Zito, G., Niere, K., Shirley, D., Emberson, J., Marschner, I. and Richardson, C. (2002) A randomised controlled trial of exercise and manipulative therapy for cervicogenic headache. *Spine*, 27, 1835–1843.

Jull, G., Kristjansson, E. and Dall'Alba, P. (2004a) Impairment in the cervical comparison of whiplash and insidious onset neck pain patients. *Manual Therapy*, 9, 89–94.

Jull, G.A., Falla, J., Sterling, M. and Oleary, S. (2004b) A therapeutic exercise approach for cervical disorders. In: *Grieve's Modern Manual Therapy – The Vertebral Column*, 3rd edn, pp. 451–470. Elsevier/Churchill Livingstone, Edinburgh.

Jull, G., Falla, D., Treleaven, J., Hodges, P. and Vicenzino, B. (2007b) Retraining cervical joint position sense: the effect of two exercise regimes. *Journal of Orthopaedic Research*, 25, 404–412.

Kay, T.M., Gross, A., Goldsmith, C., Santaguida, J., Hoving, J., Bronfort, G. and Cervical Overview Group. (2005) Exercises for mechanical neck disorders. *Cochrane Database of Systemic Reviews*, 3, CD004250.

Kennedy, C. (1998) Exercise interventions for the cervical spine. *Orthopaedic Division Review*, 13–29.

McKinney, L.A, Dornan, J.O. and Ryan, M. (1989a) The role of physiotherapy in the management of acute neck sprains following road traffic accidents. *Archives of Emergency Medicine*, 6, 27–33.

Mottram, S. (2003) In: Beeton, K. (ed.) *Manual Therapy Master Classes – The Peripheral Joints*. Elsevier, London.

Mulligan, B. (1999) *Manual Therapy 'NAGS, SNAGS, MWMS'*, 4th edn, p. 25. Plane View Services Ltd, Wellington., New Zealand.

O'Leary, S., Jull, G., Kim, M. and Vicenzino, B. (2007) Specificity in retraining craniocervical flexor muscle performance. *Journal of Orthopeadic and Sports Physical Therapy*, 37, 3–9.

Panjabi, M.M., Cholewicki, J., Nibu, K., Grauer, J., Babat, L.B. and Dvorak, J. (1998) Critical load of the human cervical spine: an in vitro experimental study. *Clinical Biomechanics*, 13, 11–17.

Rosenfeld, M., Gunnarsson, R. and Borenstein, P. (2000) Early intervention in whiplash-associated disorders. *Spine*, 25, 1782–1787.

Santana, J.C. (2000) *Functional Training: Breaking the Bonds of Traditionalism*. Optimum Performance Systems, Florida.

Sarig-Bahat, H. (2003) Evidence for exercise therapy in mechanical neck disorders. *Manual Therapy*, 8, 10–20.

Soderlund, A., Olerud, C. and Lindberg, P. (2000) Acute whiplash associated disorders: #the effect of early mobilisation and prognostic factors in long term symptomatology. *Clinical Rehabilitation*, 14, 457–467.

Steele, C. (2007) *Cervical Spine Strength/Stability/Mobility Programme*. I.R.F.U. Landsowne Road, Dublin.

Sterling, M. (2005) *Managing Cervical Spine Disorders: Research Advances and Clinical Application*. Course notes July 14th 2005. Whiplash and Neck pain Research Unit, University of Queensland, Brisbane.

Takala, E.P., Viikari Juntura, E. and Tynkkynen, E.M. (1994). Does group gymnastics at the workplace help in neck pain. *Scandinavian Journal of Rehabilitative Medicine*, 26, 17–20.

Treleaven, J. (2008) Sensorimotor disturbances in neck disorders affecting postural stability, head and eye movement control. *Manual Therapy*, 13, 2–11.

Vernon, H. and Humphries, B.K. (2007) Manual therapy for neck pain: an overview of randomised clinical trials and systemic reviews. *Europa Medicophysica*, 43, 91–118.

Viljanen, M., Malmivaara, A., Uitti, J., Rinne, M., Palmroos, P. and Laippala, P. (2003) Effectiveness of dynamic muscle training, relaxation training, or ordinary activity for chronic neck pain: randomised controlled trial. *British Medical Journal*, 327, 30.

Webb, R., Brammah, T., Lunt, M., Unwin, M., Allison, T. and Symmons, D. (2003) Prevalence and predictors of intense, chronic and disabling neck and back pain in the U.K. general population. *Spine*, 28, 1195–1202.

Wolsko, P.M., Eisenberg, D.M., Davis, R.B., Kessler, R. and Phillips, R.S. (2003) Patterns and perceptions of care for treatment of back and neck pain: results of a national survey. *Spine*, 28, 292–298.

Ylinen, J., Takala, E., Nykanen, M., Hakkinen, A., Malkia, E., Pohjolainen, T., Karppi, S.L., Kautiainen, H. and Airaksinen, O. (2003) Active neck training in the treatment of chronic neck pain in women. *Journal of the American Medical Association*, 289, 2509–2516.

Ylinen, J., Hakkinen, A., Nykanen, M., Kautianen, H. and Takala, E.P. (2007) Neck muscle training in the treatment of chronic neck pain: a three year follow up study. *Europa Medicophysica*, 43, 161–169.

The Thoracic Spine and Rib Cage

5

Fiona Wilson

SECTION 1: INTRODUCTION AND BACKGROUND

There is paucity of evidence supporting the use of exercise therapy in the management of conditions of the thoracic spine and rib cage. This could reflect the less frequent presentation to the clinician of injuries in this specific area. However, there has been increasing interest in the thoracic spine by clinicians because of several reasons: the recognition of the thoracic spine as an important source of pain; the role of thoracic curvature in determining overall spinal posture; the influence of thoracic mobility on movement patterns in other regions of the spine (Edmondston and Singer, 1997). The thorax is inherently more stable when compared with areas such as the lumbar spine. Much of the research has focused on specific conditions, notably ankylosing spondylitis (AS), scoliosis and osteoporosis. Other conditions such Scheuermann's disease, rotational instability and acute locked thoracic spine present frequently to the clinician but there is little evidence in the literature to support a particular treatment regimen. However, regional areas of the spine – that is, the cervical, thoracic and lumbar spines – should not be considered in isolation and dysfunction in any of these areas will ultimately affect adjacent structures. When considering the thoracic spine, exercises that are also applied to the lumbar spine must be considered. The reader will note that much of the lumbar spine exercise approach refers to trunk stability and thus by anatomical definition will have influence on the thoracic spine as many muscle groups will be shared by each region.

Evidence for the use of exercise in the management of disorders of the thoracic spine and rib cage

Research regarding the role of exercise in cervical and lumbar spine conditions frequently considers patients stratified into groups which are non-specific in diagnosis. However, in the case of exercise and the thoracic spine, it is common to consider the issue in terms of specific conditions, and these are reviewed below.

AS is a well-defined condition and the use of exercise in patients with AS has been consistently documented. It must, of course, be noted that the presentation of AS is not confined to the thoracic

Exercise Therapy in the Management of Musculoskeletal Disorders, First Edition. Edited by Fiona Wilson, John Gormley and Juliette Hussey.
© 2011 Blackwell Publishing Ltd

spine but that symptoms in this area are often the most notable feature of the disease, particularly in mid to early presentation. Dagfinrud *et al.* (2004) performed a Cochrane systematic review of physiotherapy interventions for AS. They compared six trials with a total of 561 participants. Two trials compared home exercises with no therapy and concluded that home exercises improved movement in the spine and fitness more than no therapy at all. The home exercises were carried out for 4–6 months and were tailored to each individual by a therapist. These programmes did not appear to have any beneficial effect on pain levels. Three other studies compared home exercises to supervised group exercise outside the home. The group exercises were found to improve movement in the spine and overall wellbeing, but did not improve fitness anymore than the home exercise programmes. The group therapy was carried out for a period of 3 weeks to 9 months and included physical training, aerobic exercise, hydrotherapy, sports activities and stretching. The final study compared two groups that both did weekly group exercises for 10 months; however, one group went to a spa resort for 3 weeks of physiotherapy. It was found that spa therapy plus group exercise improved pain, fitness and overall wellbeing more than weekly group exercises. The conclusion was that home exercises are better than no exercises and improved both movement in the spine and fitness; group exercises are better than home exercises and improve pain, stiffness, movement of the spine and overall wellbeing. It should be noted that the specific exercises were not described, although a general summary stated that exercises are helpful to people with AS.

Fernàndez De Las Peñas *et al.* (2005) evaluated the impact of a 4-month protocol of flexibility and strengthening exercises versus conventional exercises for AS. The conventional intervention consisted of 20 exercises: motion and flexibility exercises of the cervical, thoracic and lumbar spine; stretching of the shortened muscles and chest expansion exercises. The experimental protocol was based on the global posture re-education method (GPR), which employs specific stretching and strengthening exercises to improve posture. The results were monitored by changes in activity, mobility and functional capacity. Both groups showed an improvement in all measures. The intergroup comparison showed that the GPR group obtained a greater improvement than the control group in all but one of the clinical measures. The authors concluded that exercise was beneficial in the treatment of AS and that a programme specifically geared towards postural re-education may have further benefits.

Ince *et al.* (2006) investigated the effects of a 12-week exercise programme in patients with AS. Thirty patients were included in the randomised controlled trial and were assigned to either an exercise programme or the control group. The exercise programme consisted of 50 minutes of multi-modal exercise (aerobic, stretching and pulmonary exercises), three times a week for 3 months. Measurements were taken of spinal mobility and chest expansion. The spinal movements of the exercise group improved significantly but those of the control group showed no significant change. Physical work capacity and vital capacity values improved in the exercise group but decreased in the control group. The conclusion was that a multi-modal exercise programme is beneficial in the management of AS.

Exercise protocols are frequently employed in the conservative management of idiopathic scoliosis on two accounts: improvement of respiratory and musculoskeletal function. Ferraro *et al.* (1998; cited in Hawes, 2003) reported stabilisation of the spinal curvature and rib hump among 34 children with mild scoliosis over a 2-year period of treatment, which included daily taught exercises. Solberg (1996) demonstrated improved appearance and reduced spinal curvature in 10 children with mild scoliosis following a 5-month daily exercise programme. Weiss *et al.* (2003) examined the effect of exercise on the progression of idiopathic scoliosis in children. The cohort consisted of one group of untreated children and another group that received scoliosis inpatient rehabilitation, which was delivered as an individual exercise programme. The results showed that the scoliosis inpatient rehabilitation group demonstrated reduced progression of the condition in comparison with the non-exercise group.

Santos Alves *et al.* (2006) analysed the impact of a physical rehabilitation programme on respiratory function on a group of 34 patients with idiopathic scoliosis. Patients completed three weekly sessions of 60 minutes of exercise, which included stretching and aerobic exercises. Improvements were found in pulmonary capacities and volumes, and performance on a 6-minute walking test. Although this was not a specific musculoskeletal programme it demonstrates the importance and benefits of an aerobic programme to patients with this condition.

Osteoporosis is a condition that affects all the bones of the body in all population groups. While it is not the purpose of this chapter to discuss osteoporosis, specific postural changes in the thoracic spine are well documented. Exercise has been shown to generally have a positive impact. Sinaki *et al.* (2005) examined the influence of kyphotic posture associated with osteoporosis and the incidence of falls. Twelve women with osteoporosis-related kyphosis were assessed for balance and various strength measurements. This group was compared with 13 non-osteoporotic controls. The study demonstrated that the osteoporotic women had weaker back extensor and lower extremity strength, poorer balance and slower gait in comparison with the control group. This influenced their propensity to fall. The authors argued that treatment options should include exercises that address these deficits. Gold *et al.* (2004) enhanced the argument that exercises were beneficial in the management of osteoporosis based on the findings of their randomised controlled trial of 185 post-menopausal women. All women in this study had sustained at least one osteoporotic vertebral fracture. The exercises included progressive strengthening and stretching exercises. The conclusions of the study were that weak trunk extension strength and psychological symptoms associated with vertebral fractures can be improved in older women using group treatment. Katzman *et al.* (2007) demonstrated in a group of older women that kyphosis could be modified with the help of a multidimensional group exercise programme. A cohort of women with thoracic curvature of 50° or more underwent a supervised exercise programme twice a week for 12 weeks. Following the programme, significant improvements were seen such as reduced thoracic kyphosis, improved strength, improved range of motion (ROM) and physical performance.

Conditions that are seen less often in a physiotherapy department, such as spinal tuberculosis, have also been shown to benefit from physiotherapy and a rehabilitation programme. Nas *et al.* (2004) included 47 patients in a rehabilitation programme both pre- and early post-operatively. Aerobic and strengthening exercises were employed and progressed, with assessment of the patients at

regular intervals. The final outcome was that 70% of patients were independent at the end of the programme and the authors concluded that this was the result of application of an appropriate rehabilitation strategy.

Aerobic exercise

The general principles of the effect of aerobic exercise on the musculoskeletal system should be applied to all conditions affecting the thoracic spine. This is particularly important when it is noted that many conditions such as AS, which present with specific thoracic symptoms, are systemic in nature. There is little research suggesting that specific aerobic conditioning has an effect on thoracic spine conditions. There is some positive research in this area in relation to the lumbar spine and it would be logical to apply the same principles to the thoracic spine, although this is an area where further study is required.

The biomechanics of the thorax and the mechanism of respiration should be considered. The thorax is made up from a number of different types of joint, which affects the various degrees of freedom. However, in shallow respiration, movements will always occur in these joints and it is logical to conclude that the increase in respiration rate associated with increased activity would cause increased movements in the joints with associated benefits.

Muscle strength and endurance

The role of muscle endurance in postural control and activity of the trunk is discussed in depth in Chapter 6. Spinal stability and position sense theories may be applied to the thoracic spine as they are to the lumbar spine, although the thorax is more stable due to the presence of the rib cage, and the morphology and orientation of the facet joints. Postural changes in the thorax are frequently seen as an increased kyphosis and while some of these changes may be due to structural changes in the vertebrae and associated joints (as in osteoporosis and AS) some are due to poor endurance, particularly in the paraspinal muscles. None of the studies reviewed above examined the particular role of strengthening exercise in the rehabilitation of thoracic spine disorders. However, a number of the studies reviewed in the chapters examining the lumbar and cervical spine referred to the 'cervico-thoracic' spine or the 'thoraco-lumbar' spine and these should be revisited by the student.

Range of motion and flexibility

To understand the factors that limit ROM in the thoracic spine, simple biomechanics of the region need to be considered. Much of the testing of the thoracic spine has taken place on a cadaveric spine with the rib cage removed. However, to understand the contribution of the rib cage to spinal stability, there is a requirement for the unit, i.e. the spine plus intact rib cage, to be tested under conditions of loading. Watkins *et al.* (2005) demonstrated that the presence of the rib cage significantly limits motion in the thoracic spine and thus enhances stability. Testing the complete thoracic unit under conditions of loading showed that the presence of the rib cage increased the stability of the thoracic spine by 40% in flexion/extension, 35% in lateral bending and 31% in axial rotation. The most notable movement in the thoracic spine is axial rotation, which is a reflection of the coronal orientation of the facet joints particularly in the upper and middle regions. Flexion is limited by the rib cage and a prime limitation to thoracic extension is the shape of the spinous processes. Many individuals will demonstrate a very limited extension from the neutral position. Edmondston *et al.* (2007) showed that postural position has an influence on the range of motion in the thoracic spine. Testing of axial rotation in different sitting postures (neutral, end-range flexion and end-range extension) demonstrated a significant decrease in the range of thoracic rotation in flexion compared with the neutral and extended postures.

Thus, the thoracic spine is an area where ROM is limited by its structure but decreases in ROM by disorders or pain will still have a significant effect on function. Further, decreased thoracic movement, particularly at the cervico-thoracic junction and the thoraco-lumbar junction will cause increase motion demands on the cervical and lumbar spines, respectively, and may lead to a hypermobile segment or pathological changes. As noted above, thoracic extension is noted as a small movement from the neutral position and is frequently limited in patients with poor posture, poor lumbar or cervical stability

or in diseases such as osteoporosis where there are morphological changes in the vertebrae. Maintenance of thoracic extension with ROM exercises is vital to allow a neutral postural position to be achieved. Thoracic flexion is rarely limited although axial rotation is frequently noted to be limited, particularly in the presence of thoracic facet joint disease. Good thoracic and thus trunk rotation is essential for normal functioning, particularly in activities such as gait. Normal kinematics of the shoulder, cervical and lumbar joints are particularly dependent on normal thoracic biomechanics and posture (Kebaetse *et al.*, 1999) and limitation of thoracic movements have been noted as a precursor to disorders in these areas.

Balance and proprioception

The role of balance and proprioception in function in the thoracic spine is very poorly represented in literature. This is not surprising given the structural stability afforded to this region. No published studies have provided clear links between abnormal pathology in this area and proprioceptive deficits as in the cervical and lumbar spines. However, some studies have noted co-ordination patterns of the trunk which are essential for normal gait, and changes in these patterns have been associated with neurological disease such a stroke and Parkinson's disease (Kubo *et al.*, 2006). In the absence of specific evidence it may be hypothesised that deficits similar to those noted in other spinal areas would be observed, albeit in an attenuated fashion due to the structural stability of this area. Further research is required in this area.

Disorders of the thoracic spine

The most common disorders of the thoracic spine are: intervertebral joint sprain, facet joint disease or dysfunction, paraspinal muscle strain, costovertebral joint sprain, Scheuermann's disease, and osteoporosis. Less common are rib fractures, thoracic disc disorders, T4 syndrome and AS. However, cardiac, respiratory and metastatic causes of pain must also be considered (Singer, 2006).

Scheuermann's disease

Scheuermann's disease is an osteochondrosis of the spine that mainly occurs in adolescents, usually males in their last 2–3 years of growth. It is a disturbance in the normal growth of the vertebral epiphyseal ring. If the compressive forces in the spine are sufficient it may cause a wedge deformity in the vertebral body causing a kyphosis of the thoracic spine and an associated increase in lumbar lordosis.

Small disc herniations in the vertebral end plate, called Schmorl's nodes, are sometimes identified on X-rays. The condition often remains asymptomatic but can become painful after activity. Treatment usually consists of moderation of activities to minimise repetitive flexion and extension movements of the spine but with an active exercise programme. These exercises should include stretching the thoraco-lumbar fascia and hamstrings along with strengthening of the trunk muscles. Postural correction also plays a vital role in minimising the thoracic kyphosis. Aerobic exercises should be carried out to maintain general body fitness. In severe cases, if there is significant wedging of more than 5° at more than one level, a brace to restore the normal curvature of the spine may be considered.

Scoliosis

Scoliosis is a lateral deformity of the spine which is always accompanied by rotation particularly in the thoracic spine; therefore the term scoliosis is not a diagnosis but a descriptive term. In the majority of cases, a specific cause is not found and such cases are termed idiopathic, or of unknown cause. They are most commonly seen in adolescent girls.

Scoliosis can affect children from birth through to adolescence. Adolescent scoliosis is the most common type of idiopathic scoliosis. It usually starts around the time of puberty, in girls more often than boys, and may ultimately require surgery if it cannot be controlled using braces. Infantile scoliosis may resolve as the child grows but needs to be kept under observation. Pulmonary and cardiac function may be compromised if the curvature is severe, which would urgently need surgery.

Ankylosing spondylitis

Boulware *et al.* (2003) define AS as 'an inflammatory disease of unknown aetiology, characterized by prominent inflammation of spinal joints and adjacent structures, leading to progressive and ascending bony fusion of the spine'. Males are affected more than females (3:1) and the age of onset is typically from adolescence to 35 years. The disease is part of the group of disorders called seronegative spondyloarthropathies, which are characterised by the following: rheumatoid factor negativity; sacroiliitis; axial involvement; peripheral arthritis; enthesopathy; eye involvement; familial clustering and frequent presence of human leucocyte antigen (HLA) B27 (Boulware *et al.*, 2003). The patient often presents with chronic low back pain and stiffness although its inclusion in this chapter is a reflection of its common early presentation of pain and stiffness in the thoracic spine. Thoracic mobility is greatly decreased as a result of the disease with reduced respiratory expansion observed as the disease progresses. Normal curvature of the spine increases and the patient will present with a flexed, stiff and kyphotic thoracic spine. X-rays demonstrate changes which are specific to the disease with the vertebrae presenting with typical changes to a 'bamboo' appearance. The cervical spine is frequently affected at a later stage in the disease. The disease also may present with cardiac, respiratory, renal, neurological or gastrointestinal symptoms. Management of the condition is aimed at treating pain and inflammation and maintaining mobility, particularly of the thorax, which is essential for normal respiratory function. Exercise should include ROM modalities and strengthening for the thoracic spine with particular efforts towards maintaining thoracic extension and a neutral postural position of the spine. Other exercise approaches have been discussed earlier in this chapter.

SECTION 2: PRACTICAL USE OF EXERCISE

Much of the exercise approach for the management of the thoracic spine is very similar to that for the lumbar spine (Chapter 6) and thus will be referred to rather than repeated. The shoulder complex is

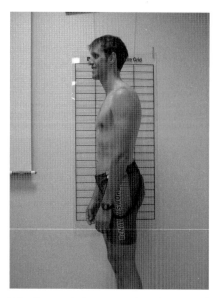

Figure 5.1 Posture being assessed and measured with a posture grid.

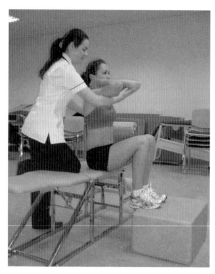

Figure 5.2 The patient's lumbar spine is fixed into flexion by flexing the hips and knees as the patient's range of thoracic extension is assessed.

also related in function to the thoracic spine and kinematics of this area should always be considered with the thoracic spine. It should also be noted that no area of the spine should be treated in isolation as its structure, by nature, demands that it is treated and considered as a continuum, albeit with localized variations.

Assessment of the patient

Posture

A number of conditions of the thoracic spine are characterized by postural changes in the thoracic spine. These include AS and osteoporosis. Postural changes, particularly those that are a result of altered morphology, will have the result of altering biomechanics in related areas such as the lumbar and cervical spines and the shoulder and hip complexes. A posture grid (Fig. 5.1) may be used to assess posture in side standing and anterior or posterior views which will give indications of kyphotic or scoliotic changes, respectively. Such a tool is a particularly useful as a simple outcome measure where disease progression and further changes may be anticipated.

Assessment of aerobic capacity

Fitness testing should be included in the assessment as aerobic exercise will be an important part of the programme. Wittink *et al.* (2000) established the Bruce treadmill test as the most valid for measuring aerobic fitness in patients with chronic low back pain, and it would be logical to use such an approach in testing patients with thoracic spine disorders. However, good practice also demands assessment of respiratory function to gain a clearer knowledge of function of the thorax.

Assessment of endurance

The endurance of the trunk musculature may be assessed using the tests described in Section 2 of Chapter 6.

Assessment of flexibility

The clinician needs to have a clear understanding of the kinematics of the thorax and associated normal movement to be able to identify limitations. It may be necessary to fix the lumbar spine into flexion (Fig. 5.2) to clearly assess the extent of thoracic extension.

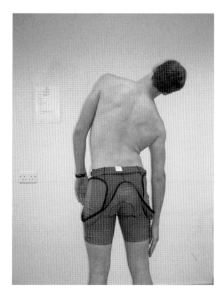

Figure 5.3 Side flexion in standing. Note the large degree of movement in the cervical and lumbar spines.

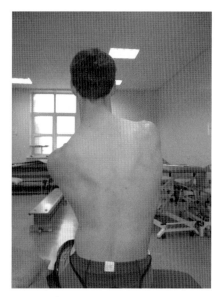

Figure 5.4 Side flexion in sitting with the cervical spine held in a neutral position allows the thoracic spine to be localised.

Assessment of movement should be confined, as far as possible, to the thoracic spine so as to achieve a clear picture of motion patterns. In standing, a great deal of side flexion takes place at the lumbar spine and cervical spine (Fig. 5.3). In sitting, the lumbar spine is less mobile and the patient is asked to keep the cervical spine in a neutral position (Fig. 5.4).

As the thorax is a stable unit, movements should be assessed simply with the addition of overpressure by the clinician (Fig. 5.5). Muscles should be assessed for length, particularly groups such as the pectorals and latissimus dorsi, which will contribute to postural changes in the thorax.

The exercise programme

Early phase

The first stage of the programme should be to establish correct posture and enhance postural control. As has been discussed earlier, many patients with thoracic spine pathology will present with hypomobility, which particularly limits extension. It may be necessary to stretch tight muscle groups and introduce mobility exercises to increase thoracic exten-

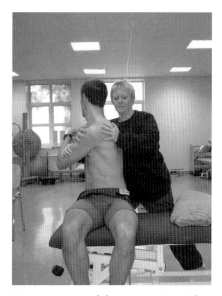

Figure 5.5 Assessment of thoracic rotation with overpressure from the clinician.

sion before the neutral posture may be achieved. Figure 5.6 shows how a patient can use a gym ball to perform a passive stretch to encourage thoracic extension.

Abdominal bracing should be taught early (see Chapter 6), although it must be ensured that thoracic spine position is not compromised. Early motor control exercises may be taught to encourage maintenance of the neutral lumbar position while introducing thoracic spine extension (Fig. 5.7).

Maintenance of a neutral spine position may also be practised with the addition of arm movement. Tightness of muscle groups around the shoulder girdle may be a limiting factor and should be addressed if necessary. Other than stretches that have been suggested so far, simple ROM exercises will address hypomobility. The gymnastic ball (Fig. 5.8) or medical exercise therapy (MET) equipment (Fig. 5.9) will help facilitate dynamic ROM exercises to improve thoracic extension, side flexion and rotation.

Aerobic exercise should be an essential part of this stage with activities such as walking (Nordic or normal) or swimming suitable in this phase (Fig. 5.10). Strengthening activities should not include specific loading in the early phase of the programme and exercises which are aimed at spinal position maintenance will suffice. Proprioceptive work will be informal and again will be an essential part of the spinal position sense work outlined above.

Intermediate phase

Postural activities and exercises (Fig. 5.11) may continue in this stage with an emphasis on loading with limb movement while maintaining good thoracic posture. Stretching and ROM exercises will continue to further enhance joint mobility and good spinal positioning and posture. Loading may be introduced with the use of the many exercises described in the lumbar spine programme. MET programmes, notably pulley-based exercises, are particularly useful in the management of the thoracic spine (Fig. 5.12).

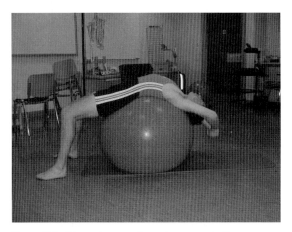

Figure 5.6 Thoracic extension using a gym ball.

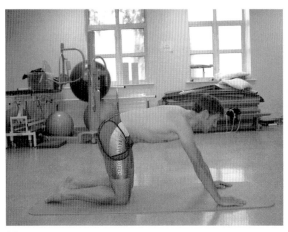

(a)

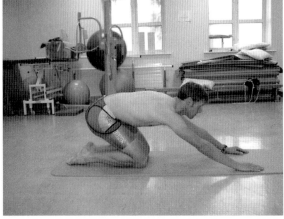

(b)

Figure 5.7 In four-point kneeling, the patient finds the neutral pelvis position (**a**) and is then asked to rock back while keeping the thoracic spine in slight extension and the lumbar spine in neutral (**b**).

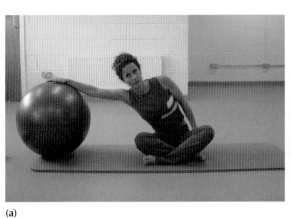

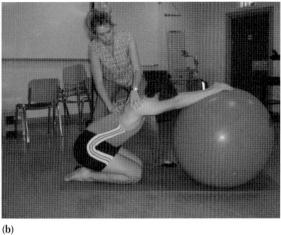

(a)   (b)

Figure 5.8 Use of the gym ball to encourage (**a**) thoracic side flexion and (**b**) thoracic extension.

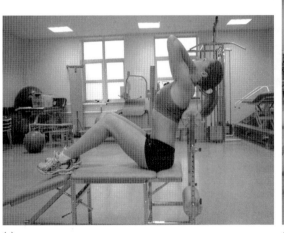

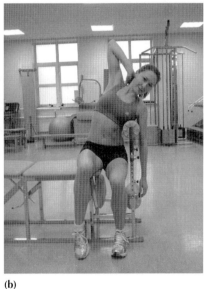

(a)   (b)

Figure 5.9 Use of MET equipment to improve (**a**) thoracic extension and (**b**) thoracic side flexion.

Particular emphasis should be placed on developing endurance of the thoracic extensors and the middle and lower trapezius muscles when there are signs of a developing thoracic kyphosis. The exercise demonstrated in Figure 5.13 is particularly useful for this. Aerobic exercise should continue in this phase with the aim to reach guideline levels of 1 hour.

Late phase

The aim of this stage should be to prepare the patient for discharge. The principles described in Chapter 6 should be considered and applied to the thoracic spine. Thus, increased loading and free weights should be added, unstable surfaces introduced, and ROM and aerobic training continued.

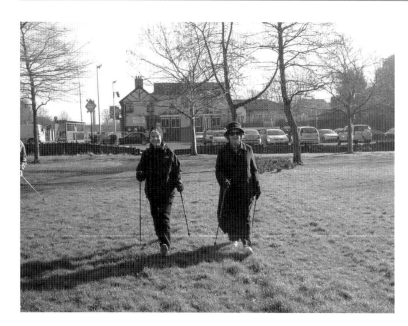

Figure 5.10   Nordic walking is a particularly suitable aerobic activity in rehabilitation of the thoracic spine as movement of this area is facilitated by the poles.

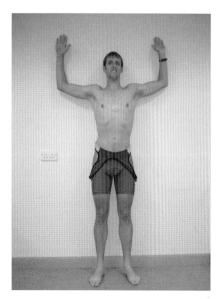

Figure 5.11   Postural activity for the thoracic spine. The patient stands against the wall with the spine in a neutral position. The hands slide up the wall and the spine position is maintained.

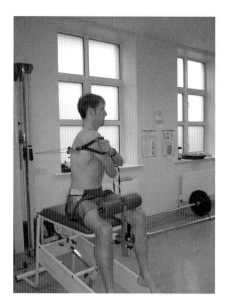

Figure 5.12   MET equipment is used to load thoracic rotation.

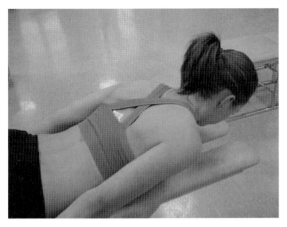

Figure 5.13 The patient lies prone and extends the thorax, placing emphasis on activating the middle and lower trapezius muscle fibres.

Functional activities which introduce high and low levels of loading should be incorporated into the regimen to ensure that the patient will be able to manage independently without the risk of re-injury, once they have been discharged. The student should read Chapter 6 for more details about this stage.

Discharge should involve development of a basic and abridged version of the programme followed to this point, which the patient may continue. Chronic diseases such as AS and osteoporosis demand that regular reviews of the exercise regimen are carried out, with alterations made in response to requirements.

SECTION 3: CASE STUDIES AND STUDENT QUESTIONS

Case study 1

A 17-year-old elite footballer complained of pain and discomfort in the thoracic region of the spine. There was an insidious onset with a gradual increase in discomfort over a number of months. There were no neurological complications but movement was restricted by discomfort and pain at the end of range movement. On examination the discomfort was described as dull rather than sharp and thoracic movements were limited, particularly extension. Postural assessment noted an increased thoracic kyphosis. Palpation was tender on both spinous and transverse processes around T–T10. Radiological investigation demonstrated that the player had Scheuermann's disease with associated Schmorl's nodes.

Management

Scheuermann's disease is a common cause of pain in preteens or adolescents and the main aim of management of this athlete should be to manage the pain and prevent progression of the postural deformity that is noted in the disease, i.e. increased thoracic kyphosis. As the patient is an elite footballer, attenuation of activity should be encouraged, with pain being the main guide to participation levels. Complete cessation of activity should not be advised except in severe cases until the pain has settled, at which time, a graduated return is advised. As this patient is already likely to be fit, aerobic activity should be encouraged from the onset of the programme. Postural correction should be addressed initially and spinal ROM exercises that particularly encourage thoracic extension should be included from the start.

Tight muscle groups, particularly the hamstrings and latissimus dorsi should be stretched, along with any others that may be compromising normal thoracic posture. Strengthening may be started as soon as the footballer can achieve a more neutral thoracic posture, with thoracic extension being the primary focus. The footballer may continue to train, provided his symptoms are well controlled, and his technique should be reviewed, with a particular emphasis on addressing postural control during activity. As good

Case study 1—cont'd

postural control is achieved and more mobility in thoracic extension is noted, the goal of the programme is to maintain gains following discharge. Specific exercises should be built into the athlete's training programme with the assistance of his coach and these will need to be adhered to on a long-term basis. Such exercises should comprise general thoracic ROM exercises, which encourage extension, postural control, particularly of the thoracic extensors, and proprioceptive training in the form of postural control under conditions of moderate loading such as match play. Discharge should take place once the ongoing programme has been established with regular follow-up as hypomobility in the thoracic spine into adulthood is a common manifestation of the disease.

Case study 2

A 30-year-old male teacher presents with insidious onset of low back pain which radiates bilaterally to the sacroiliac joints. The pain, which has a 1-year history is now radiating to the thoracic spine and chest wall. Pain and stiffness are worse in the morning, and relieved by exercise but not by rest. Physical examination shows a flattening of the lumbar lordosis, increased thoracic kyphosis and generalised hypomobility in all spinal movements as well as restricted chest expansion. Radiographic and blood investigations confirm a diagnosis of AS.

Management

The primary aims of management in this patient are to control pain and to relieve stiffness and thus maintain spinal mobility. Pharmacological input is important at an early stage, as pain that is well controlled will allow optimal benefit to be achieved from an exercise programme. The aim of the exercise programme should be to develop a protocol which will be maintained throughout life and will become part of the patient's everyday routine. ROM exercises should be started early with an aim to increase general joint function and motion, and also to achieve better posture and spine position. Exercises to improve thoracic extension are particularly important and the use of a gymnastic ball (see Section 2) is particularly suitable. All thoracic and lumbar movements should be trained with simple ROM exercises although limited attention should be paid to flexion patterns. It is important to pay attention to respiratory function, and chest expansion exercises as well as appropriate monitoring should be an integral and ongoing part of the programme.

Once an improvement in posture is noted, stability work to increase postural muscle endurance should commence with particular emphasis on lumbar control and thoracic extensor endurance; a gymnastic ball is again particularly suitable. Aerobic exercise should commence at the start of the programme with hydrotherapy showing particular benefits for the AS patient. Proprioceptive work will take the form of postural control, which will be very challenging for such a patient due to gross pathological joint activity. Progression of the programme should be aimed at increasing aerobic activity to 1 hour per day and to introduce some loading. Loading should be minimal in the form of pulleys or wrist and ankle weights, and exercise repetitions should be high to encourage endurance benefits. Loading should be aimed at increasing thoracic extension and rotational strength and trunk flexor patterns should not be emphasised. The patient should be carefully monitored for symptom aggravation and the programme altered accordingly if it is noted. ROM exercises should be continued as a fundamental lifestyle change which will be necessary for this patient. Discharge requires that the patient continues the programme daily to achieve optimal attenuation of symptoms, as the disease is chronic in nature. Best practice demands regular review of the programme. The patient may continue to work as a teacher with good ergonomic practices and inclusion of exercise in his daily routine.

Case study 3

A 12-year-old girl has been referred by an orthopaedic paediatrician for an idiopathic, structural scoliosis a result of congenital structural abnormalities. The patient has been screened and cleared of the presence of cardiac, respiratory and neuromuscular disease.

Management

Assessment of the patient and radiological investigations will establish the pattern of this patient's scoliosis and Cobb's angle, which gives an indication of the severity. Some time should be taken examining available joint ROM, endurance of trunk muscles and levels of activity. The emphasis of an exercise programme will be to improve function within the constraints of deformity. The evidence reviewed earlier in the chapter suggests that a structured exercise programme will help reduce progression of the spinal curvature and improving pulmonary function. The design of the programme will be more complex than a traditional spinal rehabilitation programme. Symmetrical exercises, both in strengthening and stretching, should not be avoided and exercise should be aimed at balancing deformity. All movements should be considered separately and emphasis should be on acquiring more equilibrium. In this patient, thoracic side flexion should emphasise one side more than the other to limit spinal concavity. The same principle should be considered with rotation, and extension should encourage the addition of side flexion away from the concavity of the curve.

Student questions

(1) What are the possible reasons for the limited research regarding the use of exercise in conditions affecting the thoracic spine?

(2) In what ways does the function and movement of the thoracic spine differ from the cervical and lumbar spines?

(3) What are the main reasons for postural changes in the thoracic spine?

(4) Why is aerobic activity important in a thoracic spine rehabilitation programme?

(5) How is respiratory function affected by musculoskeletal changes in the thorax?

(6) Outline the evidence supporting exercise in the management of AS.

(7) What are the common causes of increased thoracic kyphosis?

(8) How do principles of lumbar stability exercise relate to management of the thoracic spine?

(9) How important is proprioceptive exercise in the management of thoracic spine disorder?

(10) How does therapeutic exercise affect the progression of a chronic disease such as AS and osteoporosis?

References

Boulware, D., Arnett, F.C., Cush, J.J., Lipsky, P.E., Bennett, R.M., Mielants, H., Keyser, F. and Veys, E.M. (2003) The seronegative arthropathies. In: Koopman, W., Boulware, D.W. and Heudebert, G.R. (eds) *Clinical Primer of Rheumatology*, pp. 127–134. Lippincott, Williams & Wilkins, Philadelphia, Pennsylvania.

Dagfinrud, H., Hagen, K.B. and Kvien, T.K. (2004). Physiotherapy interventions for ankylosing spondylitis (review). *Cochrane Database of Systematic Reviews*, 4, CD002822.

Edmondston, S.J. and Singer, K.P. (1997) Thoracic spine: anatomical and biomechanical considerations for manual therapy. *Manual Therapy*, 2, 132–143.

Edmondston, S.J., Aggerholm, M., Elfving, S., Flores, N., Ng, C., Smith, R. and Netto, K. (2007) Influence of posture on the range of axial rotation and coupled lateral flexion of the thoracic spine. *Journal of Manipulative and Physiological Therapeutics*, 30, 193–199.

Fernàndez De Las Peñas, C., Alonso-Blanco, C., Morales-Cabezas, M. and Miangolarr-Page, J.C. (2005) Two exercise interventions for the management of patients with ankylosing spondylitis: a randomized controlled trial. *American Journal of Physical Medicine and Rehabilitation*, 84, 407–419.

Ferraro, C., Masiero, S. and Venturin, S. (1998) Effects of exercise therapy on mild idiopathic scoliosis. Preliminary results. *Europa Medicophysica*, 34, 25–31.

Gold, D.T., Shipp, K.M., Pieper, C.F., Duncan, P.W., Martinez, S. and Lyles, K.W. (2004) Group treatment improves trunk strength and psychological status in older women with vertebral fractures: results of a randomized clinical trial. *Journal of the American Geriatric Society*, 52, 1471–1478.

Hawes, M.C. (2003) The use of exercises in the treatment of scoliosis: an evidence-based critical review of the literature. *Paediatric Rehabilitation*, 6, 171–182.

Ince, G., Sarpel, T., Durgun, B. and Erdogan, S. (2006) Effects of a multimodal exercise program for people with ankylosing spondylitis. *Physical Therapy*, 86, 924–35.

Katzman, W.B., Sellmeyer, D.E., Stewart, A.L., Wanek, L. and Hamel, K.A. (2007) Changes in flexed posture, musculoskeletal impairments and physical performance after group exercise in community dwelling older women. *Archives of Physical Medicine and Rehabilitation*, 88, 192–199.

Kebaetse, M., McClure, P. and Pratt, N.A. (1999) Thoracic position effect on shoulder range of motion, strength, and three-dimensional scapular kinematics. *Archives of Physical Medicine and Rehabilitation*, 80, 945–950.

Kubo, M., Holt, K.G., Saltzman, E. and Wagenaar, R.C. (2006) Changes in axial stiffness of the trunk as a function of walking speed. *Journal of Biomechanics*, 39, 750–757.

Nas, K., Kemaloglu, M.S., Cevik, R., Necmioglu, S., Bukte, Y., Cosut, A., Senyigit, A., Gur, A., Sarac, A.J., Ozkan, U. and Kirbas, G. (2004) The results of rehabilitation on motor and functional improvement of the spinal tuberculosis. *Joint, Bone, Spine*, 71, 312–316.

Santos Alves, V.L., Stirbulow, R. and Avanzi, O. (2006) Impact of a physical rehabilitation program on the respiratory function of adolescents with idiopathic scoliosis. *Chest*, 130, 500–505.

Sinaki, M., Brey, R.H., Hughes, C.A., Larson, D.R. and Kaufman, K.R. (2005) Balance disorder and increased risk of falls in osteoporosis and kyphosis: significance of kyphotic posture and muscle strength. *Osteoporosis International*, 16, 1004–1010.

Singer, K. (2006) Thoracic and chest pain. In: Brukner, P. and Khan, K. (eds) *Clinical Sports Medicine*, 2nd edn, pp. 340–351. McGraw Hill, Sydney, Australia.

Solberg, G. (1996). Scoliosis: plastic changes in spinal function of pre-pubescent scoliotic children engaged in an exercise therapy programme. *South African Journal of Physiotherapy*, 52, 19–24.

Watkins, R., Watkins, R., Williams, L., Ahlbrand, S., Garcia, R., Karamanian, A., Sharp, L., Chuong, V. and Hedman, T. (2005) Stability provided by the sternum and rib cage in the thoracic spine. *Spine*, 30, 1283–1286.

Weiss, H.R., Weiss, G. and Petermann, F. (2003) Incidence of curvature progression in idiopathic scoliosis patients treated with scoliosis in-patient rehabilitation (SIR): an age and sex matched controlled study. *Paediatric Rehabilitation*, 6, 23–30.

Wittink, H., Michel, T.H., Wagner, A., Sukiennik, A. and Rogers, W. (2000) Deconditioning in patients with chronic low back pain. *Spine*, 25, 2221–2228.

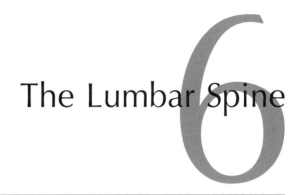

The Lumbar Spine

Fiona Wilson

SECTION 1: INTRODUCTION AND BACKGROUND

As many as 80% of all adults experience back pain at some time in their lives. Work disability caused by back pain has risen steadily despite the fact that Western economies are increasingly post-industrial with less heavy labour and more automation (Deyo, 1998). It would therefore appear that there is a positive correlation between decreasing levels of physical activity and low back pain. The purpose of this chapter is to review the evidence for exercise in both management and prevention of onset of low back pain.

Evidence for the use of exercise in the management of low back pain

The frequency of incidence of low back pain in the general population is reflected in the volume of evidence in the area. In many of the studies, however, subjects are grouped into a sample of either acute or chronic, non-specific low back pain. It is well recognised that the symptoms of low back pain are multi-pathological and that to stratify patients into these subgroups is a gross simplification. Many of the studies though are otherwise of sound methodology and provide a strong starting point.

European guidelines on low back pain include analyses of systematic reviews and existing clinical guidelines. Van Tulder *et al.* (2006) produced a set of guidelines for primary care management of *acute* non-specific low back pain following a comprehensive analysis of studies and trials that fulfilled an acceptable standard of methodological criteria. Among other recommendations, it was advised that patients with an acute episode of low back pain should avoid bed rest as treatment, stay active and continue normal daily activities if possible. It should be noted that the evidence for inclusion of specific exercises such as strengthening and stretching was not conclusive for acute pain episodes. As patients would be presenting with different pathologies under an umbrella diagnosis of non-specific low back pain, generic exercises may be inappropriate for many conditions. Trials that stratify patients by specific pain presentation patterns may present more meaningful data. It may be concluded that avoiding aggravating activity but continuing to exercise is an important management approach. Other European guidelines compiled by Airaksinen *et al.* (2006) examined current evidence for

Exercise Therapy in the Management of Musculoskeletal Disorders, First Edition. Edited by Fiona Wilson, John Gormley and Juliette Hussey.
© 2011 Blackwell Publishing Ltd

management of *chronic* non-specific low back pain. Among other recommendations, supervised exercise therapy was advised within the treatment programme. Treatments commonly adopted by many clinicians, such as electrotherapy and traction, were shown to have a poor evidence base. The authors concluded that there is moderate evidence that exercise therapy is more effective in the reduction of pain and disability than passive treatments.

Hayden *et al.* (2005) undertook a Cochrane Collaboration review of studies examining treatment of non-specific low back pain. The primary objective of the review was to assess the effectiveness of exercise therapy for reducing pain and disability in adults with non-specific acute, subacute and chronic low back pain compared with no treatment and other conservative treatments. Sixty-one randomised controlled trials met the inclusion criteria: n = 11 for acute; n = 6 for subacute and n = 43 for chronic low back pain. The authors concluded that exercise therapy appears to be slightly effective at decreasing pain and improving function in adults with chronic (longer than 12 weeks) low back pain, particularly in those visiting a health care provider. In adults with subacute (6–12 weeks) low back pain there is some evidence that a graded activity programme improves absenteeism outcomes. For patients with acute (less than 6 weeks) low back pain, exercise therapy is as effective as either no treatment or other conservative treatments. Thus the authors suggest that exercise therapy for low back pain is most effective in the chronic phase. However, this must be considered in the light of the European guidelines, which encourage activity within pain limits in the acute phase (Van Tulder *et al.*, 2006). No comment was made by any of the authors regarding this contradiction although it may be surmised that this suggests that generalised low level aerobic activity is important in the acute phase.

The UK BEAM trial (2004) aimed to measure, for patients consulting their general practitioner (GP) with back pain, the effectiveness of adding the following to general practice management of low back pain: a class-based exercise programme ('back to fitness'); a package of treatment by a spinal manipulator; or manipulation followed by exercise. The researchers also aimed to establish whether the manipulation package was more or less effective within the private setting or the National Health Service (NHS). Findings demonstrated that the most effective outcome was produced by manipulation followed by exercise and there was no significant difference between manipulation performed in a private and NHS setting. The authors did not identify what the 'back to fitness' programme specifically involved although it appears that positive benefits may be achieved even when a generic programme is delivered in a class situation.

A review of randomised controlled trials by Hayden *et al.* (2006) examined trials of suitable methodological standard which assessed the role of exercise in treatment of acute, subacute and chronic low back pain. The authors concluded that exercise is effective in improving function and reducing pain in patients with chronic low back pain. However, limited response was noted in the cases of acute and subacute pain. The authors also concluded that the most effective strategies are individually designed, supervised and performed regularly and also include conservative therapy.

Pain on movement is a primary reason for limited function in the low back pain population. This is frequently associated with lowered levels of activity and fear avoidance behaviour. Rainville *et al.* (2004) examined the influence of intense exercise-based physiotherapy on pain anticipated before and induced by physical activities. Subjects were recruited from physiotherapy programmes that used intense group-based exercise programmes as therapy. Anticipated and induced pain was measured by a visual analogue scale during six tests of back flexibility and strength and the Oswestry Low Back Pain Disability Questionnaire scores were also used as outcome measures. Subjects participated in the exercise programme three times per week (2 hours per session) for 6 weeks. The authors found that both anticipated and induced pain with physical activities reduced after the exercise programme. There were also associated improvements with global pain and disability.

Gaskell *et al.* (2007) examined the effects of a rehabilitation programme for patients with chronic low back pain. A cohort of chronic patients with low back pain (n = 877) completed a programme consisting of nine 2-hour group sessions of therapy, run over 5 weeks. The programme included an hour of exercise and an hour of education and advice. The programme proved to be effective in reducing pain, disability, anxiety and depression levels for people with chronic low back pain. Changes in outcome measures were all statistically significant.

One of the reasons that the topic of low back pain receives widespread general interest is that it is a major cause of acute and chronic disability and work absenteeism. The knock-on effect on the economy is great when measured by disability and sick payments as well as health service funding. It makes sense that treatment for back pain should not just be aimed at returning the patient to work as soon as possible but also should be economically viable on a large scale. Torstensen *et al.* (1998) examined the efficiency and cost of medical exercise therapy (MET), conventional physiotherapy and self-exercise in chronic low back pain. MET is a progressively graded programme that was developed by Norwegian physiotherapist Oddvar Holten in the early 1960s. Each patient is given their own specific programme which is tailored to their dysfunctions. Repetitions of the exercises are high and designed to improved endurance with additional aerobic exercise such as walking included as part of the programme. The MET programme allows up to five patients to be managed at one time in a specially adapted gymnasium. In a cohort of 208 chronic patient with low back pain, who were randomly assigned to one of the groups, those in the MET group demonstrated the most benefit, as measured by pain, functional activities, return to work and cost-benefit analysis. Although conventional physiotherapy also demonstrated similar benefits, patient satisfaction was highest in the MET group. This presents a useful solution for practitioners in the management of the large groups of patients presenting with chronic low back pain. While allowing a number of patients to be seen at one time, it avoids the generic-type delivery that is often seen in a class-based programme.

One of the challenges facing any patient or clinician managing back pain is that the condition often recurs. While there is a strong argument that many patients are not able to address their risk factors, the effect of introduction of a long-term exercise programme to prevent further episodes requires study. Lifestyle changes which incorporate exercise are well established in cardiac disease although there is a paucity of research in this area when low back pain is considered. Soukup *et al.* (1999) examined the effect of a combined exercise and education programme (Mensendieck's method) on the incidence of recurrent episodes of low back pain in patients with the history of the condition and who were currently working. Seventy-seven patients who had completed treatment for a low back pain episode were randomly assigned to either the exercise or control group. The exercise group received 20 group sessions over 13 weeks. At 5 and 12 month follow-up examinations, the patients were assessed for recurrence of pain, sick leave days and functional scores. The authors found that after 12 months, there was a significant reduction in recurrent episodes of low back pain in the exercise group compared with the control group. This was a small study and there is a great need for further longitudinal research in this area.

The studies that have been reviewed above focused on the general role of exercise in the management of acute and chronic low back pain. However, the design of any good rehabilitation programme must include all the components of fitness: aerobic exercise; muscle strength and endurance; range of motion (ROM) or flexibility exercises; proprioceptive and balance training. Despite this, there is a clinically observed reluctance to prescribe exercise for low back pain in this way, and the limited research examining the roles of these different fitness components is reviewed below.

Aerobic exercise

When considering rehabilitation of the patient with low back pain, the concept of aerobic training needs to be considered in two ways: generalised aerobic conditioning and localised endurance training of specific muscle groups, particularly those associated with control of posture. Generalised aerobic training has an effect of many body systems in terms of positive health benefits. However, its role in the rehabilitation of the lumbar spine is frequently overlooked by clinicians.

Chatzitheodorou *et al.* (2007) examined the efficacy of an aerobic exercise intervention in a pilot study of 25 chronic patient with low back pain. Subjects were stratified into two groups, one which underwent a 12-week, high-intensity aerobic exercise programme and a control group, which received 12 weeks of passive modalities without any form of physical activity. Data analysis identified reduction in pain, disability and psychological strain in subjects in the exercise group and no changes in subjects in the control group. This study was limited by the subject numbers, but this issue merits a larger-scale longitudinal project as the non-exercise intervention clearly reflects a treatment approach employed by many clinicians. The aerobic exercise approach presents a time-efficient and an economically efficient modality of management. Another study which had significant findings in relation to aerobic exercise and low back pain was carried out by Sculco *et al.* (2001). A cohort of 35 patients with a history of low back pain was stratified into an aerobic exercise or a non-exercise control group for a 10-week exercise programme. Subjects in the intervention group were prescribed a 10-week home-based aerobic training programme consisting of walking or cycling which they performed four times per week at 60% of maximal heart rate. Subjects in the control group were instructed to continue their normal daily routine and not to participate in any formal exercise programme for the duration of the 10-week study period. A number of outcome measures were assessed and the authors demonstrated that low to moderate aerobic exercise appears to improve mood states and work status, and reduce the need for physiotherapy referrals and pain medication for patient with low back pain under the care of a neurosurgeon. A similar small-scale study by Iversen *et al.* (2003) assessed the effectiveness of a bicycle endurance programme in older adults with chronic low back pain. Twenty-six subjects were assessed at baseline and at 6 and 12 weeks using standardised questionnaires, physical examination and endurance testing. The intervention required the subjects to exercise three times per week for 12 weeks at a set wattage. At the end of the programme, improvements were demonstrated in physical functioning and mental health and there was a decrease in chronic low back pain symptoms as assessed by a standard set of outcome measures. Despite methodological limitations, this study clearly supports the findings of those discussed previously.

The long-term benefits of aerobic exercise in the management of low back pain have been demonstrated by Mannion *et al.* (2001). One hundred and forty-eight subjects were randomly assigned to one of three groups: active physiotherapy; muscle reconditioning on training devices or; low impact aerobics. Questionnaires were used to assess pain and disability after therapy and at the 6- and 12-month follow up. All modalities were effective in reducing the intensity and frequency of pain. However, in contrast with the physiotherapy group,

the aerobics and devices groups maintained their post-treatment reductions in disability after 12 months' follow-up. The authors concluded that the larger group size and minimal infrastructure required for low-impact aerobics made it less expensive to administer and therefore the most cost-effective method of management.

Long-term management as well as prevention of low back pain depends on recognition of risk factors. Low levels of physical activity and consequent poor aerobic capacity have been noted as established risk factors for low back pain. Hartvigsen and Christensen (2007) carried out a prospective cohort study of 1387 twins over a 2-year period. The objective of the study was to examine associations between physical activity, physical function and the incident of low back pain in an elderly population. The authors found that being engaged in strenuous physical activity at baseline was strongly protective in relation to both having had any low back pain and having had low back pain lasting more than 30 days altogether during the past year at follow-up. Statistically significant dose–response associations between increasing frequency of strenuous physical activity and magnitude of this protective effect were also found. In a 25-year prospective cohort study of 640 school children, Harreby *et al.* (1997) demonstrated that there was a reduced risk of low back pain, measured as lifetime, 1-year and point prevalence of low back pain, in subjects taking physical exercise during leisure time (at least 3 hours per week) compared with the rest of the cohort.

There is a lack of consensus in the literature on the concept of deconditioning in low back pain, perhaps as a result of methodological difficulties. Most patients presenting with low back pain have no record of previous levels of fitness, i.e. a baseline measure, and studies are usually limited to measurement of changes from that point. Smeets *et al.* (2006) compared aerobic fitness in patients with chronic low back pain with matched controls. In a study of 108 patients with chronic low back pain it was noted that there was reduced aerobic fitness, especially in males, when compared with the normative population. However, Wittink *et al.* (2000a) demonstrated that levels of aerobic fitness in patients with chronic low back pain are comparable with those in healthy subjects in a study of 50 patients with chronic low back pain. Further research is required in this area.

There is considerable emphasis on individual muscle training in low back pain rehabilitation. Despite strong counter-arguments for this method of management, many clinicians concentrate on activation of, in particular, deep muscle groups to 'stabilise' the lumbar spine. This concept will be discussed later in the chapter. However, Koumantakis *et al.* (2005a) demonstrated that emphasis on specific re-training of the deep trunk muscles in conjunction with general endurance exercise is of no more benefit than general endurance exercise alone. In this randomised controlled trial, 55 recurrent patient with low back pain were randomised into either a generalised trunk muscle endurance programme enhanced with specific muscle stabilisation exercises or a generalised trunk muscle endurance programme. A series of outcome measures demonstrated equal benefits in both methods and the authors concluded that physical exercise alone and not the exercise type was the key determinant for improvement in this patient group.

Muscle strength and endurance

Much of the focus over recent years has focused on rehabilitating the patient with low back pain with specific exercises designed to enhance 'core stability'. However, this term lacks clarity and has been interpreted in many ways. It has led certain groups of clinicians to concentrate on single muscle groups in rehabilitation, while other groups, particularly those that demonstrate a depth of understanding of spinal biomechanics, would argue that this is not practically possible. This will be discussed further in this section. Stabilising muscles, by definition, have an endurance role although spinal and trunk muscles must also be able to generate power. It is necessary to have an understanding of, and to consider, the different functions of the muscles when rehabilitating the patient with low back pain. Beyond those studies which examine stability, there is little emphasis in the literature on the differing functions of the muscle groups. A problem arises when defining strength and endurance of muscles with some regarding the terms as interchangeable. When strength is regarded as the maximum force that a muscle can exert and endurance refers to the ability to maintain the force over time it would make sense that endurance plays a greater protective role for the lumbar spine (McGill, 1998).

Studies looking at general strength will be considered first.

Slade and Keating (2006) carried out a systematic review of studies examining the role of trunk strengthening exercises for chronic low back pain. Thirteen studies fulfilled the methodological criteria and their findings demonstrated that for chronic low back pain: trunk strengthening is more effective than no exercise for long-term pain; intensive trunk strengthening is more effective than less intensive strengthening in improving function. The authors found that increasing exercise intensity and adding motivation increased treatment benefits. However, they also concluded that trunk strengthening compared with aerobics or McKenzie exercises showed no clear benefit and that it was not clear whether the observed benefits were because of tissue loading or movement repetition. A very clear observation of this review and one which merits caution in its interpretation is the lack of standardisation in the exercise programmes. Many different types of exercise were used for the different muscle groups, with frequency of attendance and number of repetitions of the exercises varying a great deal between studies. Most studies appeared to include low load training with the mean number of starting repetitions at 29 and the mean number of exercise repetitions at 56. It was not clear why high load and low repetitions were only included in one study. A better planned study highlighted the importance of considering muscle *endurance* as opposed to strength. Luoto *et al.* (1995) found that poor static back endurance was a good predictor of risk for low back pain. Confusion in the literature persists with many studies not addressing endurance when strength is considered. The limited number of studies of acceptable standard in this area and the frequent use of this modality in low back pain rehabilitation, warrants more studies in this field of interest.

An area which has been widely researched, particularly in recent years is the concept of spinal stability and associated muscle recruitment patterns in patient with low back pain. Before the research is reviewed, it is necessary to define *spine stability*, *core stability* and *stabilisation exercise*. There are many different viewpoints regarding these terms, but McGill (2002) outlines a logical explanation. McGill states that:

'achieving stability is not just a matter of targeting a few muscles … Sufficient stability is a moving target that continually changes as a function of the three dimensional torques needed to support postures. It involves achieving the stiffness needed to endure unexpected loads, preparing for moving quickly, and ensuring sufficient stiffness in any degree of freedom of the joint that may be compromised from injury.'

However, recent years have seen an emphasis in by some clinicians on specific muscle groups, most notably the multifidus and transversus abdominis, in rehabilitation. This is mainly a reflection of studies that noted altered recruitment and activation patterns in these muscles following a low back pain episode (MacDonald *et al.*, 2006; Hyun *et al.*, 2007). Comerford and Mottram (2001) suggest that spinal stability is related to movement dysfunction which can present as a local or global problem. Global presentation can manifest as dysfunction of the recruitment and motor control of the deep segmental stability system resulting in poor control of the neutral joint position. The authors argue that it can also occur globally as imbalance between monoarticular stability muscles and biarticular mobility muscles. Local muscles are characterised by the fact that they are the deepest layer and appear to be biased for low load activity while global muscles are superficial and involve torque production, working at higher loads. This distinction was formalised by Bergmark (1989) and provided a focus for the early discussions on stability. In theory, rehabilitation of low back pain should recognise the role of all muscles and their contribution to stability.

Kavcic *et al.* (2004) designed a study which aimed to identify the torso muscles that stabilise the spine during different loading conditions and to identify possible mechanisms of function. Ten male university students with no history of back pain took part in the study. Spine kinematics, external forces and 14 channels of torso electromyography (EMG) were recorded for seven stabilisation exercises in order to capture the individual motor control strategies adopted by different people. The results demonstrated that a direction-dependent stabilising role was noticed in the larger, multisegmental muscles, whereas a subtle efficiency to generate stability was observed for the smaller, intersegmental muscles. This clearly supports the theory proposed by Comerford and Mottram. Kavcic *et al.* (2004) concluded that no single muscle dominated in the enhancement of spine stability

and their roles were continually changing, depending on the task. They further argued that effective clinical rehabilitation aimed at enhancing stability requires a programme aimed at improving motor patterns that incorporate many muscles rather than targeting just a few.

Biomechanical theories and findings must, of course, be applied clinically to measure efficacy and ease of practical application. Rackwitz *et al.* (2006) conducted a systematic review of randomised controlled trials that examined the role of segmental stabilising exercises in low back pain. Seven trials fulfilled the methodological criteria. It was concluded that for acute low back pain, segmental stabilising exercises are equally effective in reducing short-term disability and pain and more effective in reducing long-term recurrence of low back pain than treatment by a GP. For chronic low back pain, segmental stabilising exercises are more effective than GP treatment in the short and the long term and may be as effective as other physiotherapy treatments in reducing disability and pain. A further conclusion, however, was that segmental stabilising exercises are more effective than treatment by a GP but not more effective than other physiotherapy interventions.

Cairns *et al.* (2006) carried out a randomised controlled trial of spinal stabilisation exercises versus conventional physiotherapy for recurrent low back pain. In a cohort of 68 patients, they showed that, using a standard package of outcome measures, improvement was seen with both treatment packages to a similar degree and that no further benefit was seen following the addition of stability exercises to a conventional physiotherapy protocol. The findings of a another randomised controlled trial by Koumantakis *et al.* (2005b) were similar. This trial examined the role of trunk muscle stabilisation training plus general exercise versus general exercise only in a group of patients with recurrent, non-specific back pain. The results of the study were that a general exercise programme reduced disability in the short term to a greater extent than a stabilisation-enhanced exercise approach. Ferreira *et al.* (2007) compared the effects of general exercise, motor control exercise or spinal manipulative therapy on a cohort of 240 patients with chronic low back pain. Their results showed that the motor control exercise group had slightly better outcomes than the general exercise group at 8 weeks follow-up as did the spinal manipulative therapy group. However, this result was not sustained and all groups had similar outcomes at the 6- and 12-month follow-up. A critique of the study could be that exercise within the 'general exercise' group may be argued to include motor control demands, thus making the stratification a little vague.

Pilates has grown in popularity in the clinical setting, in recent years, primarily as a reflection of the interest in the use of spinal stability training. Pilates classes present a cost-effective method of delivery of a rehabilitation programme as a number of patients may be seen at one time. Despite this, there is still a paucity of clinical trials to reflect its growing use in the management of low back pain. Rydeard *et al.* (2006) carried out a randomised controlled trial which examined the effect of a Pilates-based exercise programme on a cohort of 39 patients with chronic low back pain. Compared with a control group, those following a 4-week programme of Pilates-based exercise, demonstrated a significantly lower level of functional disability and average pain intensity which was maintained over a 12-month follow-up period. As Pilates also includes the exercise of other components of fitness such as flexibility, it represents a comprehensive approach to rehabilitation, which also provides economic sense; however, more large-scale studies are required to demonstrate its efficacy.

Range of motion and flexibility

Despite the fact that ROM exercises are included as a matter of routine in low back pain rehabilitation programmes, there is sparse evidence to support this approach in the literature. ROM is also frequently used not only as an outcome measure but also as an assessment tool in disability screening. Furthermore, 'spinal flexibility has been shown to have little predictive value for low back pain trouble' (McGill, 1998).

A justification for including ROM exercises in the rehabilitation of low back pain has followed from the observation of altered movement patterns and ranges in patients with low back pain. Shum *et al.* (2007) found compensatory movements and altered load-sharing strategies during sit-to-stand and stand-to-sit activities in a low back pain population when compared with controls. McGregor *et al.* (1995) demonstrated that people with low back pain showed significantly reduced ROM in an antero-posterior direction compared with normal subjects. However, in McGregor *et al.*'s study of 20 patients with low back pain and 20 matched controls, no significant differences were seen in extension, lateral flexion or rotation. The difficulty in making clinical diagnoses as a result of altered ROM or movement patterns has been noted in a number of studies. Pal *et al.* (2007) noted that even in healthy individuals, movement patterns, relative contributions and kinematic characteristics of the lumbar spine and hip present conflicting results. A study of lumbar spine and hip motion during flexion and return movement in 20 healthy males confirmed the existence of kinematic and temporal variations between the two regions on movement. They also found that hip-dominant or lumbar-dominant patterns are not the same for all individuals, even in a healthy population.

The importance of ROM to spine health lacks clarity and this has been demonstrated by Poitras *et al.* (2000). In a study examining the validity of spinal ROM and velocity, it was found that kinematic variables were poor to moderately related to Oswestry questionnaire scores. It was also demonstrated that kinematic variables were also unresponsive to changes in work status and Oswestry questionnaire scores over time. A common clinical approach, particularly when a muscle balance approach is adopted is to consider altered muscle lengths and their effects on posture and ROM. A muscle group which is frequently targeted when low back pain is treated are the hamstrings. Halbertsma *et al.* (2001) investigated the extensibility and stiffness of the hamstrings in patients with non-specific low back pain. In a study of 20 patients versus 20 controls, it was found that the low back pain group showed a significant restriction in both ROM and extensibility of the hamstrings when compared with the controls. However, the danger of focusing on inclusion of ROM exercises were highlighted by Solomonow *et al.* (2003), who showed that exposure to prolonged static lumber flexion both increases the risk of further injury and exacerbates symptoms of low back pain.

Balance and proprioception

The concept of balance and proprioception and its relationship to function in the lumbar spine has generated much interest in recent years. An observation following a number of studies has been that subjects with a history of low back pain demonstrate repositioning error following specific exercises or postural perturbations. The importance of this finding is that postural control is importance for optimal biomechanical positioning, particularly in tasks such as lifting. Education of patients with low back pain is aimed at recognition of risk factors and includes ergonomic advice; poor positioning and postural control will compromise this.

O'Sullivan *et al.* (2003) examined whether individuals with lumbar segmental instability had a decreased ability to reposition their lumbar spine into a neutral position. Fifteen subjects with lumbar segmental instability were matched with 15 controls. Subjects were assisted into a neutral spine position and asked to independently reproduce this position a number of times. Lumbar repositioning error was significantly greater in subjects with segmental instability than in the control group. The authors concluded that this provided evidence of a deficiency in lumbar proprioceptive awareness among this population. A number of studies have also demonstrated that not only are repositioning deficits noted in the low back pain population when compared to controls but that the percentage error increases when a flexed posture is adopted (Wilson and Granata, 2003; Dolan and Green, 2006). Brumagne *et al.* (2000) suggest that patients with low back pain have an altered reposition sense than controls, possibly because of altered paraspinal muscle spindle afference and central processing of this afferent input. In a study of 23 patients with low back pain, who were matched with controls, repositioning accuracy was significantly lower in the low back pain group following a lumbar paraspinal muscle vibration protocol. Fatigue was also shown to amplify the error in repositioning in patients with low back pain by Taimela *et al.* (1999), which is an important consideration when considering design and loading levels in a rehabilitation programme.

A more global view of the effect of low back pain on balance has been examined in a number of studies. Henry *et al.* (2006) demonstrated decreased limits of stability in response to postural perturbations in subjects with low back pain. A study of 26 patients with low back pain measured sagittal and frontal plane displacement while standing on a force platform which was translated unexpectedly. The low back pain group had reduced and delayed sagittal plane centre of pressure responses compared with the control group. The authors concluded that the low back pain cohort had altered automatic postural co-ordination, both in terms of magnitude and timing of responses, indicating alterations in neuromuscular control. In a similar study, Volpe *et al.* (2006) also found that patients with low back pain oscillated more than controls in an antero-posterior direction when on an unstable surface. Newcomer *et al.* (2002) also carried out localised EMG measures of latency, frequency and asymmetry of muscle activation of the erector spinae, rectus abdominis, anterior tibialis and gastrocnemius in a very similar study to those outlined above. They found that significantly more subjects with low back pain had absence of firing of trunk muscles during force plate perturbations than control subjects.

Summary

While published studies clearly support the use of exercise both in prevention and management of low back pain, there is a lack of consensus regarding the type and frequency of exercise which is optimal. Although the use of aerobic exercise is quite well defined, trials that have looked at other modes of exercise were vague in their description and stratification of patients. In this case, a common sense approach would be to direct rehabilitation at restoring normal movement and thus function, using the American College of Sports Medicine (ACSM) guidelines for dosage and to include components of fitness as outlined in Chapter 2.

Lumbar spine injury

As has been mentioned previously, lumbar spine injury is rarely, if ever confined to one specific tissue. Loading stresses all tissues, albeit to different extents, and it is perhaps more appropriate to discuss injury in terms of the tissue that it affects. The reader is encouraged to examine this area further to learn more regarding specific conditions. The tissues of the lumbar spine may be described as the vertebrae, end plates, disc (annulus and nucleus), neural arch (posterior bony elements) and ligaments (McGill, 2002). Injuries to the different areas are discussed below.

Vertebrae

Fractures to vertebrae occur as a result of direct trauma or as a result of compressive loading. Unstable fractures may of course be catastrophic, resulting in paralysis as a result of spinal cord damage. Specific disease such as osteoporosis presents a major risk factor for vertebral fracture.

Neural arch

Posterior bony elements may be damaged as a result of repeated compressive loading as a result of cyclical flexion–extension cycles. Stress and occult fractures will occur at the pars interarticularis resulting in spondylolysis (unilateral fracture) or spondylolisthesis, which is a bilateral fracture associated with varying degrees of slip of the vertebra.

Disc

Damage may occur in the nucleus and/or the annulus. The annulus and nucleus work together support compressive load when the disc is subjected to bending and compression. Under compression, the nucleus pressurises, applying force to the end plates vertically and the annulus laterally. This causes the annulus fibres to bulge outwards and become tensed. If this pattern is repeated, the nucleus will penetrate the failing annulus leading to disc herniation. There are four degrees of herniation: nuclear herniation; disc protrusion; nuclear extrusion and sequestrated nucleus. The disc demonstrates dramatic changes with age, and symptoms associated with these changes are common.

Ligaments

Ligaments of the lumbar spine are well adapted to the loading and cyclical motion requirements demanded of them. However, it has been noted that lumbar ligaments avulse at lower load rates but tear in their mid-substance at higher load rates (Noyes *et al.*, 1994). Ligament damage is frequently associated with high load trauma such as road traffic accidents.

End plates

End plate damage is caused under repeated compressive loading, eventually leading to the formation of Schmorl's nodes (McGill, 2002).

Damage to all or some of the above structures can lead to the development of the number of lumbar syndromes which clinicians will be familiar with: disc disease (acute and degenerative); facet joint dysfunction (acute and degenerative); instabilities including spondylolisthesis; stenosis and other manifestations of degeneration. The reader is encouraged to read further texts to understand the epidemiology and patterns of presentation of each disorder. Co-existence of pathologies is common and good clinical practice encourages the clinician to recognise movement and functional disorder as priority when designing rehabilitation programme, rather than employing a generic treatment approach for a specific disorder.

SECTION 2: PRACTICAL USE OF EXERCISE

Assessment of the patient

It is important that a rehabilitation programme is designed to include a thorough and detailed assessment of the patient. History should not only establish the pattern and nature of the patient's pain but also assess their lifestyle, which is important to establish risk factors. Physical examination should establish postural and movement faults under both low and high load conditions. Examination of movement patterns should always be geared towards considering how exercise can improve movement both functionally and actively.

Assessment of endurance

As it is important to emphasise endurance over strength; simple tests of endurance of the trunk (flexors, extensors and lateral musculature) could include the following (from McGill, 2002).

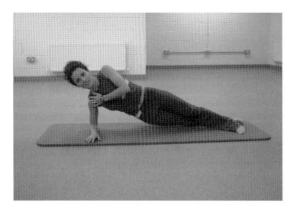

Figure 6.1   Lateral musculature test.

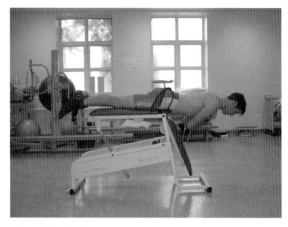

Figure 6.3   Back extensor test.

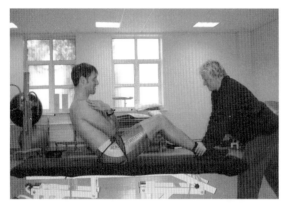

Figure 6.2   Flexor endurance test.

Lateral musculature test (Fig. 6.1)

The patient is asked to support the trunk in a side bridge, maintaining a neutral spine and straight torso. The patient is timed and failure occurs when the position can no longer be held.

Flexor endurance test (Fig. 6.2)

The patient starts leaning against a wedge with both knees and hips flexed. The wedge is pulled away from the patient and failure occurs when the patient's posture changes or they lean back against the jig.

Back extensor test (Fig. 6.3)

The patient lies over a plinth with the upper body hanging off and the feet fixed. Failure is noted when

the upper body moves from the horizontal position.

Assessment of aerobic capacity

Fitness testing should be included in the assessment as aerobic exercise will be an important part of the programme. Wittink *et al.* (2000b) established the Bruce treadmill test as the most valid for measuring aerobic fitness in patients with chronic low back pain.

Assessment of motor control

Simple tests may be performed on the patient to assess their ability to maintain their lumbar spine in a neutral position (Fig. 6.4). The neutral lumbar spine position is found when the pelvis is halfway between full anterior tilt (Fig. 6.5) and full posterior tilt (Fig. 6.6). This may then be challenged by asking the patient to move the limbs into different positions. Poor control will result in the inability to maintain the lumbar spine in neutral (Figs 6.7 and 6.8).

Assessment of proprioception

Proprioception should be examined at the initial stage using simple tests such as ability to reproduce

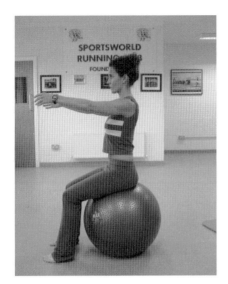

Figure 6.4 Lumbar spine neutral position.

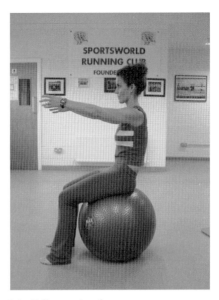

Figure 6.6 Full posterior tilt.

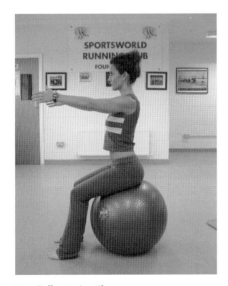

Figure 6.5 Full anterior tilt.

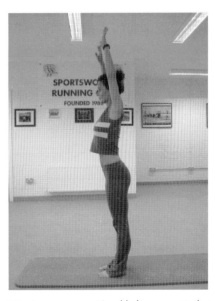

Figure 6.7 Arm movement is added, poor control results in lumbar spine movement.

postural positioning. Tools such as electrogoniometers and EMG will be useful to give some quantitative data at this stage. Electrogoniometers allow accurate measurement of the lumbar spine angles. The patient is placed into a position by the clinician. They are then allowed to move freely and asked to re-create the position (Fig. 6.9).

Assessment of flexibility

The important factor to consider when assessing flexibility in the patient with low back pain is the effect of limited ROM of joints around the lumbar spine and their effect on normal lumbar movement.

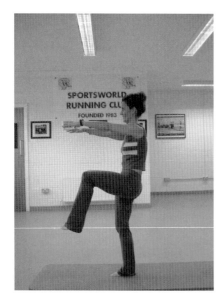

Figure 6.8 Hip flexion is added, poor control results in posterior tilting of the pelvis.

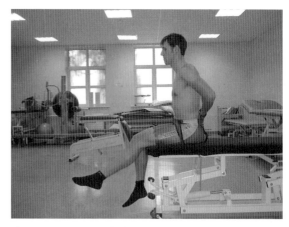

Figure 6.10 Testing for hamstring length.

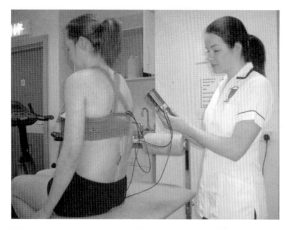

Figure 6.9 Assessment of repositioning skill using an electrogoniometer.

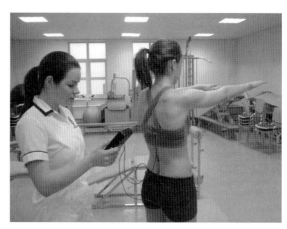

Figure 6.11 Assessment of the effect of upper limb movement on lumbar spine position.

Short hamstrings are associated with specific abnormal postural types and will frequently induce early lumbar flexion. A useful test to assess the effect of hamstring length on lumbar spine position places the patient sitting with hips and knees flexed to 90°. He or she is asked to extend the knee slowly. Hamstring tightness will result in posterior tilt of the pelvis (Fig. 6.10).

Hip, thoracic spine and even tightness around muscle groups in the shoulder will alter the biome-chanics of the lumbar spine. This may be assessed in standing with the lumbar spine in a neutral position; the patient elevates both arms slowly. If the lumbar spine moves into extension this could be caused by a combination of tight shoulder flexors, limited thoracic spine extension and poor lumbar motor control. Further localised testing is required to establish which muscle groups are affected (Fig. 6.11).

In the modified Thomas test, the patient starts with both hips and knees in flexion. One leg is lowered to allow the hip to go into extension. Tight hip flexors cause the lumbar spine to partly move into extension, resisting the efforts of the contralateral hip to maintain posterior pelvic tilt (Fig. 6.12). These tests are not an exhaustive list and thorough

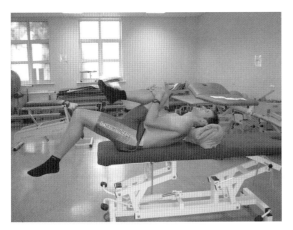

Figure 6.12 The modified Thomas test.

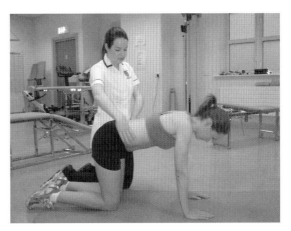

Figure 6.13 The therapist helping a patient find a neutral lumbar spine position on four-point kneeling.

postural and motion assessment will give the clinician a better focus for testing specific groups.

Design of an exercise programme

Management of patients with low back pain will frequently include modalities such as manipulation and massage but for the purposes of this text, an exercise-only approach will be described. A generic approach to programme design is strongly discouraged but general principles may be adapted according to the patient's needs. It is important that concepts are evidence based and consider the components of fitness and the ACSM's guidelines (see Chapter 2) as well as including stability and proprioceptive work throughout all stages, which are fundamental to success.

McGill (2002) emphasises the importance of training for health as opposed to performance when considering low back pain. This approach stresses the importance of:

- Muscle endurance
- Motor control perfection
- Maintenance of sufficient spine stability in all expected tasks

Strength should not be a targeted goal although strength gains will result. Training for health should also include aerobic fitness and appropriate activity levels. When elite athletes are considered, these principles will still be considered but the spine must be prepared for high stresses and loading.

Application of the principle of specificity will allow a programme of appropriate design, in terms of exercise type and loading, to be formulated.

The exercise programme will be discussed in terms of early, intermediate and late stages of management. Progression through the programme will depend on the patient's response, according to outcome measures which should be established before the programme is commenced. The programme should be carried out daily for optimum effect. This may not be possible in a clinic situation so it is important that the patients carries out an adapted programme on non clinic days. Ultimately, a lifestyle change is expected when the patient will be expected to carry out a number of components of the exercise programme, if not daily, on a regular basis.

The exercise programme

Early phase

The first stage of any programme should be to correct abnormal movement patterns, posture and to establish postural control under conditions of low load. The patient should be shown and assisted to find the position when their pelvis and spine is in a neutral position. This may be done in different positions such as sitting, standing, lying or four-point kneeling (Fig. 6.13).

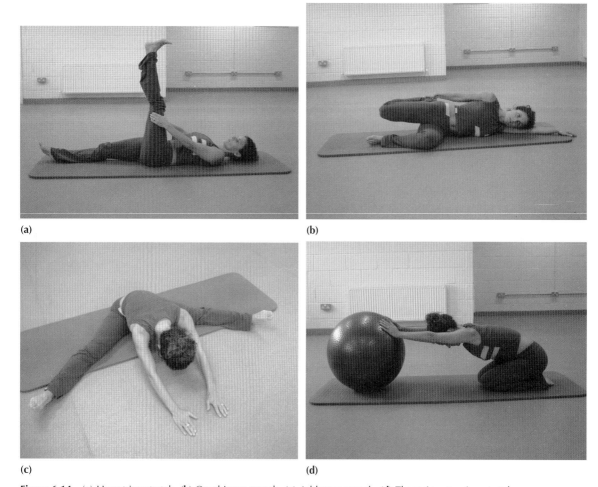

(a) (b)

(c) (d)

Figure 6.14 (**a**) Hamstring stretch. (**b**) Quadriceps stretch. (**c**) Adductor stretch. (**d**) Thoracic extension stretch.

It is common for patients with low back pain to have adopted poor posture, which may be because of a number of reasons including pain, work or sporting demands or genetically determined body type. Education and assistance by the clinician to find a more correct posture is important at this stage. It is likely that stretching or specific muscle groups will be required at this stage to allow the patient to achieve a more normal postural positioning. These muscle groups will have been identified in the assessment procedure and should be targeted early. In patients with low back pain, specific muscle groups demonstrate tightness, in particular, the hamstrings, hip flexors and the muscles of the posterior calf. Stretches appropriate for the patient with low back pain are illustrated in Figure 6.14

and should place particular emphasis on correct lumbar spine and pelvis position while carrying out the stretch.

However, an important point at this stage is that flexibility must not be overemphasised until the spine is stabilised and abnormal movement patterns are corrected. In general, at this stage, flexibility training should be aimed at those muscle groups which prevent the neutral pelvis posture being attained. It is important that movements or stretches which are already overemphasised by the patient are avoided as they may be contributing to the patient's disorder. For example, a gymnast is frequently hypermobile in lumbar extension so it would be nonsensical to emphasise this movement in rehabilitation if

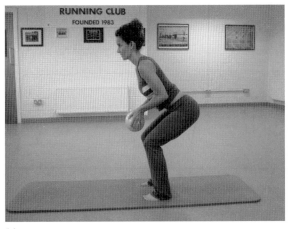
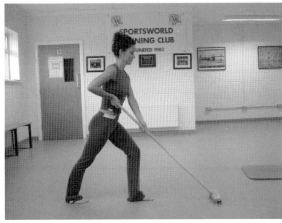

(a) (b)

Figure 6.15 Teaching simple functional activities while maintaining a neutral lumbar spine.

such a patient's pain was due to overloading in extension.

Once the patient is able to establish neutral position of the spine and improved posture, the muscles which hold the spine in this position must be trained. The first exercise is very simple and the patient is requested to hold this position in sitting, standing and other functional patterns. Such low load training is working on the endurance of the postural muscles as well as proprioception or spinal position sense. Proprioceptive training is enhanced by giving the patient feedback in the form of verbal cues, mirrors, videos, biofeedback or any other technology which has been discussed in Chapter 3. Patients often tire quickly at this stage and this must be expected. Overloading and resulting fatigue is associated with substitution of normal movement or posture to abnormal.

Once the patient is able to adopt and maintain a neutral spine in standing, simple functional movements such as squatting, flexing and extending the lumbar spine and lifting (very small and light) objects may then be introduced (Fig. 6.15). It is common at this stage to observe movement faults with position changes and the clinician must constantly correct these faults. If the patient finds any of the movements too challenging, they may not be ready to progress and control in simple standing and sitting should be reviewed.

At this stage, it is important to consider the role of the abdominal muscles in enhancing spine stability. There has been a great deal of research in this area in recent years and the reader is advised to familiarise themselves with this. McGill (2001) favours the concept of *abdominal bracing* as opposed to hollowing which is taught by some groups of clinicians. Abdominal hollowing recruits the transversus abdominis whereas bracing co-activates this muscle with the external and internal obliques, offering greater stability. McGill argues that hollowing may be used as a motor control exercise but that it does not enhance stability. Abdominal bracing requires that the abdominal wall is neither sucked in nor pushed out but contracted isometrically. Readers are encouraged to read McGill's work further to understand the mechanical concepts discussed above. Teaching abdominal bracing may present a challenge to clinicians and they should not hesitate to spend some time with the patient perfecting it (Fig. 6.16). Mental cues such as 'imagine you are about to be punched in the abdomen' may be helpful. Demonstrating isometric contractions in other joints may also be useful.

The final component of this phase is to introduce aerobic exercise. Although it may be argued that movement faults may perpetuate when such exercise is added, the patient (unless severely disabled by pain) will probably be undertaking some aerobic exercise already, such as walking. The therapist needs to make a clear clinical judgement in this case and consider whether the addition of aerobic exercise will affect movement which is already poor. If not, simple activity such as walking may be

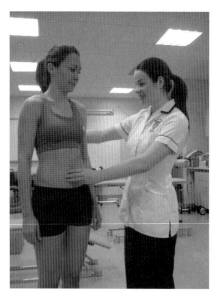

Figure 6.16 Teaching abdominal bracing.

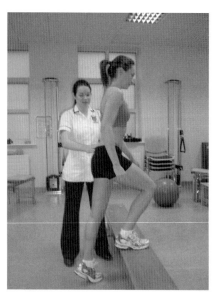

Figure 6.17 Step-ups as a warm-up activity. Note that the therapist is checking lumbar spine position.

introduced. A guideline of 30 minutes per day is the ultimate goal although for the de-trained patient, 10 minutes of walking per day may be a good starting point. The patient should be encouraged to consider postural correction exercises while walking.

Summary of the early phase

- Teach the neutral spine and spinal position sense.
- Correct postural and movement faults.
- Teach abdominal bracing.
- Minimise loading to basic functional tasks.
- Introduce low-level aerobic exercise.

Intermediate phase

This stage of the programme consolidates concepts from the first phase and introduces loading to enhance endurance. At this point it is useful to run the rehabilitation session like a conventional exercise class with a warm-up, aerobic phase and strengthening phase followed by a cool-down. Such a method of delivery works well in hospital and clinical situations and may allow a number of patients to be seen simultaneously. Reinforcing normal movement should be a constant theme

throughout the programme as an increase in loading will place stresses on proprioceptive control.

Warm-up

The warm-up should be an opportunity to consolidate normal movement and to ensure that correct motor patterns and spinal positioning is established. Light aerobic exercise to increase the heart rate could include deep knee bends while arm swinging, lunges or step-ups (Fig. 6.17). Each set of movements should be preceded by the patient establishing correct spinal position and maintaining this position throughout the movement.

ROM exercises for the spine should be introduced in the warm-up. It is important not to encourage spinal motion to extremes at this point as good stability has not yet been established. Simple exercises such as 'humping and hollowing' (Fig. 6.18), pelvic tilting (Fig. 6.19) and hip hitching (Fig. 6.20) in standing are appropriate.

Stretches may be included to incorporate those muscle groups which were highlighted as significant in initial assessment. Further stretches may be included as appropriate for any programme. As is the theme throughout the programme, stretches must be done with the spine in an optimum position.

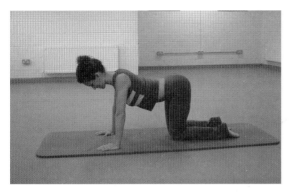

Figure 6.18 Humping and hollowing.

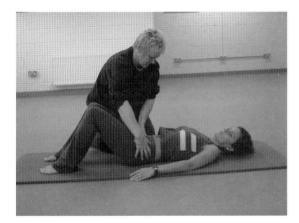

Figure 6.19 Pelvic tilting.

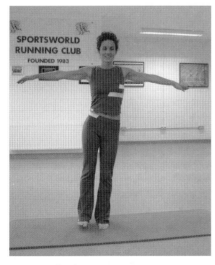

Figure 6.20 Hip hitching.

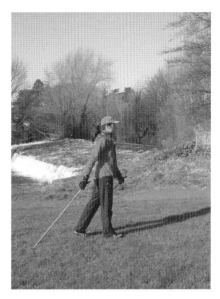

Figure 6.21 Nordic walking.

Aerobic phase

Aerobic exercise may be introduced in the form of an exercise which places minimal loading specifically on the low back but is also reproducible for the patient following discharge from the programme. Walking is particularly useful as patients are able to continue this exercise independently. Addition of spinal rotation in activities such as Nordic walking (Fig. 6.21) or using the Nordic ski track makes the activity more interesting and introduces more muscle activity. Target heart rate should be set before the activity begins and a time period of about 20 minutes is useful in a class setting. Out of a class setting, a target of up to 1 hour should be the aim. Swimming is also a useful activity to challenge the aerobic component of the programme but would be more convenient if the whole design of the class was hydrotherapy based. Activities such as rowing machines are particularly unsuitable because of the poor spine position and loading during the activity.

Strengthening phase

The aim of the strengthening phase is to enhance the endurance of the stabilising muscles. McGill (2002) identified the significant stabilisers as:

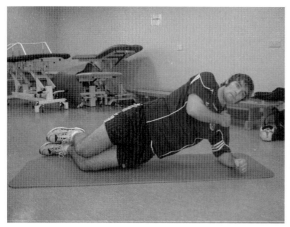
(a)

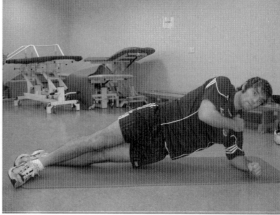
(b)

Figure 6.22   Side bridge exercise.

■ Multifidus and other extensors
■ Quadratus lumborum
■ The three layers of the abdominal wall.

A simple approach would be to train the muscles of the anterior, posterior and lateral trunk. Assessment established the holding times of the various exercises (see above) and the aim should be to increase the time that the patient is able to hold the correct position of the exercise. Repetitions as well as holding times may be increased as the patient improves. Starting position requires re-establishment of good spinal position at each repetition of the exercise. The side bridge exercise aims to improve endurance of the trunk side flexors. Figure 6.22a is an easy position with Figure 6.22b demonstrating a progression of difficulty.

The trunk curl (Fig. 6.23) aims to work the trunk flexors or muscles of the abdominal wall. The spine is held in neutral with one knee flexed to prevent pelvic rotation (McGill, 2002). It is important that the cervical spine is maintained in a neutral position throughout the exercise and the shoulders are barely raised from the supporting surface. Figure 6.24 illustrates exercises to train the trunk extensors. In four-point kneeling, the patient establishes the neutral spine position and slowly raises one arm or leg. A progression is seen when the patient raises one arm and the leg on the opposite side. The further the arm or leg is extended, the greater the loading as the lever is longer.

Exercises to challenge stability by adding limb movement may be introduced at this stage. The use

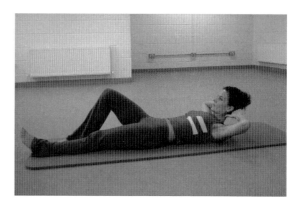

Figure 6.23   The trunk curl.

of a pressure biofeedback unit (PBU) is beneficial to give reinforcement to the patient. The PBU is placed in the lumbar lordosis; the spine is 'set' in neutral and the abdomen braced as taught in the early phase. Limb movement is introduced with the arm (Fig. 6.25) or the leg. If good stability is demonstrated, there will be no change in the spine position and thus no change in the reading on the PBU.

Cool-down

The cool-down may comprise walking or low level aerobic activity followed by proprioceptive exercises such as targeted repositioning to encourage good spinal position sense.

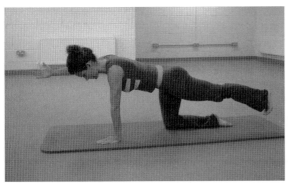

(a)

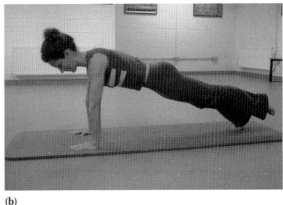

(b)

Figure 6.24 Trunk extensor exercise: (**a**) beginner to intermediate; (**b**) advanced.

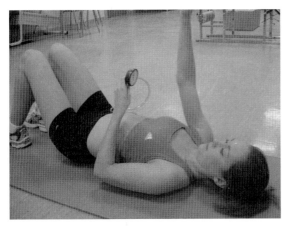

Figure 6.25 With the pressure in place and the lumbar spine in a neutral position, the patient introduces arm movement.

Summary of the intermediate phase

■ Continue to emphasise spinal position sense and good postural control.

■ Introduce exercises that challenge endurance of postural muscles.

■ Increase aerobic activity.

■ Establish a pattern of exercise that the patient will continue throughout life.

Late or advanced phase

The advanced phase of rehabilitation will be very similar in design to the previous stages but with a component of increased loading and proprioceptive challenges. Free weights, pulley weights, gym balls and wobble boards may now be introduced. Rotational movement patterns may be introduced with or without weights. As stressed throughout the text, there must continue to be strong emphasis on correct spinal positioning and control throughout movement. It is well recognised that as loading is increased, control is frequently compromised and abnormal movement patterns are observed. Speed of movement may also be increased but again movement must be observed closely for abnormality. Discharge of the patient should be considered and plans made to incorporate appropriate elements of the programme into the patient's lifestyle. It is likely that there will be a relapse in the patient's condition if recommended activity levels are not met with exercise and localised exercises are not continued. While class design is the same as that described previously, the components of the programme will change in the following ways.

Aerobic exercise

The patient should now reach the minimum requirement of 30 minutes of moderately intense exercise on 5 days of the week. The important factor is that this will continue throughout life and will be an activity or activities (variation is encouraged) that the patient may incorporate into their lifestyle such as changing the daily car commute to walking. The rehabilitation programme will only be part of this and may comprise the same exercises as those described above.

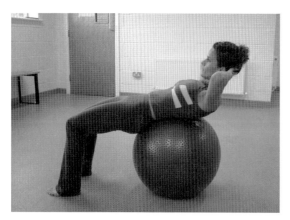

Figure 6.26   Trunk flexion curl on a gym ball.

Range of motion and flexibility training

There is a temptation at this stage to progress flexibility training to try to reach end-range or even extremes of movement. The basic functional demands of the patient must be considered and, unless they are elite athletes, conservative goals frequently suffice. If flexibility has reached the point where good posture and spinal positioning may be reached and attained and everyday activities may be carried out well, then the goal of this phase should be to maintain good movement into discharge and beyond.

Strengthening exercise

Strengthening exercise at this phase again emphasises endurance so the patient should be reaching higher exercise repetitions and longer holding capacity. Exercises may divided as above into those that work the flexors, extensors and side flexors of the trunk but rotation patterns may be added in and unstable surfaces introduced. The reader is encouraged to be imaginative and to research constantly as there are endless ideas for exercises that may be used in this phase. The following is by no means an exhaustive list but represents some basic ideas.

- *Trunk flexors:* A curl up may be performed on a gymnastic ball to add an element which challenges the proprioceptive system (Fig. 6.26). A trunk flexion exercise in standing using pulley weights adds loading (Fig. 6.27). Maintenance

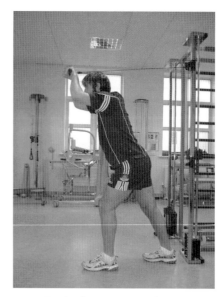

Figure 6.27   Trunk flexion in standing using pulleyed weights.

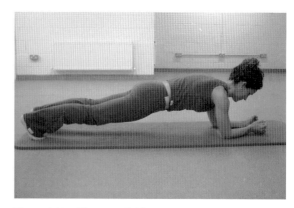

Figure 6.28   The prone bridge.

of good spinal positioning is challenging in this position and must be monitored by the therapist. The prone bridge (Fig. 6.28) works the trunk flexors to prevent the trunk sagging into extension due to gravity. However, this exercise is a very good example of a general stability exercise that facilitates co-contraction of all trunk musculature.

- *Trunk side flexors:* Two variations of the side bridge frequently seen in Pilates programmes are illustrated in Figure 6.29 and demand endurance activity in the side flexors. Figure 6.30 illustrates trunk side flexion using a pul-

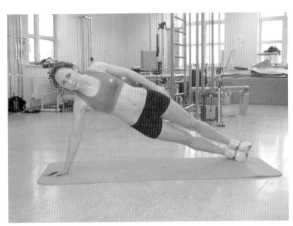

(a)

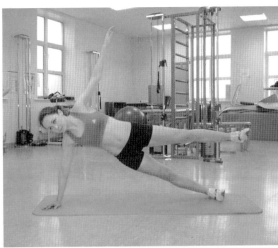

(b)

Figure 6.29   Side bridge.

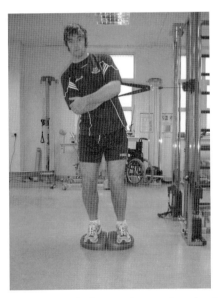

Figure 6.30   Trunk side flexion using a pulleyed weight for loading.

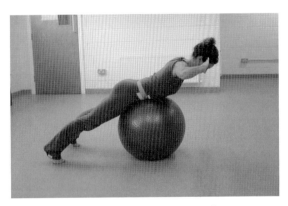

Figure 6.31   Trunk extension over a gym ball.

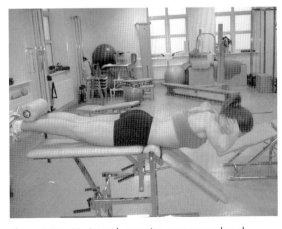

leyed weight for loading. Note that the subject is standing on an unstable surface to present a further challenge.

■ *Trunk extensors:* In Figure 6.31 the patient is performing trunk extension on an unstable surface (gym ball). In Figure 6.32 the patient is performing extension to a horizontal position

Figure 6.32   Horizontal extension over a gym bench.

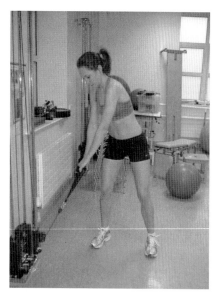

Figure 6.33   Rotation and trunk extension using a pulleyed weight.

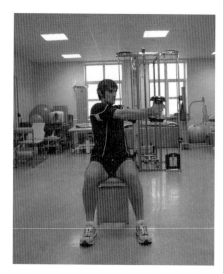

Figure 6.34   Trunk rotation using a weight.

over a gym bench. The patient may increase loading by extending the arms or placing weights in the hands.

- *Adding rotation:* The addition of rotation allows more functional patterns to be exercised. In Figure 6.33 the patient rotates and extends the trunk while pulling a pulleyed weight. An extension pattern may be worked if the patient reverses their starting position. Good spinal position sense is important in this case as loading increases with addition of torsion. In standing, the patient may rotate the trunk in a flexion to extension pattern while holding a medicine ball (Fig. 6.34). This is an advanced exercise which places high demands on control and spinal position sense.

Summary of the late phase

- Continue with postural and spinal position training with the introduction of challenges such as unstable supporting surfaces.
- Train endurance in appropriate muscles (as above) with the introduction of loading and rotational activity.

- Continue an aerobic exercise programme so that the patient completes 30 minutes of aerobic activity per day.
- Prepare and adapt the programme so that essential elements will be continued at discharge.

Discharging the patient

Criteria for discharge should have been established with the patient at commencement of the programme. It is important that the patient understands that failure to continue with exercise following discharge places them at increased risk of relapse. It is unrealistic to expect the patient to continue exercise in such an intensive way as that experienced during the rehabilitation programme. However, certain elements including aerobic exercise and endurance training of the trunk muscles will lend particular benefit if continued in the long term. The patient may be able to join a gym or exercise class which will allow them to continue exercising in a social setting.

SECTION 3: CASE STUDIES AND STUDENT QUESTIONS

Case study 1

A 72-year-old man with degenerative disc disease at L3/4 and L4/5 presents with diffuse lower back pain which radiates into the right leg. Pain is eased by walking and aggravated by prolonged sitting and gardening. The patient leads a relatively active lifestyle and is a non-smoker. Examination reveals restriction in all lumbar movements, particularly extension, flattened lumbar lordosis with poor postural control particularly when loading is added. There are no significant neurological signs.

Management

As the pathology causing this patient's pain is degenerative and, by definition, likely to demonstrate limited improvement, management should be aimed at maximising function which should has a positive effect on pain. Gardening and walking are activities that should be incorporated into the programme as the patient enjoys them. The early stage of the programme should concentrate on achieving a more normal posture in standing and sitting positions. Pelvic tilting, initially in standing should aimed at assisting the patient achieve a neutral spine position as well as increase the lumbar lordosis and increased lumbar

extension. If the patient can comfortably achieve a four-point kneeling position, the 'humping and hollowing' exercise would help mobilise the lumbar spine, which is likely to be generally hypomobile. Once a more neutral spine position is achieved, abdominal bracing may be introduced and reinforced by practising during everyday activities. Walking may be used as aerobic activity but gait should be assessed to ensure that good spine positioning is maintained. Loading may be added when the patient is able to stabilise the spine during light every day activity loading. Gardening-type exercises would be ideal for this patient to include activities such as digging, lifting light loads such as garden waste bags in simple patterns and challenging control in a kneeling position, which may add in hip flexion to simulate a weeding position.

It is hoped that normalising and mobilising spinal movements will reduce radicular pain, although many therapists may choose to add in neural tissue mobility exercises. Such exercise type is beyond the scope of this book and readers are encouraged to examine the treatment of radicular pain further. The patient's discharge programme should encourage everyday aerobic activity combined with basic spinal stability and mobility exercises which fit in well with the patient's preferred activities.

Case study 2

A 32-year-old sedentary office worker, a smoker, presents with lumbar pain due to an acute disc protrusion at L4/5. Time of presentation is 4 weeks after initial onset and initial referral into the left foot has now cleared resulting in localised pain that is aggravated by lumbar flexion and worse on rising in the morning. Examination reveals pain in early flexion and positive slump and straight leg raise on the left.

Management

This patient has presented for treatment with a number of noted risk factors for low back pain. Poor levels of activity and smoking along with the ergonomic profile of the patient's occupation must be addressed early if there is to be a successful rehabilitation programme. Smoking cessation will require the aid of an outside intervention such as

Case study 2—cont'd

a support group and nicotine replacement therapy to have optimal effect. It is likely that the patient will present with limited ROM in the lumbar spine, particularly in flexion. Simple ROM exercises into all ranges but keeping the motion very small and out of the painful range will encourage normal movement and help to reduce inflammation. Neurodynamic work may be beneficial in management as mentioned previously and the student is encouraged to read further in this area. Spinal position should be trained which may be a particular challenge to this patient as they will probably have adopted poor posture for some time. Simple stretches may be required to allow correct spinal positioning at this stage but care must be taken not to overload the spine motion as pain may be aggravated. Abdominal bracing should be taught early as it is likely that this patient's lifestyle will mean that he presents with very poor trunk control. Considerable time and effort should be spent at this stage and bracing should be assessed and practised in many different spine positions. An aerobic exercise should be introduced early but should be adapted so that the patients pain is not aggravated by the chosen activity. Once good stability in neutral positions has been achieved, some light loading may be introduced and stability may be

challenged in positions other than neutral. As the patient will be required to return to a sitting work posture, exercises must also be practised in this position. Although the patient will be advised to avoid prolonged sitting, it is not completely avoidable and good, stable sitting posture which achieves a spinal position which is as close to neutral as possible, will limit damage.

Aerobic exercise should continue with an activity that the patient will carry on following discharge. Postural control during aerobic exercise should be intermittently assessed as such exercise will also be useful for training dynamic stability of the spine. The final stage of the programme should be aimed at producing a regime that the patient will continue following discharge and will induce the lifestyle change that the patient requires for better health. Aerobic exercise should include an activity such as walking or a lunchtime swim which the patient can fit into the working day. Stability and endurance exercise may be more feasible if the patient joins a well designed Pilates programme or has a programme that may be carried out in a social gym. If the patient does not adopt the recommended lifestyle changes then it is likely that the injury will reoccur and this should be stressed on discharge.

Case study 3

A 16-year-old elite cricketer who is a bowler presents with an acute onset of right lumbar pain. X-ray reveals spondylolysis at L5/S1.

Management

Cricket bowling is commonly associated with loading in an extension pattern in the lumbar spine with particular stresses noted at the pars interarticularis. The reader is encouraged to study the biomechanics of this activity to understand further. Spondylolysis is a noted injury in cricket, particularly in elite junior players. The ultimate

aims of rehabilitation of this patient are to stabilise around the fracture and to minimise loading on return to cricket by altering biomechanics of the bowling technique. Fitness must be maintained as it is likely that the patient will already have good aerobic function. Activities such as swimming or aqua jogging will be appropriate and loading or time spent exercising should be equivalent to the time that the patient will usually spend doing daily aerobic exercise as part of their training. This level should be maintained to discharge. Early rehabilitation will be aimed at achieving stability, particularly around the affected level in the spine. Specific flexibility exercises may

Case study 3—cont'd

be required to achieve good spinal positioning or to address areas of hypomobility such as thoracic extension. Once basic stability has been achieved, loading may be introduced. However, as this patient is an athlete, the programme will require some power work as well as endurance and this should not be introduced until late rehabilitation. Early loading should include patterns which will be used during cricket, in particular, trunk rotation with arms moving from full flexion to extension as in the bowling action. Loading with the trunk in flexion and rotation as is seen in batting should also be included. Pulleys and free weights may be used to achieve these patterns with incremental loading over the progression of the programme. Proprioceptive training is particularly important as return to sport will not only place demands in this area to protect the spine but also to optimise performance.

Late stage rehabilitation should continue aerobic, proprioceptive and endurance training of the spine as described above but should also include power work. Power activities for the trunk could include pulley and free weight activities adding in high loads and speeds or activities such as throwing and catching a medicine ball with the trunk in different positions. A fundamental component of the programme which should be considered on day 1 and beyond discharge is that sporting technique should be analysed with the assistance of the coach. Abnormal movement patterns should be corrected both in sport and everyday activities and it is important that sporting activity is not resumed until patterns are normal. A graduated return to sport should be combined with continuation of the programme to address risk of re-injury. Return of symptoms may necessitate change of cricket activity to fielding rather than bowling until the spine is considered more stable, which may not be achieved until a more mature skeletal status is reached.

Student questions

(1) How does the evidence regarding management of low back pain with exercise differ for acute and chronic low back pain?
(2) What are the common criticisms of many of the exercise and low back pain trials?
(3) Why is aerobic exercise important in a low back pain rehabilitation programme?
(4) Discuss why muscle endurance rather than power is important when considering activity of the trunk muscles.
(5) Define stability and discuss its importance to the lumbar spine.
(6) How does poor proprioception and motor control in the lumbar spine contribute to low back pain?
(7) Why are common exercises such as sit-ups and lumbar extensions inappropriate and sometimes harmful to many patients with low back pain?
(8) Discuss the advantages of a custom-made and delivered exercise programme over a generic programme for patients with low back pain.
(9) Summarise the important concepts of an exercise programme for low back pain in early, intermediate and late stages.
(10) What lifestyle factors are important in long-term prevention or management of low back pain?

References

Airaksinen, O., Brox, J.I., Cedraschi, C., Hildebrandt, J., Klaber-Moffett, J., Kovacs, F., Mannion, A.F., Reis, S., Staal, J.B., Ursin, H. and Zanoli, G. (2006) Chapter 4. European guidelines for the management of chronic non-specific low back pain. *European Spine Journal*, 15(2 Suppl.), S192–S300.

Bergmark, A. (1989) Stability of the lumbar spine: a study in mechanical engineering. *Acta Orthopedica Scandinavica Supplementum*, 60, 1–54.

Brumagne, S., Cordo, P., Lysens, R., Verschueren, S. and Swinnen, S. (2000) The role of paraspinal muscle spindles in lumbosacral position sense in individuals with and without low back pain. *Spine*, 25, 989–994.

Cairns, M.C., Foster, N.E. and Wright, C. (2006) Randomised controlled trial of specific spinal stabilisation exercises and conventional physiotherapy for recurrent low back pain. *Spine*, 31, 670–681.

Chatzitheodorou, D., Kabitsis, C., Malliou, P. and Mougios, V. (2007) A pilot study of the effects of high intensity aerobic exercise versus passive interventions on pain, disability, psychological strain and serum cortisol concentrations in people with chronic low back pain. *Physical Therapy*, 87, 304–312.

Comerford, M.J. and Mottram, S.L. (2001) Movement and stability dysfunction – contemporary developments. *Manual Therapy*, 6, 15–26.

Deyo, R. (1998) Low back pain. *Scientific American*, 279, 49–55.

Dolan, K.J. and Green, A. (2006) Lumbar spine reposition sense: The effect of a 'slouched' posture. *Manual Therapy*, 11, 202–207.

Ferreira, M.L., Ferreira, P.H., Latimer, J., Herbert, R.D., Hodges, P.W., Jennings, M.D., Maher, C.G. and Refshauge, K.M. (2007) Comparison of general exercise, motor control exercise and spinal manipulative therapy for chronic low back pain. A randomised trial. *Pain*, 131, 31–37.

Gaskell, L., Enright, S. and Tyson, S. (2007) The effects of a back rehabilitation programme for patients with chronic low back pain. *Journal of Evaluation in Clinical Practice*, 13, 795–800.

Halbertsma, J.P.K., Goeken, L.N.H., Groothoff, J.W. and Eisma, W.H. (2001) Extensibility and stiffness of the hamstrings in patients with nonspecific low back pain. *Archives of Physical Medicine and Rehabilitation*, 82, 232–238.

Harreby, M., Hesselsoe, G., Kjer, J. and Neergaard, K. (1997) Low back pain and physical exercise in leisure time in 38-year old men and women: a 25-year prospective cohort study of 640 school children. *European Spine Journal*, 6, 181–186.

Hartvigsen, J. and Christensen, K. (2007) Active lifestyle protects against incident low back pain in seniors. *Spine*, 32, 76–81.

Hayden, J.A., van Tulder, M.W., Malmivaara, A. and Koes, B.W. (2005) Exercise therapy for treatment of non-specific low back pain. *Cochrane Database of Systematic Reviews*, 3, CD000335.

Hayden, J.A., van Tulder, M.W., Malmivaara, A. and Koes, B.W. (2006) Review: exercise therapy reduces pain and improves function in chronic but not acute low-back pain. *ACP Journal Club*; Jan/Feb; 144, 1.

Henry, S.H., Hitt, J.R., Jones, S.L. and Bunn, J.Y. (2006) Decreased limits of stability in response to postural perturbations in subjects with low back pain. *Clinical Biomechanics*, 21, 881–892.

Hyun, J.K., Lee, J.Y., Lee, S.J.L. and Jeon, J.Y. (2007) Asymmetric atrophy of multifidus muscle in patients with unilateral lumbosacral radiculopathy. *Spine*, 32, 598–602.

Iversen, M.D., Fossel, A.H. and Katz, J.N. (2003) Enhancing function in older adults with chronic low back pain: a pilot study of endurance training. *Archives of Physical Medicine and Rehabilitation*, 84, 1324–1331.

Kavcic, N., Grenier, S. and McGill, S. (2004) Determining the stabilising role of individual torso muscles during rehabilitation exercises. *Spine*, 29, 1254–1265.

Koumantakis, G.A., Watson, P. and Oldham, J.A. (2005a) Supplementation of general endurance exercise with stabilisation training versus general exercise only. Physiological and functional outcomes of a randomised controlled trial of patients with recurrent low back pain. *Clinical Biomechanics*, 20, 474–482.

Koumantakis, G.A., Watson, P., Oldham, J.A. (2005b) Trunk muscle stabilisation training plus general exercise versus general exercise only: randomised controlled trial of patients with recurrent low back pain. *Physical Therapy*, 85, 209–225.

Luoto, S., Heliovaara, M., Hurri, H. and Alaranta, H. (1995) Static back endurance and the risk of low back pain. *Clinical Biomechanics*, 10, 323–324.

MacDonald, D.A., Moseley, L. and Hodges, P.W. (2006) The lumbar multifidus: Does the evidence support clinical beliefs? *Manual Therapy*, 11, 254–263.

Mannion, A.F., Muntener, M., Taimela, S. and Dvorak, J. (2001) Comparison of three active therapies for chronic low back pain: results of a randomised clinical trial with one year follow up. *Rheumatology*, 40, 772–778.

McGill, S. (1998) Low back exercises: evidence for improving exercise regimens. *Physical Therapy*, 78, 755–765.

McGill, S. (2001) Low back stability: From formal description to issues for performance and rehabilitation. *Exercise and Sport Science Reviews*, 29, 26–31.

McGill, S. (2002) *Low Back Disorders, Evidence – Based Prevention and Rehabilitation*, p. 146. Human Kinetics, Windsor, Canada.

McGregor, A.H., McCarthy, I.D. and Hughes, S.P. (1995) Motion characteristics of the lumbar spine in the normal population. *Spine*, 20, 2421–2428.

Newcomer, K.L., Jacobson, T.D., Gabriel, D.A., Larson, M.S., Brey, R.H. and An, K. (2002) Muscle activation patterns in subjects with and without low back pain. *Archives of Physical Medicine and Rehabilitation*, 83, 816–821.

Noyes, F.R., De Lucas, J.L. and Torvik, P.J. (1994) Biomechanics of ligament failure. An analysis of strain rate sensitivity and mechanisms of failure in primates. *Journal of Bone and Joint Surgery, American Volume*, 56, 236.

O'Sullivan, P., Burnett, A., Floyd, A.N., Gadson, K., Logiudice, J., Miller, D. and Quirke, H. (2003) Lumbar repositioning deficit in a specific low back pain population. *Spine*, 28, 1074–1079.

Pal, P., Milosavljevic, S., Sole, G. and Johnson, G. (2007) Hip and lumbar continuous motion characteristics during flexion and return in health young males. *European Spine Journal*, 16, 741–747.

Poitras, S., Loisel, P., Prince, F. and Lemaire, J. (2000) Disability measurement in persons with back pain: A validity study of spinal range of motion and velocity. *Archives of Physical Medicine and Rehabilitation*, 81, 1395–1400.

Rackwitz, B., de Bie, R., Limm, H., von Garnier, K., Ewert, T. and Stucki, G. (2006) Segmentak stabilising exercises and low back pain. What is the evidence? A systematic review of randomised controlled trials. *Clinical Rehabilitation*, 20, 553–567.

Rainville, M.D., Hartigan, C., Jouve, C. and Martinez, M.D. (2004) The influence of intense exercise-based physical therapy program on back pain anticipated before and induced by physical activities. *Spine Journal*, 4, 176–183.

Rydeard, R., Leger, A. and Smith, D. (2006) Pilates-based therapeutic exercise: Effect on subjects with nonspecific chronic low back pain and functional disability: A randomised controlled trial. *Journal of Orthopaedic and Sports Physical Therapy*, 36, 472–484.

Sculco, A.D., Paup, D.C., Fernhall, B. and Sculco, M.J. (2001) Effects of aerobic exercise on patients with low back pain in treatment. *Spine Journal*, 1, 95–101.

Shum, G.L.K., Crosbie, J. and Lee, R.Y.W. (2007) Three-dimensional kinetics of the lumbar spine and hips in patients with low back pain during sit-to-stand and stand-to-sit. *Spine*, 32, 211–219.

Slade, S.S. and Keating, J.L. (2006) Trunk strengthening exercises for chronic low back pain: A systematic review. *Journal of Manipulative and Physiological Therapeutics*, 29, 164–173.

Smeets, R.J.E.M., Wittink, H., Hidding, A. and Knottnerus, A. (2006) Do patients with chronic low back pain have a lower level of aerobic fitness than health controls? *Spine*, 31, 90–97.

Solomonow, M., Zhou, B., Baratta, R.V. and Burger, E. (2003) Biomechanics and electromyography of a cumulative lumbar disorder: Response to static flexion. *Clinical Biomechanics*, 18, 890–898.

Soukup, M.G., Glomsrod, P.T., Lonn, J.H., Bo, K., Larsen, S., Fordyce, W.E. (1999) The effect of a mensendieck exercise programme as secondary prophylaxis for recurrent low back pain. *Spine*, 24, 1585–1597.

Taimela, S., Kankaanpaa, M. and Luoto, S. (1999) The effect of lumbar fatigue on the ability to sense a change in lumbar position. *Spine*, 24, 1322–1422.

Torstensen, T.A., Ljunggren, A.E., Meen, H.D., Odland, E., Mowinckel, P. and Geijerstam, S. (1998) Efficiency and costs of medical exercise therapy, conventional physiotherapy, and self-exercise in patients with chronic low back pain. *Spine*, 23, 2616–2624.

UK BEAM Trial Team (2004) United Kingdom back pain and manipulation (UK BEAM) randomised trial: effectiveness of physical treatments for back pain in primary care. *BMJ*, doi: 10.1136/bmj.38282.669225.AE

Van Tulder, M., Becker, A., Bekkering, T., Breen, A., Gil del Real, M.T., Hutchison, A., Koes, B., Laerum, E. and Malmivaara, A. (2006) Chapter 3. European guidelines for the management of acute non-specific low back pain in primary care. *European Spine Journal*, 15(2 Suppl.), S169–S191.

Volpe, R., Popa, T., Ginanneschi, F., Spidalieri, R., Mazzocchio, R. and Rossi, A. (2006) Changes in coordination of postural control during dynamic stance in chronic patients with low back pain. *Gait and Posture*, 24, 349–355.

Wilson, S.E. and Granata, K.P. (2003) Reposition sense of lumbar curvature with flexed and asymmetric lifting postures. *Spine*, 28, 513–518.

Wittink, H., Michel, T.H., Wagner, A., Sukiennik, A. and Rogers, W. (2000a) Deconditioning in patients with chronic low back pain. *Spine*, 25, 2221–2228.

Wittink, H., Michel, T.H., Kulich, R., Wagner, A., Sukiennik, A., Maciewicz, R. and Rogers, W. (2000b) Aerobic fitness testing in patients with chronic low back pain. *Spine*, 25, 1704–1710.

7 The Shoulder Complex

Anne S. Viser, Michael M. Reinold, Kyle J. Rodenhi and Thomas J. Gill

SECTION 1: INTRODUCTION AND BACKGROUND

The shoulder is a rather complex joint that allows the ability to perform numerous functional activities with varying combinations of speed, power and precision. A hallmark of the shoulder region is its large freedom of movement, yet poor static stability, given its minimal bony congruency and thin, flexible capsulo-ligamentous structures. All shoulder motion, from simple arm elevation to high-velocity throwing, requires considerable strength and precise interaction of the surrounding musculature to achieve dynamic stabilization. As our understanding of these processes has evolved, so has our approach to shoulder rehabilitation.

Evidence of role of exercise in shoulder rehabilitation

Therapeutic exercise is a well-established component of shoulder rehabilitation. A variety of shoulder exercise and rehabilitation programmes have been shown to be effective in improving function in patients with impingement (Bang and Deyle, 2000; Roy et al., 2008), shoulder pain (Ginn et al., 1997; Ludewig and Borstad, 2003) and adhesive capsulitis (Carette et al., 2003). Studies have also shown shoulder stretching and strengthening exercises to be effective at improving faulty posture (Kluemper et al., 2006) and mechanics (Wang et al., 1999).

The purpose of this chapter is to discuss the role of exercise in the rehabilitation of shoulder injuries and it will provide an overview of exercise principles that address impairments of mobility, strength, dynamic stability and proprioception. a functional exercise progression will be outlined based on these principles and which includes a gradual and full return to daily and recreational activities.

Range of motion and flexibility exercise

Several studies (Ginn et al., 1997; Ludewig and Borstad, 2003; McClure et al., 2004) have attempted to assess the effectiveness of stretching and strengthening programmes in reducing pain and improving function in patients with various shoulder pathologies. The results of the studies suggest that pro-

Exercise Therapy in the Management of Musculoskeletal Disorders, First Edition. Edited by Fiona Wilson, John Gormley and Juliette Hussey.
© 2011 Blackwell Publishing Ltd

grammes of this nature can benefit shoulder pain and function. An understanding of the anatomy and biomechanics of the shoulder can help guide proper exercise prescription.

Adequate range of motion (ROM) and soft tissue mobility is essential for proper function of the shoulder girdle. The shoulder exhibits extreme mobility in all planes of motion. Full shoulder mobility requires proper physiological and accessory motion of the glenohumeral, scapulothoracic, acromioclavicular and sternoclavicular joints. Due to the shoulder's complex range of motion sequence, restrictions within any of these joints can significantly impact the biomechanics of the entire kinetic chain. It is important to understand the normal arthrokinematics of the shoulder and its capsular restraints to best assess and treat ROM restrictions.

Humerothoracic motion can be divided into three main components (Rockwood *et al.*, 2004). The first component is the articular surface of the glenohumeral ball and socket joint. The remaining two components are the bursal-lined surfaces known as the humeroscapular motion interface (HSMI) and the scapulothoracic motion interface (STMI).

Aside from bony surface changes that can occur with fracture or osteoarthritis, there are four major factors that can cause shoulder stiffness. The first factor is contractures of the glenohumeral joint capsule and ligaments. This can significantly restrict shoulder motion by reducing the normal glide of the humerus within the glenoid (arthrokinematic motion). Secondly, contractures of muscle–tendon units crossing the glenohumeral joint can reduce the roll of the humerus within the glenoid (physiological motion). The third factor involves the necessary gliding of the tendons of the rotator cuff and biceps. Adhesions between the tendon surfaces and adjacent soft tissues can limit this gliding and reduces glenohumeral motion. The fourth factor involves any adhesions or soft tissue restriction of the scapulothoracic joint, as this can limit the three-dimensional motion of the scapula.

The capsulo-ligamentous restraints of the glenohumeral joint have received a lot of attention due to its significant role in maintaining an important balance between stability and mobility. There is little capsular tension in the midranges of shoulder motion. However, as motion approaches end range, capsular tension increases. This helps to protect the rotator cuff tendons from excessive tensile loads (Rockwood *et al.*, 2004). In the presence of asym-

metrical capsular tightness, where one aspect of the capsule becomes tight and restricted, the humeral head migrates away from the area of restriction.

Specific areas of the glenohumeral joint capsule (with its closely related ligaments) are responsible for limiting physiological motion and checking excessive translation. Knowledge of these biomechanical factors can help the clinician accurately assess the cause of motion restrictions and develop a treatment programme designed to specifically address certain aspects of the joint. The rotator cuff interval, coracohumeral ligament and superior glenohumeral ligament act to limit flexion, extension and external rotation with the arm at 0° of abduction. The middle glenohumeral ligament tightens at the end range of external rotation at approximately 45° of abduction. The three portions of the inferior glenohumeral ligament complex each have independent roles. The anterior portion serves to limit external rotation at 90° of abduction. The middle portion of the inferior glenohumeral ligament complex tightens with end-range abduction and flexion. Finally, the posterior portion checks internal rotation at 90° of abduction. The posterior capsule serves to limit internal rotation from 0° to 45° of abduction (Rockwood *et al.*, 2004).

This information is extremely valuable when assessing the ROM restrictions and can help guide proper stretching and joint mobilization techniques. It is necessary to assess each patient's available ROM to determine which planes of motion may be limited. For example, a patient who has difficulty performing overhead reaching activities and exhibits adequate external rotation of the glenohumeral joint at 0° and 45° of abduction but limited external rotation at 90° may benefit from joint mobilization and stretching techniques designed to improve mobility of the inferior glenohumeral ligament complex, specifically the anterior band (Fig. 7.1). The information can also help guide exercise interventions aimed at restoring shoulder ROM. By placing stress on structures limiting shoulder ROM, tissue remodelling in ligament, tendon and muscle can be influenced. This can be accomplished with a variety of ROM exercises, capsular and muscular stretches.

Strengthening exercise

The efficacy of shoulder strengthening programmes is difficult to evaluate. Several studies (Ginn *et al.*,

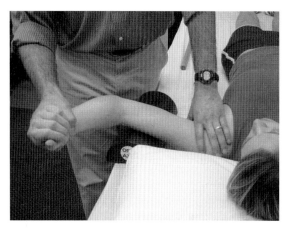

Figure 7.1 Passive external rotation stretching at 90° of abduction in the scapular plane.

1997; Ludewig and Borstad, 2003; McClure *et al.*, 2004; Andersen *et al.*, 2008; Roy *et al.*, 2008) have attempted to assess the effect of strengthening programmes on various pathologies; however results vary and may be limited to the inability to control a study of this magnitude. Several studies that have attempted to determine the most effective exercise to perform for specific musculature based on electromyographic (EMG) activity and biomechanical modelling will be discussed.

Rehabilitation programmes for the shoulder joint often focus on restoring strength and muscular balance, particularly of the rotator cuff and scapulothoracic joint. The majority of research regarding shoulder biomechanics has focused on quantifying the EMG activity of particular muscles during common rehabilitation exercises, the goal of which is to determine the most optimal exercise to recruit specific muscle activity.

Of 17 exercises studied by Townsend *et al.* (1991), the authors recommend the following exercises be included in shoulder rehabilitation programmes, on the basis of the high EMG activity of each muscle examined: (1) elevation in the scapular plane, (2) shoulder flexion, (3) prone horizontal abduction with external rotation, and (4) press-up. It should be noted that the study did not include statistical analysis of muscle activity between exercises; for example, the supraspinatus activity during the empty-can and full-can exercises. Therefore, comparison of muscle activity cannot be considered conclusive. Many studies have since expanded on the work of Townsend *et al.* In particular, studies

have sought to compare the effectiveness of several exercises for the external rotators, supraspinatus and scapulothoracic musculature. The following sections will discuss each one in detail.

External rotators

Several studies have been published to document the EMG activity of the glenohumeral musculature during specific shoulder exercises (Moynes *et al.*, 1986; Blackburn *et al.*, 1990; Greenfield *et al.*, 1990; Kronberg *et al.*, 1990; Bradley and Tibone, 1991; Townsend *et al.*, 1991; Worrell *et al.*, 1992; Ballantyne *et al.*, 1993; McCann *et al.*, 1993; Malanga *et al.*, 1996). Variations in experimental methodology have resulted in conflicting outcomes and controversy in exercise selection.

Exercises in the 90° of abduction position are often incorporated to simulate the position and strain on the shoulder during overhead activities such as throwing. This position produced moderate activity of the external rotators but also increased activity of the deltoid and supraspinatus to stabilise the shoulder. It appears that the amount of infraspinatus and teres minor activity progressively decreases as the shoulder moves into an abducted position, while activity of the supraspinatus and deltoid increases. This may imply that as the arm moves into a position of less shoulder stability, the supraspinatus and deltoid are active to assist in the external rotation movement while providing some degree of glenohumeral stability through muscular contraction.

While standing, external rotation at 90° of abduction may have a functional advantage over 0° of abduction and in the scapular plane due to the close replication of this position in sporting activities, the combination of abduction and external rotation places strain on the shoulder's capsule, particularly the anterior band of the inferior glenohumeral ligament (O'Brien *et al.*, 1990; Scovazzo *et al.*, 1991). When the arm is not in an abducted position, external rotation places less strain on this portion of the joint capsule. Therefore, although muscle activity was low to moderate during external rotation at 0° of abduction, this rehabilitation exercise may be worthwhile when strain of the inferior glenohumeral ligament is of concern. Side lying may be the most optimal exercise to strengthen the external rotators, based on the highest amount of EMG activity observed during this study.

Supraspinatus and deltoid

Numerous investigations have studied the EMG activity of the supraspinatus during rehabilitation exercises ,and controversy exists regarding the optimal exercise to elicit muscle activity. Clinically, many authors have suggested that the empty-can exercise may provoke pain in many patients by encroaching on the soft tissue within the subacromial space during this impingement type manoeuvre. Numerous authors have since compared the empty-can exercise with several other common supraspinatus exercises to determine if exercises that place the shoulder in less of a disadvantageous position elicit similar amounts of supraspinatus activity.

The effect of increased deltoid activity during arm elevation is a concern to rehabilitation specialists, especially when rehabilitating a patient with subacromial impingement or rotator cuff pathology. Morrey *et al.* (1998) examined the resultant force vectors of the deltoid and supraspinatus during arm elevation at various degrees of motion. Deltoid activity alone exhibited a superiorly orientated force vector from 0° to 90°, and a compressive force on the glenohumeral joint at 120–150°. Conversely, the supraspinatus muscle produced a consistent compressive force throughout the range of elevation. In patients with inefficient subacromial impingement, weak posterior rotator cuff muscles, inefficient dynamic stabilisation, and/or rotator cuff pathology, exercises that produce high levels of deltoid activity may be detrimental due to the amount of superior humeral head migration observed when the rotator cuff does not efficiently compress the humeral head within the glenoid fossa. Therefore, exercises are often chosen to minimise the opportunity for the deltoid to overpower the rotator cuff musculature during arm elevation.

Biomechanically, Poppen and Walker (1978) examined the resultant force vectors of the glenohumeral joint during elevation with the arm position in neutral, internal rotation ('empty can' position) and external rotation ('full can' position). The authors report that at angles below 90° of abduction, the empty-can position resulted in a superiorly orientated force vector while the full-can position produced a compressive force from 0° to 120°. These results may correlate well with the previously mentioned studies reporting increased deltoid activity, and thus superior humeral head migration, during the empty can exercise.

Therefore, based on the numerous EMG investigations, the full-can exercise may be the best exercise for the supraspinatus due to the moderate amounts of muscle activity with the least amount of pain provocation and surrounding muscle activation.

Subscapularis

The subscapularis provides anterior stabilization and assists the posterior rotator cuff with compression of the humeral head in the glenoid fossa during overhead and throwing activities (Glousman *et al.*, 1988; Scovazzo *et al.*, 1991; Wilk *et al.*, 1997). While many shoulder rehabilitation programmes integrate internal rotation strengthening in the neutral position, recent evidence suggests that this may not be the most effective exercise for selectively strengthening the subscapularis. Several EMG studies have identified exercises and shoulder positions that elicit the most muscle activity and may be important to consider in developing rehabilitation programmes (Decker *et al.*, 2003; Suenaga *et al.*, 2003).

Decker *et al.* (2003) evaluated EMG data for seven shoulder exercises with 15 healthy subjects in seven muscles including both upper and lower portions of the subscapularis. They found that the push-up with a plus and a diagonal exercise moving from flexion, abduction and external rotation to extension, adduction and internal rotation, consistently elicited the most subscapularis activity in both the upper and lower portions. Furthermore, they found that the upper and lower portions of subscapularis may function independently. Upper subscapularis activity was greater during internal rotation at 90° of abduction while the lower portion was more active at neutral abduction.

Suenaga *et al.* (2003) examined subscapularis activity during isometric and active internal rotation at 0° and 90° of abduction. Using fine wire EMG, they report subscapularis activity at 12.1% of maximum voluntary contraction (MVC) at 90° of abduction compared to 2.0% at 0° of abduction. In addition, pectoralis major activity was greater than all other internal rotators for active and isometric contractions at 0° abduction. The results of this study suggest that larger muscle groups, such as the pectoralis, latissimus dorsi, and anterior

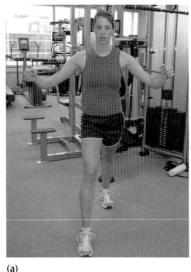
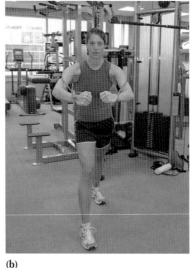

(a)   **(b)**

Figure 7.2 Dynamic hug exercise. Using resistance, patient horizontally adducts the shoulder at 60° of elevation while protracting the scapula.

deltoid, are likely have a greater effect on glenohumeral internal rotation at 0° of abduction.

The aforementioned studies indicate that internal rotation exercises at 90° of abduction may be the most advantageous position to strengthen the subscapularis while minimising contributions from larger muscle groups. Functional exercises such as the diagonal and push-up plus exercises should be considered at the appropriate stage of rehabilitation to strengthen the subscapularis and enhance glenohumeral stability.

Scapulothoracic musculature

The function of the scapulothoracic joint is critical for normal shoulder function. Several authors have noted that weakness or muscle imbalance of the scapular musculature can lead to altered scapular position and dyskinesis, which may be a factor in shoulder dysfunction such as glenohumeral instability and shoulder impingement (Ludewig and Cook, 2000; Cools *et al.*, 2003; Kibler and McMullen, 2003). The lower scapular stabilisers such as the serratus anterior, rhomboids, and middle and lower trapezius are the most commonly weak or inhibited muscles, and are often targeted in shoulder rehabilitation (Voight and Thomson, 2000).

The EMG activity of the scapulothoracic musculature has also been investigated. Moseley *et al.*

(1992) examined eight muscles, including the upper, middle and lower trapezius, levator scapula, rhomboids, pectoralis minor, and middle and lower serratus anterior, during 16 commonly performed exercises in nine healthy subjects. The authors reported the peak EMG activity for each muscle and noted that the majority of the muscles assisted in more than one scapular function. Based on the results of the study, the authors recommended a core programme of scapular strengthening exercises that included shoulder scaption, prone rowing, push-ups with a plus, and press-ups.

Serratus anterior

Decker *et al.* (1999) looked more specifically at the EMG activity of the serratus anterior during eight common scapulohumeral exercises in 20 healthy subjects. The authors selected exercises that are typically performed below 90° of humeral elevation, a range of motion deemed safe for most patients with shoulder pathology. The exercises that elicited the greatest amount of serratus activity included the push-up with a plus, dynamic hug (Fig. 7.2), and a standing serratus anterior punch exercise (Fig. 7.3).

Ekstrom *et al.* (2003) studied EMG activity of the trapezius and serratus anterior during 10 different exercises in 30 subjects. The authors identified two exercises that yielded the most significant EMG

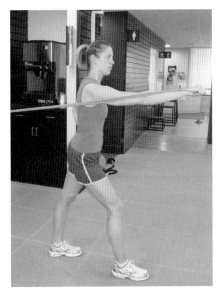

Figure 7.3 Serratus anterior punch. The patient elevates the arm to 90° and protracts the scapula against resistance.

activity in the serratus anterior: (1) a diagonal exercise with a combination of shoulder and horizontal flexion, and (2) external rotation and standing shoulder scaption above 120°. EMG activity was greater for both exercises than with traditional straight plane scapular protraction, suggesting that strengthening programmes for serratus anterior should incorporate an element of protraction combined with elevation.

Lower trapezius

Exercises designed to strengthen the lower trapezius are often desired in rehabilitation settings. One of the most effective exercises is the prone horizontal abduction with full glenohumeral external rotation. This exercise is often performed at 100–110° of abduction. However, Ekstrom *et al.* (2003) identified, with EMG analysis, the prone arm raise in line with the fibres of lower trapezius as the most effective exercise to recruit the lower trapezius. Thus it is important to watch the patient perform the exercise with direct visualisation of the scapula to determine the specific angle of lower trapezius insertion.

Cools *et al.* (2007) investigated the balance ratio of the scapular musculature during 12 commonly used shoulder strengthening exercises. The authors aimed to determine which exercise optimally recruited the lower trapezius, middle trapezius and serratus anterior with minimal participation of the upper trapezius. Based on the EMG analysis, the following exercises were suggested for high activation of the lower and middle trapezius with low activation of the upper trapezius: side lying external rotation, side lying forward flexion, prone horizontal abduction with external rotation and prone extension.

Proprioception

The efficacy of proprioceptive training has received much attention in the orthopaedic community, demonstrating the ability to effectively enhance proprioception after injury and surgery in various joints (Lephart *et al.*, 1997; Mendelsohn *et al.*, 2004; Fu and Hui-Chan, 2005; Risberg *et al.*, 2007; Panics *et al.*, 2008). While the lower extremity has been the subject of the bulk of the research in this area, there have been some studies on proprioception of the shoulder (Lephart *et al.*, 1992; Swanik *et al.*, 2002; Barden *et al.*, 2004) that have shown positive results. In order to train the proprioceptive system, it is important to first understand the static and dynamic functions of shoulder stability and how they relate to shoulder function.

Functional stability of the glenohumeral joint is achieved through the precise interaction of both static and dynamic stabilisers. Due to the anatomical configuration of the glenohumeral joint, static stability is compromised to allow for an increase in functional activities of the upper extremity. This compromise results in an increased demand of the dynamic shoulder stabilisers to control joint arthrokinematics.

Static stabilisers

Several passive mechanisms provide static stability of the glenohumeral joint (Wilk *et al.*, 1997). The first mechanism is the osseous articulation between the humeral head and the glenoid fossa. The convex surface of the humeral head is approximately three to four times the size of the concave glenoid fossa, resulting in a significant amount of available glenohumeral rotation and translation, with minimal bony congruency (Soslowsky *et al.*, 1992). The second mechanism of static stability involves the glenoid labrum, which serves to deepen the glenoid fossa and enlarge the contact area of glenohumeral articulation. The labrum also serves as an attachment site of the glenohumeral joint capsule and ligaments, the third mechanism of static stability. The joint capsule is enhanced with fibrous thickenings which form the glenohumeral ligaments and serve to reinforce the capsular tissue (Wilk *et al.*, 1997).

The last two mechanisms of static stabilisation are intra-articular pressure and joint cohesion. The glenohumeral joint capsule is sealed airtight with negative intra-articular joint pressure and a small amount of joint fluid providing passive stabilisation by a vacuum effect of viscous and intermolecular forces (Kumar and Balasubramaniam, 1985; Browne *et al.*, 1990; Matsen *et al.*, 1990; Gibb *et al.*, 1991; Habermeyer *et al.*, 1992; Wilk *et al.*, 1997).

Several pathological conditions may compromise the static stability of the glenohumeral joint. Most common among athletes are capsulolabral injuries including labral degeneration, detachment of the superior labrum near the biceps tendon attachment (SLAP lesions), loose or redundant capsules, and Bankart lesions (Bison and Andrews, 1998; Meister, 2000; Wilk *et al.*, 2002). Any of these pathologies may have an effect of the static stability of the shoulder and may occur concomitantly with one another.

Dynamic stabilisers

Dynamic stabilisation of the glenohumeral joint is achieved through the interaction of several active mechanisms. The muscles primarily responsible for dynamic stabilisation are the rotator cuff (infraspinatus, supraspinatus, teres minor, and subscapularis), deltoid and long head of the biceps brachii (Wilk *et al.*, 1997, 2002). Secondary stabilisers include the pectoralis major, latissimus dorsi, and the scapulothoracic musculature (trapezius, rhomboids, serratus anterior, and pectoralis minor, and levator scapulae) (Wilk *et al.*, 1997).

The first mechanism of dynamic stabilisation is the interaction of glenohumeral joint force couples. Inman *et al.* (1996) described two force couples of the glenohumeral joint. The first force couple involves the subscapularis and the posterior rotator cuff, the infraspinatus and teres minor. The second force couple of the glenohumeral joint involves the deltoid and the entire rotator cuff complex. These forces couples are active throughout the entire range of shoulder motion and serve to provide a dynamic symmetry of joint forces (Wilk *et al.*, 1993).

The role of the surrounding glenohumeral musculature in dynamic stabilisation is multifactorial. The precise interaction of the anterior and posterior rotator cuff musculature as well as the prime movers and the stabilising rotator cuff musculature is vital for normal glenohumeral joint arthrokinematics. The rotator cuff musculature also provides dynamic stabilisation through blending of the musculotendinous tissue within the shoulder capsule, the second component of dynamic stabilisation (Clark and Harryman, 1992). Therefore, contraction of the rotator cuff produces tension within the joint capsule, centring the humeral head within the glenoid.

The third component to active glenohumeral joint stability is neuromuscular control of the shoulder. Neuromuscular control may be defined as the efferent or motor, output in reaction to afferent, or sensory, input (Lephart *et al.*, 1997; Wilk *et al.*, 1997; Myers and Lephart, 2000). Thus, afferent input is comprised of the ability to detect glenohumeral joint position (proprioception) and motion (kinaesthesia) in space, with subsequent efferent output to produce dynamic joint stabilisation.

The component of neuromuscular control appears to be critical in normal function, and thus drills designed to enhance proprioception, kinaesthesia, and dynamic stabilisation are emphasised when designing rehabilitation programmes. Furthermore, exercises to promote muscular endurance may also assist in preventing abnormal glenohumeral joint translation by minimising muscle fatigue.

Aerobic exercise

It is important to consider aerobic exercises for the general health of any patient with shoulder pathology. After a shoulder injury, patients are generally recommended to remain active with activities such as walking, riding a bike or jogging.

SECTION 2: PRACTICAL USE OF EXERCISE

Functional rehabilitation of the shoulder: Clinical application of dynamic stabilisation

The rehabilitation process for shoulder injuries must include the restoration of ROM, muscular strength, muscular endurance, as well as a gradual restoration of proprioception, dynamic stability and neuromuscular control. As the patient advances, functional or sport-specific drills are emphasised to prepare for a gradual return to activity. Neuromuscular control drills are performed throughout and advanced as the patient progresses to provide continuous challenge to the neuromuscular control system. The following section provides an overview of a functional rehabilitation progression for patients following injury or operative procedure. The programme is divided into four separate phases with specific goals and criteria for advancement for each phase. The use of a criteria-based rehabilitation programme allows for its individualisation for each patient and specific pathology or surgical procedure. Alterations in exercise activities, positioning and rate of progression are based on the type of injury, surgical procedure performed, healing constraints involved and the tissues that are being stressed during rehabilitation.

Acute phase

The acute phase of rehabilitation begins immediately following injury or surgery. The duration of the acute phase is dependent on the healing constraints of the involved pathological tissues. Rehabilitation precautions will vary based on the exact pathology and any postoperative limitations. The initial goals of the acute phase are to diminish pain and inflammation, and progress to include the normalization of motion and muscular balance, and the restoration of baseline proprioceptive and kinaesthetic awareness.

ROM exercises are performed immediately in a restricted ROM, based on the theory that motion assists in the enhancement and organisation of col-

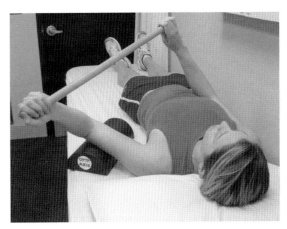

Figure 7.4 Active-assist range of motion with external rotation at 45° of abduction in the scapular plane.

lagen tissue and the stimulation of joint mechanoreceptors, and may assist in the neuromodulation of pain. The rehabilitation programme should allow for progressive applied loads, beginning with gentle passive range of motion. Active-assisted ROM exercises are instructed to the patient including cane or L-Bar (Breg Corporation, Vista, CA, USA) range of motion for flexion, external rotation, and internal rotation (Fig. 7.4). As the patient advances, flexion progresses as tolerated and shoulder rotation ROM is progressed from 0° of abduction to 30° and 45° of abduction. Also, pendulum, and rope and pulley, exercises are used as needed.

Self-capsular stretches may be performed for the anterior, posterior, and inferior glenohumeral joint complex as appropriate. Also, gentle joint mobilization and contract-relax or hold-relax stretching techniques may be performed during the early stages of rehabilitation for pain modulation and to maintain symmetrical capsular mobility.

Strengthening begins with submaximal, pain-free isometrics for shoulder flexion, extension, abduction, external rotation, internal rotation, and elbow flexion. Isometrics are used to retard muscular atrophy and restore voluntary muscular control, while avoiding detrimental shoulder forces. Isometrics should be performed at multiple angles throughout the available range of motion, with particular emphasis on contraction at the end of the currently available range of motion.

Manual rhythmic stabilisation drills are performed for the shoulder internal and external rotators with the arm in the scapular plane at 30° of

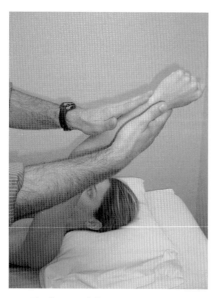

Figure 7.5 Rhythmic stabilisation at 120° of elevation.

abduction. Alternating isometric contractions are performed to facilitate co-contraction of the anterior and posterior rotator cuff musculature. Rhythmic stabilisation drills may also be performed with the patient supine and arm elevated to approximately 90–100° and 10° of horizontal abduction. This position is chosen for the initiation of these drills due to the combined centralised line of pull of both the rotator cuff and deltoid musculature at this angle, causing a humeral head compressive force during muscle contraction. The rehabilitation specialist employs alternating isometric contractions in the flexion, extension, horizontal abduction, and horizontal adduction planes of motion. As the patient progresses, the drills can be performed at variable degrees of elevation such as 45° and 120° (Fig. 7.5).

Active ROM activities are permitted when adequate muscular strength and balance has been achieved. Active motion is initiated in the acute phase with joint reproduction exercises. With the patient's eyes closed, the rehabilitation specialist passively moves the upper extremity in the planes of flexion, external rotation and internal rotation, pauses, and then returns the extremity to the starting position. The patient is then instructed to actively reposition the upper extremity to the previous location. The rehabilitation specialist may perform these joint repositioning activities in vari-

able degrees throughout the available range of motion and notes the accuracy of the patient.

Also performed during the acute phase is weight-bearing, or axial compression exercises. Initial exercises are performed below shoulder level, such as weight-bearing on a table while standing. The patient may perform weight shifts in the anterior/posterior and medial/lateral directions. Rhythmic stabilisations may also be performed during weight shifting. As the patient progresses, a medium-sized ball may be placed on the table and weight shifts may be performed on the ball. Weight-bearing exercises are progressed from the table to the quadruped position.

Once the acute pain has subsided, the patient may begin aerobic exercise such as walking, or riding on a stationary bike at low resistance. This can be progressed in intensity and duration according to the patient's tolerance. Modalities including ice, high-voltage stimulation, ultrasound and non-steroidal anti-inflammatory medications may also be employed as needed to control pain and inflammation.

Intermediate phase

The intermediate phase begins once the patient has regained near-normal passive motion and sufficient balance of strength of the shoulder musculature. Baseline proprioception, kinaesthesia, and dynamic stabilisation are also needed before progressing, as emphasis will now be placed on regaining these sensory modalities throughout the patient's full ROM, particularly at end range. The goals of the intermediate phase are to enhance functional dynamic stability, re-establish neuromuscular control, restore muscular strength and balance, and to regain and maintain full ROM.

ROM exercises are continued and the athlete is encouraged to perform active-assisted ROM with a cane or L-bar to maintain motion. External and internal ROM may be performed at 90° of abduction. Joint mobilisations and self-capsular stretches are performed as necessary to prevent asymmetrical glenohumeral joint capsular tightness.

Strengthening exercises are advanced to include external and internal rotation with exercise tubing at 0° of abduction and active ROM exercises against gravity. These exercises initially include

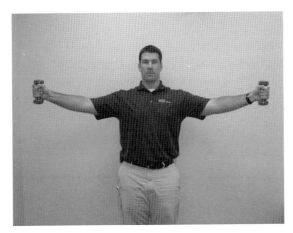

Figure 7.6 Full-can: standing scaption with external rotation.

standing scaption in external rotation (full can) (Fig. 7.6), standing abduction, side lying external rotation, and prone rowing. As strength returns, the program may be advanced to a programme that includes full upper extremity strengthening with emphasis on posterior rotator cuff and scapular strengthening

Isolated rhythmic stabilisation exercises are performed during the early part of the intermediate phase. Drills performed in the acute phase may be progressed to include stabilisation at end ranges of motion and with the patient's eyes closed. Proprioceptive neuromuscular facilitation (PNF) patterns are performed in the patient's available ROM and progressed to include full arcs of motion. Rhythmic stabilisations may be incorporated in various degrees of elevation during the PNF patterns to promote dynamic stabilisation.

Also performed during the intermediate phase is manual resistance to external rotation. By applying manual resistance to specific exercises, the rehabilitation specialist can vary the amount of resistance throughout the range of motion and incorporate concentric and eccentric contractions, as well as rhythmic stabilisations at end range (Fig. 7.7). The application of manual resistance assists in the reinforcement of proper resistance, form, and cadence based on the symptoms of each patient. As the patient regains strength and neuromuscular control, external and internal rotation with tubing may be performed at 90° of abduction (Fig. 7.8). All stabilization drills may be advanced by removing the patient's visual stimulus.

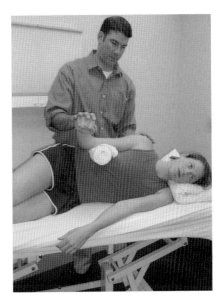

Figure 7.7 Manual resistance of external rotation both concentrically and eccentrically at patient's side.

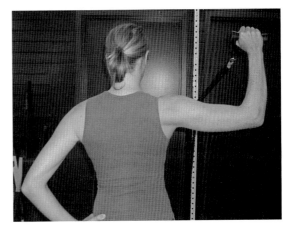

Figure 7.8 External rotation with tubing at 90° of abduction.

Scapular strengthening and neuromuscular control are also critical to regaining full dynamic stability of the glenohumeral joint. The scapular functions to provide a stable base of support for distal upper extremity movement and serves as a site of attachment for the stabilizing musculature of the shoulder. Thus exercises are performed to enhance scapulothoracic function. Isotonic exercises for the scapulothoracic joint are performed as

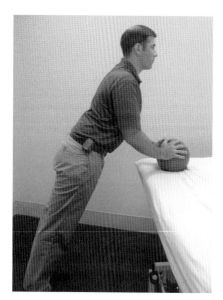

Figure 7.9 Push-up on ball.

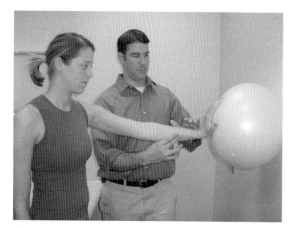

Figure 7.10 Axial compression of the upper extremity on a ball versus the wall. The therapist applies alternating rhythmic stabilisation to the upper extremity.

well as manual resistance prone rowing. Also, neuromuscular control drills and PNF patterns may be applied to the scapular.

Axial compression exercises are also advanced. Weight shifting on a ball is progressed to a push-up on a ball or unstable surface on a tabletop (Fig. 7.9). Rhythmic stabilisations can be performed by the rehabilitation specialist at the upper extremity as well. Wall stabilisation drills are performed with the patient's hand on a small ball (Fig. 7.10). Further axial compression exercises include table

and quadruped exercises using a towel around the hand, slide board or unstable surface.

Aerobic exercise can be progressed to moderate intensity exercises such as jogging or exercising on a cross-training machine such as an elliptical trainer. The patient may find it more comfortable to start on the elliptical with the arms stabilized, working the legs only. The upper extremities can be gradually incorporated into the exercise according to the patient's tolerance.

Advanced phase

The third phase of a functional rehabilitation programme, the advanced phase, is designed to advance the patient through a series of progressive strengthening and neuromuscular control activities, while preparing the patient to begin a gradual return to full activity. Criteria to enter this phase include minimal pain and tenderness, full ROM, symmetrical capsular mobility, good (4/5 on manual muscle testing) strength and endurance of the upper extremity and scapulothoracic musculature, and sufficient dynamic stabilisation.

Full motion and capsular mobility are maintained through ROM and self-stretching techniques. These include manual stretching and L-bar exercises. Specific emphasis on soft tissue mobility of the posterior musculotendinous structures should be made through exercises such as horizontal adduction stretching while stabilising the scapula (Fig. 7.11).

Strengthening exercises for the entire shoulder complex as well as exercises for the lower extremities and trunk are continued with a gradual increase in resistance. Exercises such as internal and external rotation with exercises tubing at 90° of abduction may be progressed to also incorporate eccentric and higher speed contractions. Aggressive strengthening of the upper body may also be initiated depending on the needs of the individual patient. Common exercises include isotonic weight machine exercises such as bench press, seated row, and latissimus pull downs within a restricted ROM. During bench press and seated row, the patient is instructed to not extend the upper extremities beyond the plane of the body to minimise stress of the shoulder capsule. Latissimus pull downs are performed in front of the head and the patient is instructed to avoid full

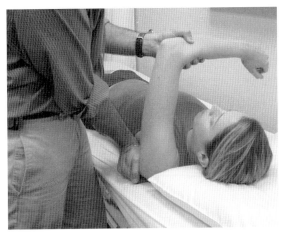

Figure 7.11 Horizontal adduction stretch of posterior soft tissue. The therapist manually stabilises the scapula from moving during stretch.

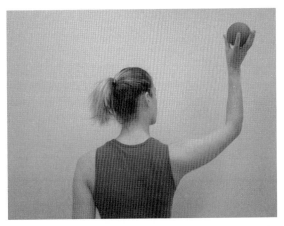

Figure 7.12 Wall dribbling. One-handed plyometrics in the 90/90 position.

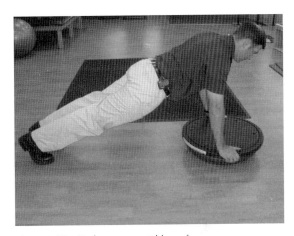

Figure 7.13 Push-up on unstable surface.

extension of the arms to minimise the amount of traction force applied to the upper extremities.

Plyometric activities for the upper extremity may be initiated during this phase as well to train the upper extremity to produce and dissipate forces. Plyometric exercises are initially performed with two-hands. Specific exercises include a chest pass, overhead throw, and alternating side-to-side throw with a 1–2 kg (or 3–5 lb) medicine ball. Two-hand drills are progressed to one-hand drills as tolerated by the athlete, usually between 10 and 14 days following the initiation of two-hand drills. Specific one-hand plyometrics include baseball style throws in the 90/90 position with a 1 kg (or 2 lb) ball (Fig. 7.12) and stationary and semi-circle wall dribbles. Wall dribbles are also beneficial to increase upper extremity endurance while overhead and may be progressed to include dribbles in the 90/90 position.

Axial compression exercises are progressed to include the quadruped and tripled positions. Rhythmic stabilisations of the involved extremity as well as at the core and trunk may be applied. Unstable surfaces, such as tilt boards, foam, large exercise balls, or the Biodex stability system (Biodex Corp., Shirley, NY, USA) may be incorporated to further challenge the patient's stability system while in the closed chain position (Figs 7.13 and 7.14).

Rhythmic oscillations may also be incorporated into the exercise programme through the use several tools such as the Bodyblade (Hymanson Inc., Playa Del Ray, CA, USA), Thera-Band® Resistance Bar (Thera-Band, Akron, OH, USA), or other manufactured or self-made devices. Rhythmic oscillations can be incorporated into exercise tubing and manual resistance exercises to develop stability and muscular endurance in a variety of positions. Oscillations may also be performed during quadruped or tripled exercises using the uninvolved extremity.

Dynamic stabilisation and neuromuscular control drills are progressed to include reactive neuromuscular control drills and functional, sport-specific positions. Concentric and eccentric manual resistance may be applied as the patient performs external rotation with exercise tubing with the arm at 0° of abduction. Rhythmic stabilisations may be

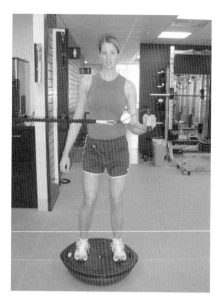

Figure 7.14 External rotation with exercise tubing at side while standing on an unstable surface for added trunk and lower extremity stabilisation.

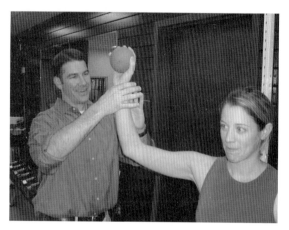

Figure 7.15 Rhythmic stabilization in sports-specific position (90°/90°).

included at end range to challenge the patient to stabilise against the force of the tubing as well as the therapist. This exercise may be progressed to the 90/90 position to require the patient to stabilise the shoulder at end range in a more sport-specific position (Fig. 7.15). Also, rhythmic stabilisations may be applied at end range during the 90/90 wall dribble exercise. The patient performs a predetermined number of repetitions before the therapist implies a series of rhythmic stabilisations at exter-

nal rotation end range. These drills are designed to impart a sudden perturbation to the throwing shoulder at near end range to develop the athlete's ability to dynamically stabilise the shoulder to prevent the shoulder from translating into excessive ranges of motion.

Near the end of the advanced phase, the patient may begin basic sport-specific drills. Various activities such as underweight and overweight ball throwing or swinging for baseball, golf, and tennis players may be performed. Upper extremity aerobic activities such as swimming or rowing can be initiated.

Return to activity phase

Upon the completion of the previously outlined rehabilitation programme and the successful evaluation of the injured shoulder, the patient may begin the final phase of the rehabilitation programme, the return to activity phase. Specific criteria during the clinical exam that needs to be met to begin an interval return to work or sport programme include minimal complaints of pain or tenderness, full ROM, balanced capsular mobility, adequate proprioception, dynamic stabilisation, and neuromuscular control, and full muscular strength and endurance based on an isokinetic examination.

Several authors have advocated an interval return to sport activities (Axe *et al.*, 1996; Ellenbecker and Mattalino, 1997; Axe *et al.*, 2001; Wilk *et al.*, 2001; Reinold *et al.*, 2002). Interval sport programmes are designed to gradually return motion, function and confidence in the upper extremity after injury or surgery by slowly progressing through graduated sport-specific activities. These programmes are intended to gradually return the overhead athletes to full athletic competition as quickly and safely as possible. An athlete is allowed to begin an interval sport programme following a satisfactory clinical examination.

Conclusion

The shoulder joint complex is inherently unstable and must interact with the neuromuscular control system to perform optimally while minimising the risk for injury. Based on a sound understanding of the anatomy and biomechanics of the shoulder joint, comprehensive rehabilitation should include proprioception, dynamic stabilisation, and neuromuscular control drills to establish full range of motion, balanced capsular mobility, and maximal muscular strength and endurance. A functional approach to rehabilitation, using activity-specific exercises, minimises injury risk and ensures a gradual return to activity.

SECTION 3: CASE STUDIES AND STUDENT QUESTIONS

Case study 1

Impingement

A 35-year-old man presents with a complaint of right shoulder pain and stiffness following a weekend of home redecorating and painting 3 weeks ago. During the week he works at a computer for the majority of the day. Examination reveals a forward head posture with increased thoracic kyphosis and protracted, anterior-tilted scapula, superior pain with end range right shoulder flexion, weak and painful right full-can and external rotator strength (4/5) and decreased strength of the scapular retractors and upward rotators (4/5). Flexibility testing reveals decreased length of the pectoral muscles and anterior cervical musculature. Cervical mobility is within normal limits and pain-free.

Management

This patient presents with clinical findings suggestive of impingement syndrome, with symptoms exacerbated by a weekend of intense and repetitive upper extremity activity. The early stage of rehabilitation should include postural retraining with exercise activities to address cervico-thoracic and scapular alignment, stretching of the pectoral muscles, and initiation of basic rotator cuff strengthening. Patient education should focus on proper reach technique to avoid provoking positions/activities. Other modalities such as ice, ultrasound, electrical stimulation or non-steroidal anti-inflammatories may be used for symptom management.

As the acute reactivity calms and full pain-free ROM returns, the patient moves into the intermediate phase of rehabilitation, during which rotator cuff and scapular strengthening is advanced with increased level of resistance and position from neutral to shoulder height and above. Focus is placed on proper postural alignment and scapulohumeral rhythm during each exercise activity. Emphasis is placed on strengthening the external rotators and lower trapezius.

The advanced phase of rehabilitation should focus on strength and control through functional ranges for tasks such as overhead reaching, lifting, pushing and pulling. PNF D2 patterns may be helpful in engaging multiple muscle groups, including supportive trunk musculature. The patient should be observed performing overhead tasks with attention paid to postural alignment and proper scapulohumeral control.

As the patient gradually returns to his normal daily and recreational activities, he should continue a basic exercise regimen to minimise return of symptoms or a re-injury.

Case study 2

Instability

An 18-year-old female cheerleader presents with recurrent anterior glenohumeral subluxations, which limits her ability to participate in cheerleading. She has had three subluxations over the past year. Examination reveals excessive ROM in all directions with multi-directional glenohumeral joint laxity. She is also systemically hypermobile. She has decreased external rotation and flexion strength (4–/5) and poor scapular stability with scapular winging at rest, which is increased with upper extremity weight-bearing and resisted shoulder testing.

Management

Early treatment of this patient needs to address her issues of rotator cuff and peri-scapular muscle control. Postural education with a focus on activation of middle and lower trapezius to achieve neutral scapular positioning can be initiated in side lying. Stabilization and activation of these muscles can be progressed into manually resisted PNF diagonal patterns. Rhythmic stabilisation exercises for internal/external rotators can be performed with manual resistance in supine with the shoulder in resting position (scapular plane, 30° of abduction). Similarly, rhythmic stabilisation can be performed in elevation (supine 100° of flexion, slight horizontal abduction). An impor-

tant consideration throughout this patient's rehab is the strength and control of her core trunk and lower extremities. Initially any strength deficits can be worked on in isolation, but must be integrated with the shoulder in the later stages of treatment.

Once the patient is able to consistently stabilise her scapula and humeral head, resistance can increase to isotonic exercises in standing, side lying and prone. Weight and elastic resistance can be progressed as tolerated. Initial focus of this phase, however, should be on form and control with lower load and higher repetition.

Weight-bearing exercises can also be initiated at this point to further challenge the patient's stability while recruiting multiple large and small muscle groups around the shoulder and creating axial compression. These exercises should start below shoulder height on a stable surface but need to be progressed to and above shoulder height. Decreasing the stability of the surface and/or adding manual resistance can add further challenge.

The final phase of rehabilitation for this patient needs to prepare her for a return to sports. Strengthening exercises from earlier phases can be progressed in terms of resistance (with decreased repetitions), but they also must be taken through larger ROMs (e.g. PNF shoulder diagonals). The patient should gradually resume individual activities in practice and eventually progress to full participation with other team members.

Case study 3

Proximal humeral fracture

A 72-year-old woman presents with a right proximal humeral fracture following a fall on ice 6 weeks ago. Examination reveals limited active and passive range of motion of the shoulder in all planes and increased kyphotic posture and forward head. She appears guarded with basic mobility tasks using her right upper extremity.

Full shoulder strength testing deferred given fracture status but rotator cuff appears intact (negative drop arm and lag tests).

Management

The patient is referred to physiotherapy, following a period of prolonged immobilization in a sling.

Case study 3—cont'd

During this period the patient performed gentle elbow motion out of the sling to minimize stiffness and frequent ball squeezes to promote circulation.

During the initial phase of rehabilitation and mobilisation the patient is instructed in pendulum exercises and scapular retraction with sternal elevation exercises. Passive ROM exercises are initiated with caution regarding pain and the principles of bony healing, given patient's age, severity of fracture and location of fracture site. Joint mobilisations are also avoided at this point for the same reason. Flexion, external rotation and internal rotation are the primary motions of focus during this phase.

During the intermittent phase (usually determined by bony healing via X-ray) the focus is shifted to active-assist and active ROM with an emphasis on functional tasks to increase the patient's confidence and use of the right extremity for activities of daily living. Interventions can range from supine active-assistive exercises (similar to passive exercises) to side lying and standing active motions. Patient position is manipulated to vary the effect of gravity on the arm in order to increase or decrease the challenge to the shoulder musculature. To further improve the functional benefit of these types of exercises, the patient can be given objects or targets to reach and/or grasp towards the limits of her ROM. The use of PNF diagonals can also be helpful in this regard.

During the advanced phase, once good bony healing has occurred, basic rotator cuff and scapular strength is initiated. Attention should be paid to scapular alignment and mechanics to optimise available upper quarter motion. These exercises are begun at the patient's side and progressed to elevated positions as the patient's control and tolerance improves. Depending on the extent of pain or weakness, these exercises may need to be progressed from isometric to isotonic exercises. PNF patterns with manual resistance, and eventually band or weight resistance, may also be beneficial.

Student questions

(1) Describe the three components of humerothoracic motion and one specific pathology or impairment that could impact each.

(2) List the capsule-ligamentous structures of the glenohumeral joint and the respective motions that excessive tightness in each would restrict.

(3) Describe an appropriate intervention for tightness in each of the capsular regions of the glenohumeral joint.

(4) Describe factors that would influence clinical decision making around in the intensity of ROM/stretching exercise.

(5) Why is the 'full-can' exercise preferable to the 'empty-can' exercise?

(6) List exercises most effective in eliciting the external rotators of the shoulder.

(7) List strengthening exercises that optimise a proper balance ratio of the peri-scapular musculature.

(8) List the static and dynamic stabilisers of the shoulder.

(9) Describe important force couples of the shoulder.

(10) Outline goals and treatment progression of an overhead athlete in the return to activity phase of rehabilitation.

References

Andersen, L.L., Jorgensen, M.B., Blangsted, A.K., Pedersen, M.T., Hansen, E.A. and Sjogaard, G. (2008) A randomized controlled intervention trial to relieve and prevent neck/shoulder pain. *Medicine and Science in Sports and Exercise*, 40, 983–990.

Axe, M.J., Snyder-Mackler, L., Konin, J.G. and Strube, M.J. (1996) Development of a distance-based interval throwing program for little league-aged athletes. *American Journal of Sports Medicine*, 24, 594–602.

Axe, M.J., Wickham, R. and Snyder-Mackler, L. (2001) Data-based interval throwing programs for little league, high school, college, and professional baseball pitchers. *Sports Medicine Arthroscopy Reviews*, 9, 24–34.

Ballantyne, B.T., O'Hare, S.J., Paschall, J.L., Pavia-Smith, M.M., Pitz, A.M., Gillon, J.F. and Soderberg, G.L. (1993) Electromyographic activity of selected shoulder muscles in commonly used therapeutic exercises. *Physical Therapy*, 73, 668–677.

Bang, M.D. and Deyle, G.D. (2000) Comparison of supervised exercise with and without manual physical therapy for patients with shoulder impingement syndrome. *Journal of Orthopaedic and Sports Physical Therapy*, 30, 126–137.

Barden, J.M., Balyk, R., Rasco, V.J., Moreau, M. and Bagnall, K. (2004) Dynamic upper limb proprioception in multidirectional shoulder instability. *Clinical Orthopaedics and Related Research*, 420, 181–189.

Bison, L.J. and Andrews, J.R. (1998) Classification and mechanics of shoulder injuries in throwers. In: Andrews, J.R., Zarins, B. and Wilk, K.E. (eds) *Injuries in Baseball*, pp. 47–56. Lippincott-Raven Publishing, Philadelphia.

Blackburn, T.A., McLeod, W.D. and White, B. (1990) EMG analysis of posterior rotator cuff exercises. *Athletic Training*, 25, 40–45.

Bradley, J.P. and Tibone, J.E. (1991) Electromyographic analysis of muscle action about the shoulder. *Clinics in Sports Medicine*, 10, 789–805.

Browne, A.O., Hoffmeyer, P. and An, K.N. (1990) The influence of atmospheric pressure on shoulder stability. *Orthopaedic Transactions*, 14, 259–263.

Carette, S., Moffet, H., Tardif, J., Bessette, L., Morin, F., Fremont, P., Bykerk, V., Thorne, C., Bell, M., Bensen, W. and Blanchette, C. (2003) Intraarticular corticosteroids, supervised physiotherapy, or a combination of the two in the treatment of adhesive capsulitis of the shoulder: a placebo-controlled trial. *Arthritis and Rheumatism*, 48, 829–838.

Clark, J.M. and Harryman, D.T. (1992). Tendons, ligaments, and capsule of the rotator cuff. Gross and microscopic anatomy. *Journal of Bone and Joint Surgery, American Volume*, 74, 713–725.

Cools, A.M., Witvrouw, E.E., Declercq, G.A., Danneels, L.A. and Cambier, D.C. (2003) Scapular muscle recruitment patterns: trapezius muscle latency with and without impingement symptoms. *American Journal of Sports Medicine*, 31, 542–549.

Cools, A.M., Dewitte, V., Lanszweert, F., Notebaert, D., Roets, A., Soetens, B., Cagnie, B. and Witvrouw, E.E. (2007) Rehabilitation of scapular muscle balance: which exercises to prescribe? *American Journal of Sports Medicine*, 35, 1744–1751.

Decker, M.J., Hintermeister, R.A., Faber, K.J. and Hawkins, R.J. (1999) Serratus anterior muscle activity during selected rehabilitation exercises. *American Journal of Sports Medicine*, 27, 784–791.

Decker, M.J., Tokish, J.M., Ellis, H.B., Torry, M.R. and Hawkins, R.J. (2003) Subscapularis muscle activity during selected rehabilitation exercises. *American Journal of Sports Medicine*, 31, 126–134.

Ekstrom, R.A., Donatelli, R.A. and Soderberg, G.L. (2003) Surface electromyographic analysis of exercises for the trapezius and serratus anterior muscles. *Journal of Orthopaedic and Sports Physical Therapy*, 33, 247–258.

Ellenbecker, T.S. and Mattalino, A.J. (1997) *The Elbow in Sport*. Human Kinetics, Champaign, Illinois.

Fu, A.S. and Hui-Chan, C.W. (2005) Ankle joint proprioception and postural control in basketball players with bilateral ankle sprains. *American Journal of Sports Medicine*, 33, 1174–1182.

Gibb, T.D., Sidles, J.A., Harryman, D.T., McQuade, K.J. and Matsen, F.A. (1991) The effect of capsular venting on glenohumeral laxity. *Clinical Orthopaedics and Related Research*, 268, 120–127.

Ginn, K.A., Herbert, R.D., Khouw, W. and Lee, R. (1997) A randomized, controlled clinical trial of a treatment for shoulder pain. *Physical Therapy*, 77, 802–809.

Glousman, R., Jobe, F., Tibone, J., Moynes, D., Antonelli, D. and Perry, J. (1988) Dynamic electromyographic analysis of the throwing shoulder with glenohumeral instability. *Journal of Bone and Joint Surgery, American Volume*, 70, 220–226.

Greenfield, B.H., Donatelli, R., Wooden, M.J. and Wilkes, J. (1990) Isokinetic evaluation of shoulder rotational strength between the plane of scapula and the frontal plane. *American Journal of Sports Medicine*, 18, 124–128.

Habermeyer, P., Schuller, U. and Wiedemann, E. (1992) The intra-articular pressure of the shoulder: an experimental study on the role of the glenoid labrum in stabilizing the joint. *Arthroscopy*, 8, 166–172.

Inman, V.T., Saunders, J.B. and Abbott, L.C. (1996) Observations of the function of the shoulder joint. 1944. *Clinical Orthopaedics and Related Research*, 330, 3–12.

Kibler, W.B. and McMullen, J. (2003) Scapular dyskinesis and its relation to shoulder pain. *Journal of the American Academy of Orthopaedic Surgeons*, 11, 142–151.

Kluemper, M., Uhl, T. and Hazelrigg, H. (2006) Effect of stretching and strengthening shoulder muscles on forward shoulder posture in competitive swimmers. *Journal of Sport and Rehabilitation*, 15, 58–70.

Kronberg, M., Nemeth, G. and Brostrom, L.A. (1990) Muscle activity and coordination in the normal shoulder. An electromyographic study. *Clinical Orthopaedics and Related Research*, 76–85.

Kumar, V.P. and Balasubramaniam, P. (1985) The role of atmospheric pressure in stabilising the shoulder. An experimental study. *Journal of Bone and Joint Surgery, British Volume*, 67, 719–721.

Lephart, S.M., Warner, J.J., Borsa, P.A. and Fu, F.H. (1992) Proprioception of the shoulder joint in healthy, unstable, and surgically repaired shoulders. *Journal of Bone and Joint Surgery, American Volume*, 74, 713–725.

Lephart, S.M., Pincivero, DM., Giraldo, J.L. and Fu, F.H. (1997) The role of proprioception in the management and rehabilitation of athletic injuries. *American Journal of Sports Medicine*, 25, 130–137.

Ludewig, P. and Borstad, J. (2003) Effects of a home exercise programme on shoulder pain and functional status in construction workers. *Occupational and Environmental Medicine*, 60, 841–849.

Ludewig, P.M. and Cook, T.M. (2000) Alterations in shoulder kinematics and associated muscle activity in people with symptoms of shoulder impingement. *Physical Therapy*, 80, 276–291.

Malanga, G.A., Jenp, Y.N., Growney, E.S. and An, K.N. (1996) EMG analysis of shoulder positioning in testing and strengthening the supraspinatus. *Medicine and Science in Sports and Exercise*, 28, 661–664.

Matsen, F.A., Thomas, S.C. and Rockwood, C.A. (1990) Anterior glenohumeral instability. In: Rockwood, C.A. and Matsen, F.A. (eds) *The Shoulder*. W.B. Saunders, Philadelphia, Pennsylvania.

McCann, P.D., Wootten, M.E., Kadaba, M.P. and Bigliani, L.U. (1993) A kinematic and electromyographic study of shoulder rehabilitation exercises. *Clinical Orthopaedics and Related Research*, 288, 179–188.

McClure, P.W., Bialker, J., Neff, N., Williams, G. and Karduna, A. (2004) Shoulder function and 3-dimensional kinematics in people with shoulder impingement syndrome before and after a 6-week exercise program. *Physical Therapy*, 84, 832–848.

Meister, K. (2000) Injuries to the shoulder in the throwing athlete. Part one: Biomechanics/pathophysiology/classification of injury. *American Journal of Sports Medicine*, 28, 265–275.

Mendelsohn, M.E., Overend, T.J. and Petrella, R.J. (2004) Effect of rehabilitation on hip and knee proprioception in older adults after hip fracture: a pilot study. *American Journal of Physical Medicine and Rehabilitation*, 83, 624–632.

Morrey, B.F., Itoi, E. and An, K.N. (1998) Biomechanics of the shoulder. In: Rockwood, C.A. and Matsen, F.A. (eds) *The Shoulder*, 2nd edn, pp. 233–276. W.B. Saunders, Philadelphia, Pennsylvania.

Moseley, J.B. Jr, Jobe, F.W., Pink, M., Perry, J. and Tibone, J. (1992) EMG analysis of the scapular muscles during a shoulder rehabilitation program. *American Journal of Sports Medicine*, 20, 128–134.

Moynes, D.R., Perry, J., Antonelli, D.J. and Jobe, F.W. (1986) Electromyographic motion analysis of the upper extremity in sports. *Physical Therapy*, 66, 1905–1911.

Myers, J.B. and Lephart, S.M. (2000) The role of the sensorimotor system in the athletic shoulder. *Journal of Athletic Training*, 35, 351–363.

O'Brien, S.J., Neves, M.C., Arnoczky, S.P., Rozbruck, S.R., Dicarlo, E.F., Warren, R.F., Schwartz, R. and Wickiewicz, T.L. (1990) The anatomy and histology of the inferior glenohumeral ligament complex of the shoulder. *American Journal of Sports Medicine*, 18, 449–456.

Panics, G., Tallay, A., Pavlik, A. and Berkes, I. (2008) Effect of proprioception training on knee joint position sense in female team handball players. *British Journal of Sports Medicine*, 42, 472–476.

Poppen, N.K. and Walker, P.S. (1978) Forces at the glenohumeral joint in abduction. *Clinical Orthopaedics and Related Research*, 165–170.

Reinold, M.M., Ellerbusch, M.T. and Barrentine, S.W. (2002) Electromyographic analysis of the supraspinatus and deltoid muscles during rehabilitation exercises. *Journal of Orthopaedic and Sports Physical Therapy*, 32, A43.

Risberg, M.A., Holm, I., Myklebust, G. and Engebretsen, L. (2007) Neuromuscular training versus strength training during first 6 months after anterior cruciate ligament reconstruction: a randomized clinical trial. *Physical Therapy*, 87, 737–750.

Rockwood, C., Matsen, F., Wirth, M. and Lippitt, S. (2004) *The Shoulder*, 3rd edn. W.B. Saunders, Philadelphia, Pennsylvania.

Roy, J.S., Moffet, H., Hebert, L.J. and Lirette R. (2008) Effect of motor control and strengthening exercises on shoulder function in persons with impingement syndrome: A single-subject study design. *Manual Therapy*, 14, 180–188.

Scovazzo, M.L., Browne, A., Pink, M., Jobe, F.W. and Kerrigan, J. (1991) The painful shoulder during freestyle swimming. An electromyographic cinematographic analysis of twelve muscles. *American Journal of Sports Medicine*, 19, 577–582.

Soslowsky, L.J., Flatow, E.L., Bigliani, L.U., Pawluk, R.J., Ateshian, G.A. and Mow, V.C. (1992) Quantitation of in situ contact areas at the glenohumeral joint: a biomechanical study. *Journal of Orthopaedic Research*, 10, 524–534.

Suenaga, N., Minami, A. and Fujisawa, H. (2003) Electromyographic analysis of internal rotational motion of the shoulder in various arm positions. *Journal of Shoulder and Elbow Surgery*, 12, 501–505.

Swanik, K.A., Lephart, S.M., Swanik, C.B., Lephart, S.P., Stone, D.A. and Fu, F.H. (2002) The effects of shoulder plyometric training on proprioception and selected muscle performance characteristics. *Journal of Shoulder and Elbow Surgery*, 82, 579–586.

Townsend, H., Jobe, F.W., Pink, M. and Perry, J. (1991) Electromyographic analysis of the glenohumeral muscles during a baseball rehabilitation program. *American Journal of Sports Medicine*, 19, 264–272.

Voight, M.L. and Thomson, B.C. (2000) The role of the scapula in the rehabilitation 1060 of shoulder injuries. *Journal of Athletic Training*, 35, 364–372.

Wang, C.H., McClure, P., Pratt, N.E. and Nobilini, R. (1999) Stretching and strengthening exercises: their effect on three-dimensional scapular kinematics. *Archives of Physical Medicine and Rehabilitation*, 80, 923–929.

Wilk, K.E., Andrews, J.R., Arrigo, C.A., Keirns, M.A. and Erber, D.J. (1993) The internal and external rotator strength characteristics of professional baseball pitchers. *American Journal of Sports Medicine*, 1, 61–66.

Wilk, K.E., Arrigo, C.A. and Andrews, J.R. (1997) Current concepts: the stabilizing structures of the glenohumeral joint. *Journal of Orthopaedic and Sports Physical Therapy*, 25, 364–379.

Wilk, K.E., Reinold, M.M. and Andrews, J.R. (2001) Postoperative treatment principles in the throwing athlete. *Sports Medicine Arthroscopy Reviews*, 9, 69–95.

Wilk, K.E., Meister, K. and Andrews, J.R. (2002) Current concepts in the rehabilitation of the overhead throwing athlete. *American Journal of Sports Medicine*, 30, 136–151.

Worrell, T.W., Corey, B.J., York, S.L. and Santiestaban, J. (1992) An analysis of supraspinatus EMG activity and shoulder isometric force development. *Medicine and Science in Sports and Exercise*, 24, 744–748.

The Elbow and Forearm Complex

8

Bill Vicenzino, Michelle Smith and Leanne Bisset

SECTION 1: INTRODUCTION AND BACKGROUND

It is essential that the elbow and forearm complex, an important link in the upper kinetic chain, functions optimally in order to enable participation in activities of work, sport, leisure and daily living. This region is more commonly afflicted by overuse or insidious injuries of the soft tissues (e.g., tennis elbow, medial ulnar collateral ligament (UCL) instability) than by fractures and dislocations. However, it is noteworthy to consider that the latter can be very debilitating and challenging to rehabilitate.

Restoration of function and participation in activities of daily living following any injury to the elbow and forearm are largely achieved through exercise therapy. The successful application of exercise therapy is reliant upon the selection of specific exercises to bring about adaptations that are commensurate with goals of rehabilitation that have been agreed on by the patient and practitioner. Exercise therapy for the elbow and forearm can be compartmentalised using an outcome-based perspective (schema) into the following categories: (1) exercises geared at improving general aerobic fitness; (2) exercises that aim to restore muscle length and joint range of motion; (3) exercises that aim to improve endurance, strength and power of elbow and forearm muscles; and (4) exercises that seek to normalise elbow and forearm co-ordination and proprioception.

Regardless of the focus of the exercise, there are some fundamental principles that must be followed for effective application of exercise therapy. An initial assessment is mandatory in order to establish baseline measures of performance and to identify specific deficits and impairments that need to be addressed. This requires assessment of local and regional muscle performance as well as global function and work/sport specific skills. For example, optimal assessment of a tennis player may require analysis of the different tennis strokes to identify muscle weakness and/or problems with co-ordination that can be addressed with exercise therapy. Continual assessment must also occur throughout the rehabilitation programme to ensure correct exercise performance and to determine the need for exercise progression or modification. At both the initial and follow-up assessments, it is important to ascertain the phase of healing and degree of severity of the condition in terms of impairments in the neuro-musculoskeletal and sen-

Exercise Therapy in the Management of Musculoskeletal Disorders, First Edition. Edited by Fiona Wilson, John Gormley and Juliette Hussey.

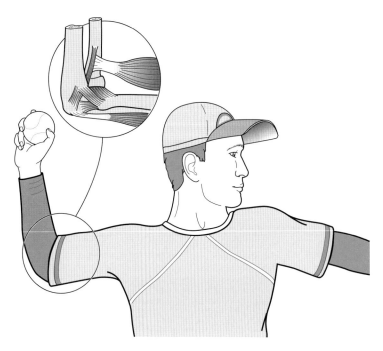

Figure 8.1 Schematic of the anatomy of the elbow (pitcher with inset). Based on a drawing by Timothy Salmond.

sorimotor systems. These factors are critical in planning, implementing and monitoring exercise prescription and progression. All exercises should be pain-free and performed with correct trunk and upper limb alignment. If these criteria are not met, exercises must be adjusted by altering exercise parameters such as the amount of resistance, degree of difficulty and patient position.

Interestingly, as opposed to the spine, there appears to be little emphasis on the benefits of general aerobic exercises for individuals with elbow and forearm conditions. Notwithstanding this, it is important to consider general body fitness (i.e. aerobic, anaerobic) as well as forequarter fitness (i.e., strength, endurance, posture) when managing patients with isolated injuries to the elbow and forearm.

The prescription of exercises for musculoskeletal disorders of the elbow and forearm complex requires the practitioner to be cognisant of salient elbow and forearm anatomy (Fig. 8.1). In brief, the elbow comprises three distinct articulations: the radiocapitellar (radiohumeral), ulnotrochlear (ulnohumeral), and proximal radioulnar joints. The two principal arcs of motion are flexion (135–145°)/extension (0–5°) and supination (85°)/pronation (75°) (Oatis, 2004; Lockard, 2006). In day-to-day function most people only use 30–130° of extension/flexion and 50° pronation/supination; however, athletes often require much more (Morrey *et al.*,

1981; Wilk *et al.*, 1993). The elbow is an inherently stable joint due to the congruency of its articulations. The primary restraints of the elbow include the ulnohumeral joint and collateral ligaments, and the secondary restraints include the radial head, flexor pronator origin, common extensor origin and joint capsule (Saati and McKee, 2004). The UCL provides approximately 54% of the elbow's resistance to valgus forces, followed by the articulation of the radial head with the capitellum and proximal ulna (Morrey and An, 1983; Cook and McKee, 2003).

In order to cover exercise therapy for musculoskeletal conditions of the elbow and forearm complex, it is instructive to discuss a range of disorders from acute traumatic injuries of the bone and ligaments through to overuse injuries of the soft tissues. This chapter will review the epidemiology, aetiology, neuro-musculoskeletal and pain system impairments, and evidence for exercise therapy for fracture and dislocation of the elbow, ligament injures and tennis elbow. Impairments that relate to these conditions and are relevant to exercise will be highlighted. In brief, the sequelae of the acute management of fracture/dislocations, which requires some period of immobilisation, will require exercises that focus on regaining range of motion and strength. In contrast, overuse/insidious onset injuries will focus less on range of motion and more on restoring muscle strength, endurance and power, and retraining co-ordination and proprioception. Thus, this chapter will provide practical guidelines for exercise prescription for post fracture/dislocation of the elbow, ligamentous instability of the elbow and tennis elbow.

Acute traumatic injuries of bone and ligaments

The elbow is the second most commonly dislocated joint in adults (Sobel and Nirschl, 1996) and the most commonly dislocated joint in children (Sobel and Nirschl, 1996; O'Driscoll, 2000), with dislocation typically occurring in a posterior or posterolateral direction. Elbow dislocations are most prevalent in sports such as cycling, gymnastics, football and wrestling (Sobel and Nirschl, 1996), and are commonly caused by a fall on the outstretched hand, hyperextension of the elbow, or a combination of valgus, supination and external rotation of the forearm during axial loading (Sheps et al., 2004). The structures involved in an elbow dislocation vary (Sheps et al., 2004) and may include rupture or avulsion of the collateral ligaments, tearing of the capsule or brachialis muscle and fracture of the medial epicondyle (Mehlhoff et al., 1988; Hotchkiss, 1997; O'Driscoll, 2000). Isolated dislocation of the radial head is unlikely, although subluxation of the radial head may present in young children (Sobel and Nirschl, 1996). To optimise outcomes, the specific structures damaged must be taken into consideration when planning rehabilitation.

A radial head fracture is the most common fracture in the elbow (Herbertsson et al., 2005; Bano and Kahlon, 2006). The mechanism of injury for fractures is similar to that for dislocations (e.g. a fall on the outstretched hand with forearm in pronation) (Herbertsson et al., 2005; Bano and Kahlon, 2006). Radial fractures in the presence of an elbow dislocation are often accompanied by a fracture of the coronoid process and damage to the collateral ligaments (Regan and Morrey, 1989). Appropriate management of this injury is essential to avoid chronic instability (Bano and Kahlon, 2006). In adolescents, a valgus stress from a fall or muscle contraction may result in a fracture through the epiphyseal plates of the medial epicondyle. Diagnosis of a fracture is confirmed by radiographs.

Although there is a dearth of studies outlining the best practice approach to managing acute elbow injuries, it is generally agreed that a stable reduction post-dislocation and/or a stable fracture site is best managed conservatively (i.e. casting/bracing), and unstable injuries are best managed with open reduction and internal fixation (Case and Hennrikus, 1997; Frankle et al., 1999; Ross et al., 1999; Liow et al., 2002; Saati and McKee, 2004; Sheps et al., 2004; Bano and Kahlon, 2006).

The long-term sequelae of acute traumatic injuries of the elbow include loss of range of motion (particularly extension), decreased force production, recurrent instability, heterotopic ossification, neurovascular problems and chronic pain (Protzman, 1978; Case and Hennrikus, 1997; Frankle et al., 1999; Liow et al., 2002; Sheps et al., 2004; Casavant and Hastings, 2006). The degree of loss of motion is related to the duration of elbow immobilisation (Protzman, 1978). Heterotopic ossification in soft tissues is more common following a severe injury with concomitant neural or thermal injuries, and presents with progressive loss of range of motion and/or difficulty in regaining range of motion (Casavant and Hastings, 2006). Although there is a lack of quality clinical trials examining the most appropriate management of heterotopic ossification, there is some evidence to suggest that it is not exacerbated by early movement (Wharton and Morgan, 1970; Stover et al., 1975).

The evidence for exercise therapy post-dislocation and fracture

The evidence base for the rehabilitation of elbow dislocations is limited to non-randomised case series and review papers. It suggests that early active/active-assisted range of motion exercises are essential for the restoration of elbow function (Ross et al., 1999) and are associated with good long-term results and low risk of re-injury (Mehlhoff et al., 1988).

An early range of motion protocol is also considered to be optimal for stable fractures that have been managed non-operatively and fractures in which a congruous reduction and stable fixation have been attained. Early active mobilisation is imperative to avoid complications associated with immobilisation, such as pain and loss of motion

(Hotchkiss, 1997; Liow *et al.*, 2002; Bano and Kahlon, 2006). Indeed, a randomised clinical trial that compared immediate mobilisation and cast immobilisation in traumatically induced effusion of the elbow found improvements in short-term pain and range of motion in individuals who were mobilised (Henriksen *et al.*, 1995). Another randomised clinical trial in children with open reduction and internal fixation of a supracondylar humeral fracture showed that a pragmatic physiotherapy programme following cast immobilisation led to improved range of motion at 12–18 weeks than cast immobilisation without physiotherapy intervention (Keppler *et al.*, 2005).

Overuse injuries of elbow ligaments

Injury to the UCL is common in sports that involve repetitive valgus stress to the elbow (Safran and Baillargeon, 2005a; Safran *et al.*, 2005b,c; Nassab and Schickendantz, 2006) (e.g. baseball pitchers due to the large valgus forces incurred when the arm moves from humeral external rotation and elbow flexion to humeral internal rotation and elbow extension during the late cocking and early acceleration phases of throwing) (Callaway *et al.*, 1997; Azar *et al.*, 2000; Cain *et al.*, 2003; Nassab and Schickendantz, 2006). Apart from the UCL, valgus stress may also result in trauma to other structures, such as ulnar nerve, medial head of the triceps, insertion of the wrist flexor and forearm pronator muscles and medial epicondyle (Safran and Baillargeon, 2005a; Safran *et al.*, 2005b,c; Nassab and Schickendantz, 2006). Laxity of the UCL has been shown to alter the articulation between the posteromedial trochlea and olecranon and lead to the development of osteophytes and loose bodies (Ahmad and ElAttrache, 2004a; Ahmad *et al.*, 2004b).

Physical examination of the athlete with an UCL injury typically reveals palpable tenderness approximately 2 cm distal to the medial epicondyle (Safran and Baillargeon, 2005a; Safran *et al.*, 2005c) and a positive valgus stress test (Hyman *et al.*, 2001). Radiography and arthroscopy may also assist in the diagnosis of an UCL injury; but their diagnostic accuracy is questionable in baseball and team handball players, because non-injured elbows may also exhibit significant wider medial elbow

joint space (Popovic *et al.*, 2001; Sasaki *et al.*, 2002), joint effusions and loose bodies (Popovic *et al.*, 2001).

The evidence for exercise therapy in unstable elbows

The majority of articles on UCL injuries are clinical commentaries that recommend initial conservative management, followed by surgical intervention if unsuccessful (Field and Savoie, 1998; Hyman *et al.*, 2001; Cain *et al.*, 2003; Safran *et al.*, 2005b; Nassab and Schickendantz, 2006). Rettig *et al.* (2001) evaluated a conservative rehabilitation programme that involved rest, splinting/bracing (protecting against valgus stress and elbow extension), anti-inflammatory medication, ice, active and passive range of motion exercises for the flexor and pronator muscles, strengthening of the upper extremity muscles and progressive throwing. They found that 42% of athletes were able to return their pre-injury level of competition.

Tennis elbow

Tennis elbow is largely a clinical diagnosis characterised by pain over the lateral elbow that is typically aggravated by gripping activities. It tends to occur in the dominant upper limb, most commonly in those aged between 40 and 50 years and of either gender, being most prevalent in jobs requiring repetitive manual tasks (as high as 35–64% of all cases) (Kivi, 1982; Dimberg, 1987; Feuerstein *et al.*, 1998). Most importantly, it is one of the most costly of all work-related illnesses (Kivi, 1982; Dimberg, 1987; Feuerstein *et al.*, 1998) and restricts function in all aspects of life.

The nomenclature and underlying pathology of tennis elbow are intertwined and impact on the concepts of treatment (Vicenzino and Wright, 1996; Khan *et al.*, 2002). Tennis elbow has been called lateral epicondylitis, lateral epicondylosis and extensor tendinosis. The term epicondylitis infers inflammation, which is inaccurate in this condition, as a number of studies have found no signs of inflammation (Nirschl and Pettrone, 1979; Regan *et al.*, 1992; Potter *et al.*, 1995; Kraushaar and

Nirschl, 1999; Alfredson *et al.*, 2000). Terms with the suffix 'osis' infer a degenerative change, and while the changes exhibit elements of degeneration/disarray or break down of collagen fibrils in the tendon (Regan *et al.*, 1992; Kraushaar and Nirschl, 1999), it is not known how these morphological changes relate to the pain and dysfunction experienced by patients with tennis elbow (Khan and Cook, 2000). It appears that the condition is far more complex than these terms suggest (Vicenzino and Wright, 1996). For example, the condition is characterised by a constellation of changes in the extensor carpi radialis brevis and common extensor tendon mechanism, such as signs of neurogenic involvement (Ljung *et al.*, 2004) in the form of pain-provoking chemical mediators located in myelinated sensory fibres (e.g. substance P and calcitonin gene-related peptide) (Ljung *et al.*, 1999, 2004), increased levels of excitatory amino acids (glutamate) (Alfredson *et al.*, 2000) and associated neovascularisation (Zeisig *et al.*, 2006). Thus, the current preferred term for this condition is lateral epicondylalgia or tendinopathy, which infer some level of abnormality (possibly in the pain system or in the tendon, respectively) without categorically defining pathology.

The evidence for exercise in tennis elbow

A number of systematic reviews have identified that studies generally lack high methodological quality and standardised outcomes, which make it difficult to determine the efficacy of exercise (Bisset *et al.*, 2005; Woodley *et al.*, 2007). The literature on exercise in tennis elbow appears to focus on two forms of exercise: a combination of isometric, concentric and eccentric contractions and eccentric-only exercise. Programmes that involve isometric, concentric and eccentric exercises for the forearm muscles are usually accompanied by other physical therapy interventions such as friction massage, manipulation or ultrasound. As such, it is difficult to determine how much of the treatment effects are due solely to exercise. Our recent randomised clinical trial in 198 subjects studied the efficacy of a physiotherapy programme of manual therapy and exercise compared with a corticosteroid injection and a wait-and-see approach (Bisset *et al.*, 2006a).

This study showed that the physiotherapy programme was superior to the wait-and-see approach and similar to corticosteroid injections in the short term (6 weeks) (Hay *et al.*, 1999; Smidt *et al.*, 2002). However, an important finding in our study was that over a 12-month period, physiotherapy was responsible for far fewer recurrences, fewer consultations to medical practitioners and increased grip strength compared with corticosteroid injections (Bisset *et al.*, 2006a), a finding consistent with the suggestion of a protective effect of exercise (Pienimaki *et al.*, 1996, 1998). Pienimaki *et al.* (1996) compared the effects of a graduated progressive exercise programme of strengthening and stretching to ultrasound over 6–8 weeks in 36 patients with chronic tennis elbow that was recalcitrant to many other treatments including physiotherapy and corticosteroid injections. This study reported a statistically significant but small beneficial effect of exercise on resting pain. A recent systematic review of eccentric-only exercise concluded that due to the small number of trials and very large confidence intervals, it was difficult to draw any conclusions on the efficacy of eccentric exercise in tennis elbow (Woodley *et al.*, 2007).

A number of impairments affecting the neuromuscular and sensorimotor systems have been identified in people with tennis elbow including: reduced pain-free gripping capacity; bilateral abnormal wrist posture during these gripping tasks; bilateral deficits in reaction time and speed of movement of the upper limb; and abnormal motor control of the forearm muscles in a tennis back hand stroke (Kelley *et al.*, 1994; Pienimaki *et al.*, 1997a; Bisset *et al.*, 2006b). These deficits and abnormalities can be addressed with specific exercise prescription.

SECTION 2: PRACTICAL USE OF EXERCISE

Practical guidelines for exercise therapy post-dislocation and fracture

Range of motion and flexibility

Active-assisted range of motion exercises can begin as early as pain and inflammation allow (usually

1–5 days post-reduction/operation). These exercises typically start with elbow flexion/extension through pain-free range of motion with the forearm in neutral supination/pronation. This can often be best achieved in a gravity-eliminated position. For example, elbow flexion can be done in supine and elbow extension can be done in sitting. A general guideline for prescription is 5–10 repetitions every 2–3 hours with progression to 15–20 repetitions hourly. Range of motion exercises for the uninvolved joints of the upper limb should also be performed.

Within the first week, exercises should be progressed to active range of motion against gravity. If the elbow remains unstable or required open-reduction with internal fixation, the patient may be required to exercise within a valgus-restricting brace. In the presence of lateral instability due to associated soft tissue injury, exercises should be performed in forearm pronation to provide maximum stability and avoid excessive load on the radiocapitellar joint (Chinchalkar and Szekeres, 2004; Sheps *et al.*, 2004). When the elbow is stable, active-assisted supination/pronation can be commenced with the elbow positioned in 90° flexion. At approximately 4 weeks, range of motion exercises can be progressed to low load stretches sustained for 20 seconds and repeated 4–5 times (Davila and Johnston-Jones, 2006); however, this should be initiated after strengthening is underway to minimise applying a stretch overload to healing tissue. Proprioceptive neuromuscular facilitation stretching (e.g., hold-relax, contract-relax) can also be used to improve flexibility of muscles at this point.

Strengthening

The progression of strength training can be divided up into a number of phases based on tissue healing and stability of the elbow joint. Early in the programme, exercises will focus on improving or maintaining strength in adjacent joints (i.e. the shoulder, scapula and wrist) with gradual addition of the exercises at the elbow.

Early resolution phase (0–4 weeks)

Shoulder and scapular strengthening, isometric wrist flexion/extension and radial/ulnar deviation can begin within the first 2 weeks. Isometric exercises should be performed at multiple points

Table 8.1 Exercise prescription guidelines to improve muscle endurance, strength and power

Desired adaptation (goal)	Prescription: guiding principle
Endurance	15–20 RM × 1–3 sets; 30–60 seconds rest between sets
Strength	3–8 RM × 3–5 sets; 3–5 minutes rest between sets
Power	1–3 RM × 3–5 sets; 5–8 minutes rest between sets; explosive tempo

RM = repetition maximum.
Bird *et al.*, 2005.

through available range of motion. Contractions should be pain-free and sub-maximal with slow onset and offset.

Consolidation phase (4–8 weeks)

Initially exercises will be isometric with progression to isotonic exercises and gradual addition of load in 0.5–1 kg increments. Submaximal isometric elbow exercises can begin at 3–4 weeks if the elbow is stable or at 4–6 weeks if it is unstable. Once bone healing is deemed adequate (usually around 4–8 weeks), resistive exercises can be commenced. Initial prescription of approximately 1–3 sets of 15–20 repetition maximum (RM) daily will promote endurance adaptations (Table 8.1) while avoiding overload to the injured tissues. Examples of appropriate strengthening exercises for the biceps and triceps muscles are shown in Figures 8.2 and 8.3, respectively. Light throwing activities may also be commenced at approximately 6 weeks in an athlete with a stable medial epicondyle fracture (Davila and Johnston-Jones, 2006).

Restoration phase (8–12 weeks)

Exercises can be progressed by increasing resistance and speed to improve strength and power (Table 8.1), and closed kinetic chain exercises, such as wall or floor push-ups (Fig. 8.4) can be introduced. Different types of resistance can be used including free weights (Figs 8.2 and 8.3), pulleys, elastic

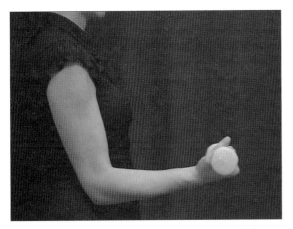

Figure 8.2 Concentric/eccentric contraction of biceps muscle using a free weight. The patient is standing with the elbow extended at her side. The elbow is flexed to full flexion range of motion (mid-position shown) and returned to the starting position.

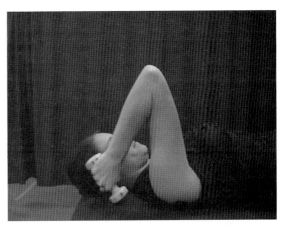

Figure 8.3 Concentric/eccentric contraction of the triceps muscle using a free weight. The starting position is shown (i.e. the patient is in supine with the shoulder in 90° flexion and the elbow pointing towards the ceiling). The elbow is extended so the arm is vertical and then returned to the starting position.

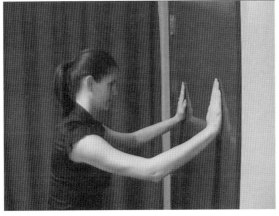

(a)

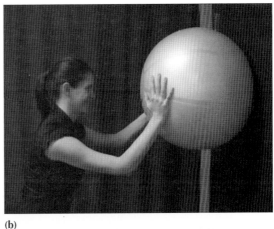

(b)

Figure 8.4 Wall push-ups to strengthen triceps, shoulder and scapular muscles. The patient stands with the hands against the wall shoulder-width apart or slightly wider and elbows near extension. The elbows are flexed and the body approaches the wall (**a**). To increase the challenge to the sensorimotor system this exercise can be performed on a ball (**b**) or two rubber discs (**c**), and to increase the amount of load applied through the upper limb, the feet can moved further way from the wall or the push-up can be performed against the floor.

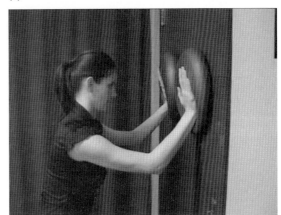

(c)

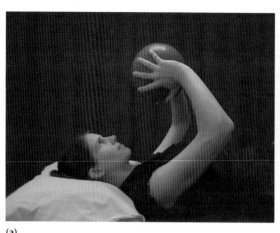
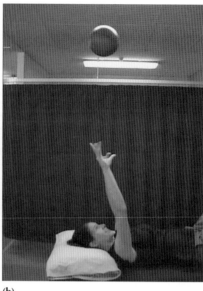

(a)   (b)

Figure 8.5   Chest passes with a medicine ball. Ball is held in from of chest with elbows bent (**a**) and arms are extended as ball is released (**b**). This exercise can be repeated in quick succession to train power.

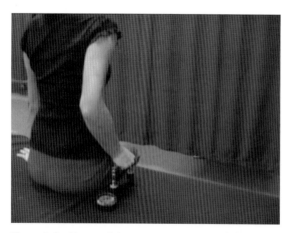

Figure 8.6   Concentric/eccentric contraction of the triceps muscle using body-weight resistance and a grip dynamometer. The starting position is shown (i.e. the patient is sitting weight-bearing through a grip dynamometer on the affected side). The elbow is extended to lift the patient off the bed and then flexed to return to the starting position.

tubing, medicine balls (Fig. 8.5) and grip dynamometers (Fig. 8.6). Elastic tubing can assist in the simulation of functional and/or sport-specific skills such as throwing a ball, serving in tennis or golfing. An arm ergometer or stationary bike with moveable handholds can also be used during this stage of rehabilitation to improve upper limb endurance.

Work and/or sport-specific phase

Once range of motion and strength are within 10% of the unaffected side, training of sport-specific activities can commence (Davila and Johnston-Jones, 2006). During these exercises, taping or bracing may be used to protect the joint from unexpected stress or overload. Exercises to prepare the individual to return to work should replicate specific work requirements, such as lifting, carrying, pushing, pulling and use of tools.

Practical guidelines for exercise therapy in unstable elbows

Strengthening

Protection of the UCL is a priority in the initial stages of rehabilitation. This can be achieved with taping or bracing to protect the UCL and elbow from unwanted stress, restricting activities that

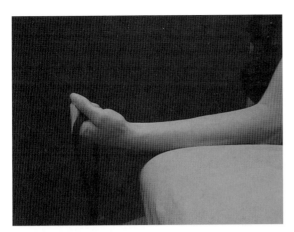

Figure 8.7 Concentric/eccentric contraction of the wrist flexor muscles using rubber tubing resistance. The forearm is positioned in supination. The wrist starts in extension and is flexed until full pain-free flexion range motion is attained before returning to the starting position (i.e. extension).

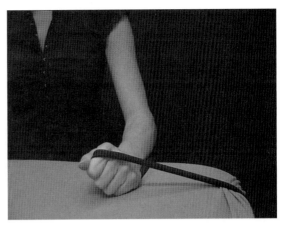

Figure 8.9 Concentric/eccentric contraction of the pronator teres and pronator quadratus muscles using rubber tubing resistance. The forearm starts in supination or neutral (i.e. mid-supination/pronation) and pronated until full pain-free pronation range motion is attained before returning to the starting position. The rubber tubing can be placed on the medial, rather than lateral, side of the arm to perform exercises for supination.

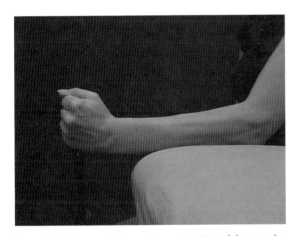

Figure 8.8 Concentric/eccentric contraction of the muscles that cause radial deviation of the wrist using rubber tubing resistance. The forearm is positioned in neutral (i.e. mid-supination/pronation). The wrist starts in ulnar deviation and is radial deviated until full pain-free radial deviation range motion is attained before returning to the starting position (i.e. ulnar deviation). The rubber tubing can be attached above, rather than below, the arm to perform exercises for ulnar deviation.

apply a valgus strain to the elbow and by avoiding passive elbow motion (Armstrong *et al.*, 2000).

Exercises for the musculoskeletal system should involve muscles that provide medial stability to the elbow joint, such as flexor carpi radialis (Figs 8.7 and 8.8) and pronator teres (Fig. 8.9 and see also

8.12 below), as well as muscles that primarily act at the elbow joint, such as biceps brachii (see Fig. 8.2) and triceps brachii (see Fig. 8.3), and muscles in adjacent areas (i.e. the shoulder, scapula and trunk). Exercises for these muscles may initially be isometric and progression to isotonic with gradual addition of resistance using free weights (see Figs 8.2 and 8.3) or elastic tubing (Figs 8.7–8.9). The amount of resistance used and number of times the exercise is repeated will depend on the goal of the exercise (see Table 8.1) and what the patient is able to perform without producing pain.

Exercises are relatively simple initially, but as the integrity of the ligament and elbow joint improves exercises are progressed to become more complex and achieve concurrent strength, power and sensorimotor adaptations. For example, medicine ball throws (see Fig. 8.5) and high-speed humeral rotations (Fig. 8.10) train strength and power of the upper limb muscles, stability of the scapula and trunk, and proprioception. Eventually the focus turns to function and return to work and/or sport. Exercises to prepare athletes for return to sport may include throwing and tennis strokes (i.e. serving, forehand and backhand) of progressively increased distance and speed and altered predictability. Examples of exercise progressions from simple to

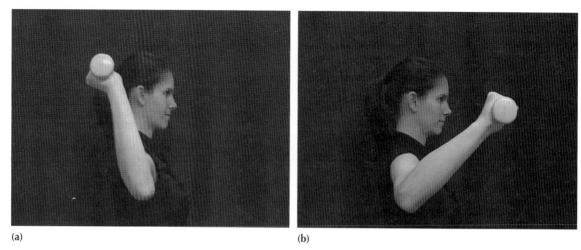

(a)   (b)

Figure 8.10   (**a**) External and (**b**) internal rotation of the shoulder using a free weight. The shoulder is rotated between maximal external and internal rotation. Position of the shoulder, scapula and trunk is monitored and should be held static. This exercise can be progressed by increasing load, speed or predictability of movement.

more complex to functional for a throwing athlete are outlined in Table 8.2.

Proprioception

In contrast to the considerable evidence from other areas of the body implicating joint position sense deficits (Willems *et al.*, 2002; Bonfim *et al.*, 2003) and muscle reaction time impairments (Konradsen and Ravn, 1991; Bonfim *et al.*, 2003) following ligament injuries, there is a lack of similar evidence following an UCL injury. Not surprisingly then, proprioceptive retaining is commonly lacking from conservative management approaches.

There is evidence to suggest that activation of the wrist and forearm muscles is altered in athletes with UCL injuries, for example reduced activity of the flexor and pronator muscles (Glousman *et al.*, 1992; Hamilton *et al.*, 1996) and increased extensor muscle activity (Glousman *et al.*, 1992) with valgus stress at the elbow during throwing. As these muscles contribute to medial elbow stability (Hamilton *et al.*, 1996), we recommend retraining activation of these muscles.

Exercises for the sensorimotor system should include closed-kinetic chain exercises to increase neural input to the area, joint position sense and muscle reaction time retraining. Closed kinetic chain exercise may simply involve weight-bearing

through the affected limb, and difficultly can be increased by altering surface compliance/ predictability (i.e. firm surface, foam surface or ball), increasing load (i.e. leaning against a wall, four-point kneeling or a floor push-up position), adding movement (i.e. rolling a ball or performing a push-up) and increasing speed of movement (Fig. 8.4). Joint position sense retraining involves the therapist positioning the athlete's limb in a certain position (i.e. 70° of elbow flexion) and then the athlete relocating this position independently. This should be performed with the athlete's eyes closed, and measuring the difference between the target and achieved position can assess accuracy. This retraining can be progressed by altering amount of external input (i.e. supine with the arm on a bed or standing with the arm unsupported), shoulder position and speed of movement.

Practical guidelines for exercise in tennis elbow

A graduated progressive exercise programme is essential to resolve symptoms, as well as prevent chronicity and recurrence (Pienimaki *et al.*, 1996; Pienimaki *et al.*, 1998). The key to success is early management of overall load at the involved muscles and tendons. This requires the practitioner to

Table 8.2 Possible exercises for an UCL injury progressing from early post-injury (i.e. simple) to return to sport (i.e. functional)

Simple
Isometric exercises for upper limb muscles
Isotonic exercises with addition of 20 RM load to improve muscular endurance of upper limb muscles (Figs 8.2, 8.3, 8.7–8.9, 8.11 and 8.12)
Isotonic exercises with addition of 8 RM load to improve muscular strength of upper limb muscles
Unloaded exercises for scapular control
Motor control retraining for stability of the trunk
Weight-bearing against wall (Fig. 8.4)
Joint position sense retraining
More complex
Weight-bearing against wall on ball ± moving ball up and down wall (Fig. 8.4)
Push-ups on wall/floor ± with hands on unstable surface (i.e. foam, ball, disc) (Fig. 8.4)
Medicine ball throws (Fig. 8.5)
Resisted small-range humeral internal and external rotation with elbow at 90° flexion with increasing velocity (Fig. 8.10)
Functional (throwing example)
Throwing action with tubing resistance
Throwing: short distance and slow speed with increasing repetitions
Throwing: gradual progression of distance and speed
Throwing: altered predictability of direction

RM = repetition maximum.

balance up the demands of the exercise programme with those outside rehabilitation, such as in the workplace, sport, leisure and activities of daily living. In some cases, loading of the extensor muscles and tendons while gripping during work or sport-related tasks may have to be reduced or modified if painful. Tasks may be modified to reduce load and pain by lifting objects with a less forceful grip, having the forearm supinated rather than pronated and ensuring that the overall posture of the forequarter is such that the forearm extensors are not being used inappropriately (e.g. if the upper limb is held in internal rotation) (Vicenzino, 2003).

Strengthening

The management of tennis elbow can be divided into two phases: the restoration of pain-free muscle performance (i.e. strength and endurance) and the restoration of functional performance. The muscle performance restoration phase involves reduction of pain and improvement of pain-free grip strength to within approximately 80% of the unaffected side. Once pain is absent or difficult to exacerbate, the rehabilitation program focuses on higher order strengthening exercises and functional tasks. The functional restoration phase will improve strength to that of the unaffected side (or >110% if affected side is dominant) and incorporate specific functional activities.

Restoration of pain-free muscle performance (approximately 6–8 weeks)

Due to the intricately involved pain system in tennis elbow, it is our contention that exercise should be conducted without reproduction of the patient's pain. Within the confines of this caveat, the goal is to improve strength and endurance of the forearm muscles. The loads recommended to optimally improve strength (i.e., 3–5 sets of 3–8 RM) (Bird *et al.*, 2005) will probably provoke pain in most individuals with tennis elbow, so in the first instance a lower load with a higher number of repetitions is used (i.e. 1–3 sets of 15–20 repetitions). This exercise prescription lends itself to improvements in muscle endurance and size (Bird *et al.*, 2005). The exercises that are usually performed at this stage are for the forearm flexor/extensor (Figs 8.7 and 8.11), supinator/pronator (Figs 8.9 and 8.12) and radial/ulnar deviator (Fig. 8.8) muscles. The exercises should be performed slowly over about 8 seconds for each repetition when the exercise includes both concentric and eccentric contractions. Isometric

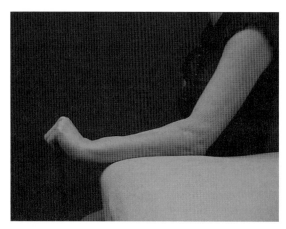

Figure 8.11 Concentric/eccentric contraction of the wrist extensor muscles using rubber tubing resistance. The forearm is positioned in pronation. The wrist starts in flexion and is extended until full pain-free extension range motion is attained before returning to the starting position (i.e. flexion).

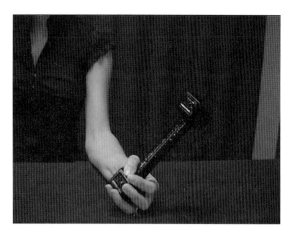

Figure 8.12 Concentric/eccentric contraction of the forearm pronator and supinator muscles using a hammer or free weight. The forearm starts in a neutral position (i.e. mid-supinaton/pronation). It is taken into full pain-free supination range motion (shown in figure) and then full pain-free pronation range motion.

contractions are used when resistance (e.g. tubing, weights) is unavailable or when the concentric and eccentric contractions are pain provocative.

Initially, forearm exercises can be performed with the elbow in a flexed position as this is usually least pain provocative. However, as grip strength is greatest when the elbow is extended (Kuzala and Vargo, 1992), it is important to progress doing the exercises with the elbow in an extended position.

This may initially necessitate a reduction in load to ensure pain-free exercise performance. Throughout this phase of rehabilitation the unaffected forearm should be maximally exercised, as this will afford some adaptation to the affected side (Bonato *et al.*, 1996; Stinear *et al.*, 2001). We strongly believe that regular visits to a physiotherapist at least once a week for the initial 6–8 weeks is essential for a successful outcome. These sessions allow the therapist to check the exercises and evaluate progress (i.e. pain-free grip strength), which facilitates adherence to the exercise programme and allows for programme modifications such as the progression of load and addition of exercises (Vicenzino, 2003).

Restoration of functional performance

The strengthening exercises in this phase of rehabilitation use higher loads to maximise strength gains (Table 8.1). We find that eccentric only protocols are beneficial at this point when there is minimal pain and a reasonable level of extensor muscle strength. When there is no pain and work/sport activities require explosive and ballistic actions, there may be a need to use weekly exercises performed with increased movement speed to address muscular power (Table 8.1). In contrast, some work specific tasks require prolonged isometric gripping under heavy load, such as the need to lift and hold a nail-gun up above the horizontal. Training for these types of tasks requires sustained functional isometric exercises that can be progressed by moving the upper limb into various positions of elevation and adding load. An example is gripping a dynamometer to a designated level of force (e.g. 40% 1 RM) and elevating the upper limb against a load using pulleys or resistance tubing. The exercise prescribed and duration of this phase will vary according to the individual's work or sport requirements.

Flexibility and stretching

As flexibility impairments occur less frequently in tennis elbow than impairments in pain and muscle performance (i.e. strength and endurance), our clinical approach is to prescribe stretching only to those who have reduced extensibility of the forearm muscles and/or decreased elbow and wrist joint motion.

Proprioception

It has previously been identified that people with unilateral tennis elbow have reduced sensorimotor function and abnormally flexed wrist postures during gripping in both the unaffected and affected upper limbs (Kelley *et al.*, 1994; Pienimaki *et al.*, 1997b; Bisset *et al.*, 2006b). These data suggest that wrist posture should be observed during a spontaneous grip test and corrected as necessary to maintain the wrist in slight extension during gripping tasks. In addition, exercises that challenge the sensorimotor system could be included in the programme to improve awareness of wrist posture. Examples of exercises include spontaneously gripping objects and weight-bearing through an exercise ball. These exercises can be progressed by altering the size, texture and density of the objects/ball, performing tasks with the eyes closed and using a weight-scale to control load through the wrist and forearm muscles during weight-bearing.

Conclusion

This chapter has highlighted the evidence for three major injury types for the elbow and forearm. The three examples cover impairments of the bone, joint, ligament, muscle, sensorimotor and pain systems, and thus serve as a basis on which the reader may approach the treatment of any elbow and forearm condition with exercise therapy. The key to successful exercise therapy resides in a sound clinical assessment to identify the stage of injury/condition, impairments across all involved systems and level of disability, as well as an understanding of possible adaptations following various exercises. The planning, implementation, modification and progression of the exercise programme can then occur on a pragmatic case-by-case basis.

SECTION 3: STUDENT QUESTIONS

As this chapter is so condition specific, no case studies have been included and the reader should refer to the text for examples for treating various disorders.

Student questions

(1) Identify the key issues in planning and implementing an exercise programme for the elbow and forearm.

(2) Once an elbow dislocation is reduced and deemed stable, when should an exercise rehabilitation programme commence?

(3) Design an exercise programme for a volleyball player who has undergone reduction of an elbow dislocation and open reduction internal fixation of a medial epicondylar fracture 2 days ago. Include the progression of exercises from the early post-operative period through to return to sport. List the expected timeline and outcome measures that would be used to determine the progression of exercises.

(4) Describe exercises that can be used to train the sensorimotor system in a tennis player with an UCL injury. Identify progression of these exercises from the early phase of rehabilitation to return to playing tennis.

(5) What exercise prescription would you use if your goal was to improve strength of the flexor carpi radialis muscle? How would you modify this prescription if your goal was to improve endurance?

(6) Describe several exercises that can be used to train both the musculoskeletal and sensorimotor systems. Also provide an explanation of your exercise selection.

(7) List the likely impairments in a patient with tennis elbow.

(8) Describe the role of isometric, concentric and eccentric exercises in the management of tennis elbow.

(9) Compare and contrast the application of exercise therapy at the elbow for a dislocation, an instability and tennis elbow.

(10) Does aerobic exercise have a role in the management of elbow disorders?

References

Ahmad, C.S. and ElAttrache, N.S. (2004a) Valgus extension overload syndrome and stress injury of the olecranon. *Clinics in Sports Medicine*, 23, 665–676.

Ahmad, C.S., Park, M.C. and ElAttrache, N.S. (2004b) Elbow medial ulnar collateral ligament insufficiency alters posteromedial olecranon contact. *American Journal of Sports Medicine*, 32, 1607–1612.

Alfredson, H., Ljung, B.O., Thorsen, K. and Lorentzon, R. (2000) In vivo investigation of ECRB tendons with micro-dialysis technique – no signs of inflammation but high amounts of glutamate in tennis elbow. *Acta Orthopaedica Scandinavica*, 71, 475–479.

Armstrong, A.D., Dunning, C.E., Faber, K.J., Duck, T.R., Johnson, J.A. and King, G.J. (2000) Rehabilitation of the medial collateral ligament-deficient elbow: an in vitro bio-mechanical study. *Journal of Hand Surgery*, 25, 1051–1057.

Azar, F.M., Andrews, J.R., Wilk, K.E. and Groh, D. (2000) Operative treatment of ulnar collateral ligament injuries of the elbow in athletes. *American Journal of Sports Medicine*, 28, 16–23.

Bano, K. and Kahlon, R. (2006) Radial head fractures – advanced techniques in surgical management and rehabilitation. *Journal of Hand Therapy*, 19, 114–135.

Bird, S.P., Tarpenning, K.M. and Marino, F.E. (2005) Designing resistance training programmes to enhance muscular fitness: a review of the acute programme variables. *Sports Medicine*, 35, 841–851.

Bisset, L., Paungmali, A., Vicenzino, B. and Beller, E. (2005) A systematic review and meta-analysis of clinical trials on physical interventions for lateral epicondylalgia. *British Journal of Sports Medicine*, 39, 411–422.

Bisset, L., Beller, E., Jull, G., Brooks, P., Darnell, R. and Vicenzino, B. (2006a) Mobilisation with movement and exercise, corticosteroid injection, or wait and see for tennis elbow: randomised trial. *British Medical Journal*, 333(7575), 939.

Bisset, L.M., Russell, T., Bradley, S., Ha, B. and Vicenzino, B.T. (2006b) Bilateral sensorimotor abnormalities in unilateral lateral epicondylalgia. *Archives of Physical Medicine and Rehabilitation*, 87, 490–495.

Bonato, C., Zanette, G., Manganotti, P., Tinazzi, M., Bongiovanni, G., Polo, A. and Fiaschi, A. (1996) 'Direct' and 'crossed' modulation of human motor cortex excitability following exercise. *Neuroscience Letters*, 216, 97–100.

Bonfim, T.R., Jansen Paccola, C.A. and Barela, J.A. (2003) Proprioceptive and behaviour impairments in individuals with anterior cruciate ligament reconstructed knees. *Archives of Physical Medicine and Rehabilitation*, 84, 1217–1223.

Cain, E.L. Jr., Dugas, J.R., Wolf, R.S. and Andrews, J.R. (2003) Elbow injuries in throwing athletes: a current concepts review. *American Journal of Sports Medicine*, 31, 621–635.

Callaway, G.H., Field, L.D., Deng, X.H., Torzilli, P.A., O'Brien, S.J., Altchek, D.W. and Warren, R.F. (1997) Biomechanical evaluation of the medial collateral ligament of the elbow. *Journal of Bone and Joint Surgery, American Volume*, 79, 1223–1231.

Casavant, A. and Hastings, H. (2006) Heterotopic ossification about the elbow: a therapist's guide to evaluation and management. *Journal of Hand Therapy*, 19, 255–266.

Case, S. and Hennrikus, W. (1997) Surgical treatment of displaced medial epicondyle fractures in adolescent athletes. *American Journal of Sports Medicine*, 25, 682–686.

Chinchalkar, S. and Szekeres, M. (2004) Rehabilitation of elbow trauma. *Hand Clinics*, 20, 363–374.

Cook, R.E. and McKee, M.D. (2003) Techniques to tame the terrible Triad: unstable fracture dislocations of the elbow. *Operative Techniques in Orthopaedics*, 13, 130–137.

Davila, S. and Johnston-Jones, K. (2006) Managing the stiff elbow: operative, nonoperative, and postoperative techniques. *Journal of Hand Therapy*, 19, 268–281.

Dimberg, L. (1987) The prevalence and causation of tennis elbow (lateral humeral epicondylitis) in a population of workers in an engineering industry. *Ergonomics*, 30, 573–580.

Feuerstein, M., Miller, V.L., Burrell, L.M. and Berger, R. (1998) Occupational upper extremity disorders in the federal workforce – prevalence, health care expenditures, and patterns of work disability. *Journal of Occupational and Environmental Medicine*, 40, 546–555.

Field, L.D. and Savoie, F.H. (1998) Common elbow injuries in sport. *Sports Medicine*, 26, 193–205.

Frankle, M., Koval, K., Sanders, R. and Zuckerman, J. (1999) Radial head fractures associated with elbow dislocations treated by immediate stabilization and early motion. *Journal of Shoulder and Elbow Surgery*, 8, 355–360.

Glousman, R.E., Barron, J., Jobe, F.W., Perry, J. and Pink, M. (1992) An electromyographic analysis of the elbow in normal and injured pitchers with medial collateral ligament insufficiency. *American Journal of Sports Medicine*, 20, 311–317.

Hamilton, C.D., Glousman, R.E., Jobe, F.W., Brault, J., Pink, M. and Perry, J. (1996) Dynamic stability of the elbow: electromyographic analysis of the flexor pronator group and the extensor group in pitchers with valgus instability. *Journal of Shoulder and Elbow Surgery*, 5, 347–354.

Hay, E.M., Paterson, S.M., Lewis, M., Hosie, G. and Croft, P. (1999) Pragmatic randomised controlled trial of local corticosteroid injection and naproxen for treatment of lateral epicondylitis of elbow in primary care. *British Medical Journal*, 319, 964–968.

Henriksen, B., Gehrchen, P., Jørgensen, M. and Gerner-Smidt, H. (1995) Treatment of traumatic effusion in the elbow joint: a prospective, randomized study of 62 consecutive patients. *Injury*, 26, 475–478.

Herbertsson, P., Josefsson, P., Hasserius, R., Karlsson, C., Besjakov, J. and Karlsson, M. (2005) Displaced mason type 1 fractures of the radial head and neck in adults: a fifteen to thirty-three year follow-up study. *Journal of Shoulder and Elbow Surgery*, 14, 73–77.

Hotchkiss, R. (1997) Displaced fractures of the radial head: internal fixation or excision? *Journal of the American Academy of Orthopedic Surgeons*, 5, 1–10.

Hyman, J., Breazeale, N.M. and Altchek, D.W. (2001) Valgus instability of the elbow in athletes. *Clinics in Sports Medicine*, 20, 25–45.

Kelley, J.D., Lombardo, S.J., Pink, M., Perry, J. and Giangarra, C.E. (1994) Electromyographic and cinematographic analysis of elbow function in tennis players with lateral epicondylitis. *American Journal of Sports Medicine*, 22, 359–363.

Keppler, P., Salem, K., Schwarting, B. and Kinzl, L. (2005) The effectiveness of physiotherapy after operative treatment of supracondylar humeral fractures in children. *Journal of Pediatric Orthopaedics*, 25, 314–316.

Khan, K.M. and Cook, J.L. (2000) Overuse tendon injuries: Where does the pain come from? *Sports Medicine and Arthroscopy Review*, 8, 17–31.

Khan, K.M., Cook, J.L., Kannus, P., Maffulli, N. and Bonar, S.F. (2002) Time to abandon the 'tendinitis' myth – painful, overuse tendon conditions have a non-inflammatory pathology. *British Medical Journal*, 324, 626–627.

Kivi, P. (1982) The etiology and conservative treatment of humeral epicondylitis. *Scandinavian Journal of Rehabilitation Medicine*, 15, 37–41.

Konradsen, L. and Ravn, J.B. (1991) Prolonged peroneal reaction time in ankle instability. *International Journal of Sports Medicine*, 12, 290–292.

Kraushaar, B.S. and Nirschl, R.P. (1999) Tendinosis of the elbow (tennis elbow). Clinical features and findings of histological, immunohistochemical, and electron microscopy studies. *Journal of Bone and Joint Surgery, American Volume*, 81, 259–278.

Kuzala, E.A. and Vargo, M.C. (1992) The relationship between elbow position and grip strength. *American Journal of Occupational Therapy*, 46, 509–512.

Liow, R., Cregan, A., Nanda, R. and Montgomery, R. (2002) Early mobilisation for minimally displaced radial head fractures is desirable. A prospective randomised study of two protocols. *Injury*, 33, 801–806.

Ljung, B.O., Forsgren, S. and Friden, J. (1999) Substance P and calcitonin gene-related peptide expression at the extensor carpi radialis brevis muscle origin: Implications for the etiology of tennis elbow. *Journal of Orthopaedic Research*, 17, 554–559.

Ljung, B.O., Alfredson, H. and Forsgren, S. (2004) Neurokinin 1-receptors and sensory neuropeptides in tendon insertions at the medial and lateral epicondyles of the humerus–Studies on tennis elbow and medial epicondylalgia. *Journal of Orthopaedic Research*, 22, 321–327.

Lockard, M. (2006) Clinical biomechanics of the elbow. *Journal of Hand Therapy*, 19, 72–80.

Mehlhoff, T., Noble, P., Bennett, J. and Tullos, H. (1988) Simple dislocation of the elbow in the adults. Results after closed treatment. *Journal of Bone and Joint Surgery, American Volume*, 70, 244–249.

Morrey, B. and An, K. (1983) Articular and ligamentous contributions to the stability of the elbow joint. *American Journal of Sports Medicine*, 11, 315–319.

Morrey, B., Askew, L. and An, K. (1981) *A biomechanical study of* normal functional elbow motion. *Journal of Bone and Joint Surgery, American Volume*, 63, 872–877.

Nassab, P.F. and Schickendantz, M.S. (2006) Evaluation and treatment of medial ulnar collateral ligament injuries in the throwing athlete. *Sports Medicine and Arthroscopy Review*, 14, 221–231.

Nirschl, R. and Pettrone, F. (1979) Tennis Elbow: The surgical treatment of lateral epicondylitis. *Journal of Bone and Surgery*, 61, 832–839.

Oatis, C. (2004) *The Mechanics and Pathomechanics of Human Movement*. Lippincott & Williams and Wilkins, Philadelphia, Pennsylvania.

O'Driscoll, S. (2000) Elbow dislocations. In: Morrey, B. (ed.) *The Elbow and its Disorders*, 3rd edn, pp. 409–420. W.B. Saunders, Philadelphia, Pennsylvania.

Pienimaki, T., Tarvainen, T., Siira, P. and Vanharanta, H. (1996) Progressive strengthening and stretching exercises and ultrasound for chronic lateral epicondylitis. *Physiotherapy*, 82, 522–530.

Pienimaki, T., Siira, P. and Vanharanta, H. (1997a) Muscle function of the hand, wrist and forearm in chronic lateral epicondylitis. *European Journal of Physical Medicine and Rehabilitation*, 7, 171–178.

Pienimaki, T.T., Kauranen, K. and Vanharanta, H. (1997b) Bilaterally decreased motor performance of arms in patients with chronic tennis elbow. *Archives of Physical Medicine and Rehabilitation*, 78, 1092–1095.

Pienimaki, T., Karinen, P., Kemila, T., Koivukangas, P. and Vanharanta H. (1998) Long-term follow-up of conservatively treated chronic tennis elbow patients. A prospective and retrospective analysis. *Scandinavian Journal of Rehabilitation Medicine*, 30, 159–166.

Popovic, N., Ferrara, M.A., Daenen, B., Georis, P. and Lemaire, R. (2001) Imaging overuse injury of the elbow in professional team handball players: a bilateral comparison using plain films, stress radiography, ultrasound, and magnetic resonance imaging. *International Journal of Sports Medicine*, 22, 60–67.

Potter, H.G., Hannafin, J.A., Morwessel, R.M., DiCarlo, E.F., O'Brien, S.J. and Altchek, D.W. (1995) Lateral epicondylitis: correlation of MR imaging, surgical, and histopathologic findings. *Radiology*, 196, 43–46.

Protzman, R. (1978) Dislocation of the elbow joint. *Journal of Bone and Joint Surgery, American Volume*, 60, 539–541.

Regan, W. and Morrey, B. (1989) Fractures of the coronoid process of the ulna. *Journal of Bone and Joint Surgery, American Volume*, 71, 1348–1354.

Regan, W., Wold, L.E., Coonrad, R. and Morrey, B.F. (1992) Microscopic histopathology of chronic refractory lateral epicondylitis. *American Journal of Sports Medicine*, 20, 746–749.

Rettig, A.C., Sherrill, C., Snead, D.S., Mendler, J.C. and Mieling, P. (2001) Nonoperative treatment of ulnar collateral ligament injuries in throwing athletes. *American Journal of Sports Medicine*, 29, 15–17.

Ross, G., McDevitt, E., Chronister, R. and Ove, P. (1999) Treatment of simple elbow dislocation using an immediate motion protocol. *American Journal of Sports Medicine*, 27, 308–311.

Saati, A. and McKee, M. (2004) Fracture-dislocation of the elbow: diagnosis, treatment and prognosis. *Hand Clinics*, 20, 405–414.

Safran, M.R. and Baillargeon, D. (2005a) Soft-tissue stabilizers of the elbow. *Journal of Shoulder and Elbow Surgery*, 14(1 Suppl. S), 179S–185S.

Safran, M.R., Ahmad, C.S. and Elattrache, N.S. (2005b) Ulnar collateral ligament of the elbow. *Arthroscopy*, 21, 1381–1395.

Safran, M.R., McGarry, M.H., Shin, S., Han, S. and Lee, T.Q. (2005c) Effects of elbow flexion and forearm rotation on valgus laxity of the elbow. *Journal of Bone and Joint Surgery, American Volume*, 87, 2065–2074.

Sasaki, J., Takahara, M., Ogino, T., Kashiwa, H., Ishigaki, D. and Kanauchi, Y. (2002) Ultrasonographic assessment of the ulnar collateral ligament and medial elbow laxity in college baseball players. *Journal of Bone and Joint Surgery, American Volume*, 84, 525–531.

Sheps, D., Hildebrand, K. and Boorman, R. (2004) Simple dislocations of the elbow: evaluation and treatment. *Hand Clinics*, 20, 389–404.

Smidt, N., van der Windt, D., Assendelft, W.J.J., Deville, W., Korthals-de Bos, I.B.C. and Bouter, L.M. (2002) Corticosteroid injections, physiotherapy, or a wait-and-see policy for lateral epicondylitis: a randomised controlled trial. *Lancet*, 359, 657–662.

Sobel, J. and Nirschl, R. (1996) Elbow injuries. In: Zachazewski, J.E. and Quillen, W.S. (eds) *Athletic Injuries and Rehabilitation*, pp. 543–583. W.B. Saunders, Philadelphia, Pennsylvania.

Stinear, C.M., Walker, K.S. and Byblow, W.D. (2001) Symmetric facilitation between motor cortices during con-traction of ipsilateral hand muscles. *Experimental Brain Research*, 139, 101–105.

Stover, S., Hataway, C. and Zeiger, H. (1975) Heterotopic ossification in spinal cord-injured patients. *Archives of Physical Medicine and Rehabilitation*, 56, 199–204.

Vicenzino, B. (2003) Lateral epicondylalgia: A musculoskeletal physiotherapy perspective. *Manual Therapy*, 8, 66–79.

Vicenzino, B. and Wright, A. (1996) Lateral epicondylalgia: A review of epidemiology, pathophysiology, aetiology and natural history. *Physical Therapy Reviews*, 1, 23–34.

Wharton, G. and Morgan, T. (1970) Ankylosis in the paralyzed patient. *Journal of Bone and Joint Surgery, American Volume*, 52, 105–112.

Wilk, K., Arrigo, C. and Andrews, J. (1993) Rehabilitation of the elbow in the throwing athlete. *Journal of Orthopedic and Sports Physical Therapy*, 17, 305–317.

Willems, T., Witvrouw, E., Verstuyft, J., Vaes, P. and De Clercq, D. (2002) Proprioception and muscle strength in subjects with a history of ankle sprains and chronic instability. *Journal of Athletic Training*, 37, 487–493.

Woodley, B.L., Newsham-West, R.J., Baxter, G.D., Kjaer, M. and Koehle, M.S. (2007) Chronic tendinopathy: effectiveness of eccentric exercise. *British Journal of Sports Medicine*, 41, 188–198.

Zeisig, E., Ohberg, L. and Alfredson, H. (2006) Extensor origin vascularity related to pain in patients with Tennis elbow. *Knee Surgery Sports Traumatology Arthroscopy*, 14, 659–663.

The Wrist and Hand

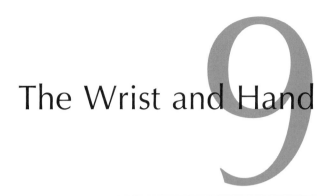

Mandy Johnson

SECTION 1: INTRODUCTION AND BACKGROUND

The wrist and hand is a complex system of inter-related joints and soft tissues that play a major role in all aspects of activity. Injuries to the wrist and hand are common due to the constant involvement of the hand in most activities of daily living and sporting pursuit. Many of these injuries are a result of trauma, particularly in a physical occupation or sport, but there are a number of overuse conditions which can have a debilitating effect on the patient. There is a tendency to underestimate the importance of injuries to the wrist and hand but even the simplest injury, if not treated correctly, can have a disabling effect on not just sporting activities but activities of daily living.

Evidence for the use of exercise in the rehabilitation of wrist and hand injuries

There is limited evidence that exercise regimens have a positive effect in the rehabilitation of any wrist or hand injury. Theoretically, the use of therapeutic exercise is essential for a number of reasons.

Exercises help to prevent contractures, which can cause limitation in some elements of motion. Range of movement exercises should be reintroduced as early as possible to ensure that joint mobility is restored. These movements can be active, active-assisted or passive, depending on the status of the patient. Strengthening exercises will be required later in rehabilitation so the patient can achieve the best functional outcome possible.

In patients following an uncomplicated fracture of the distal radius, a regimen of prescribed home exercises has been shown to be adequate rehabilitation. In contrast, in patients at risk of a poor outcome, individualised physiotherapy has been found to increase the range of flexion and extension of the wrist at 6 months post-injury (Wakefield and McQueen, 2000). A Cochrane review in this area (the effect of rehabilitation following fractures of the distal radius) concluded that there was not enough evidence to establish the effectiveness of rehabilitation interventions in patients with distal fractures of the radius (Handoll *et al.*, 2006). The review included 15 randomised or quasi-randomised trials, involving 746, mainly female and older patients, which evaluated interventions such as active and passive mobilisation exercises, training for activities of daily living and rehabilitation interventions that could be carried out by the patient themselves or in combination with clinicians. Initial

Exercise Therapy in the Management of Musculoskeletal Disorders, First Edition. Edited by Fiona Wilson, John Gormley and Juliette Hussey.
© 2011 Blackwell Publishing Ltd

treatment was identified as being conservative, involving plaster cast immobilisation (in all but 27 participants whose fractures were fixed surgically). One trial showed that there was weak evidence of improved hand function with hand therapy in the days after plaster cast removal, and beneficial effects continued for 1 month later. Another trial showed weak evidence of improved hand function in the short term, but not in the longer term (3 months), for early occupational therapy whereas another study showed no difference in outcome between supervised and unsupervised exercises. Four trials examined formal rehabilitation, two trials investigated passive movements, ice or pulsed electromagnetic field (one trial), or whirlpool immersion (one trial). Weak evidence of short-term benefits was found for continuous passive motion (CPM), intermittent pneumatic compression, ultrasound, and also to support better short-term hand function in patients given physiotherapy compared with patients given exercises by surgeons.

Thien *et al.* (2004) reviewed studies examining rehabilitation of flexor tendon injuries following surgery. Six randomised controlled and quasi-randomised controlled studies were identified, with 464 participants. However the exercise regimens varied and studies included a traditional passive movement regimen, a CPM protocol, early controlled mobilisation using rubber band traction, static and dynamic splinting for the thumb, and controlled passive flexion with active extension and controlled passive mobilisation. The only study that showed a significant effect was that comparing passive mobilisation to CPM, with the CPM regimen having a favourable outcome. However, due to differences in surgical techniques it was difficult to compare interventions. Generally it appears that to regain full function, the majority of tendon injuries should undergo surgical intervention followed by rehabilitation. In the initial stages this should be limited to active-assisted movements and passive movements with no resistance. Tensile loading is gradually increased with some functional movements to re-establish neurological patterns and this is progressed with an emphasis on eccentric loading, plyometric activity, and co-contractions of agonist/antagonist force couples and gradual reintroduction of sporting activities or activities of daily living (Kibler, 1997).

Strength in the hand and wrist is relevant to each individual. The demands of the patient in normal everyday life needs to be known to fully assess the strength requirements in the rehabilitation programme. The benefits of strength training in this area are supported by the results of a study examining the effect of unilateral upper limb strength training on finger pinch force in older men (Keogh *et al.*, 2007). The strength training group exercised twice a week for 6 weeks whereas controls maintained normal activities. The strength training group achieved significantly greater increases in finger pinch force, biceps curl and wrist flexion strength (Keogh *et al.*, 2007). Another recent study compared the effect of an intensive hand exercise programme with a conservative protocol in patients with rheumatoid arthritis (Ronningen and Kjeken, 2008). After 2 and 14 weeks the there were significant differences between the groups in terms of pinch strength (2 weeks) and grip strength (14 weeks) in favour of the intensive exercise programme.

Injuries to the wrist and hand

Fractures, dislocations and ligament injuries

The two most common fractures at the wrist are Colles' and Smith's fractures. Both occur at the distal end of the radius. Colles' fracture occurs as a result of a fall on the outstretched arm and results in the distinctive 'dinner fork' deformity. Smith's fracture can be referred to as a reverse Colles' fracture and is as a result of a direct blow or fall on a flexed wrist. Fracture reduction is followed by immobilisation in a cast for approximately 6 weeks. It is important that active range of movement exercises are commenced for the shoulder and elbow during the period of immobilisation. Following a period of immobilisation for the wrist, active range of movement exercises should be commenced for all movement patterns with particular attention to extension and supination. Active exercises should be gradually progressed to strengthening exercises, which can be carried out using light hand springs, therapeutic putty, various elastic bands and small hand weights. This is followed by a gradual reintroduction of functional and sporting activities.

Dislocations and ligament injuries are usually treated by splinting the injured finger to the next finger but it is important that a full range of movement is regained following the injury and that there are no avulsion fractures present which may influence the range of movement after full healing has occurred. Injury to the ulna collateral ligament often occurs as a result of a fall on the outstretched hand with the thumb forced into abduction and extension, which creates tension in the ligament. The ulnar side of the thumb will be tender and sometimes swollen with pain and weakness on grasping or pinching movements. For treatment purposes the injuries are usually divided into two categories depending on the integrity of the ligament, which is tested by stressing the accessory and ulnar collateral ligaments (as the critical stress point to cause complete rupture is approximately 30° of abduction). Initially a short opponens splint or thumb spica cast may be required to rest the ulna collateral ligament for approximately 3 weeks. This is then replaced by a splint that can be removed for mobility and strengthening exercises, which should be commenced at approximately 8 weeks. It is essential that no abduction forces are applied to the joint for the first 6 weeks. If the ligament is not intact, surgery is required. A Stener lesion occurs if there is a complete disruption of the ulnar collateral ligament which then protrudes beneath the adductor aponeurosis. After surgery the thumb should be immobilised in a cast for 3 weeks. This cast can then be replaced with a splint for a further 2–3 weeks; the splint can be removed for exercise purposes.

Tendinopathy

Tendon pathology used to be referred to as tendinitis but the preferred term is tendinopathy. Rest and pain-relieving modalities are used in the initial stages. Resting the tendon does not necessarily mean immobilisation but may entail the avoidance of movements that cause pain.

Exercise therapy is an important aspect of the rehabilitation of tendinopathy and related conditions but it is essential that the appropriate exercise therapy is introduced at the correct time or the condition may be exacerbated. Flexibility exercises are usually the first type of exercise to be reintroduced but eccentric exercise followed by concentric strengthening exercises are the major components of an exercise programme. Evidence for the effectiveness of the various exercise modalities is poor due to the lack of well-designed trials.

Tendon rupture can occur following a traumatic incident involving undue force through a tendon. The initial symptoms are severe pain and loss of function and these could lead to permanent disability if untreated. Depending on the site and severity of the rupture, treatment could be conservative or surgical. Tendons on the flexor aspect of the hand and wrist have synovial sheaths but extensor tendons do not. The most common cause of tendon ruptures of the wrist and hand are caused by lacerations due to injuries or a forcible impact to the fingers causing a hyperflexion or extension of the digits. These latter injuries are common in sport particularly in cricket, volleyball and basketball. There is often an avulsion fracture where the tendon is pulled off the bone and in these cases surgical intervention may be required to reattach the tendon and bone fragment. There are differences in the rehabilitation protocols for ruptures of extensor tendons and of flexor tendons in the hand and wrist. This is mainly due to the strong pulley system that exists within the flexor tendons. The extensor tendon is more passive in function, but disruption of this tendon can be as debilitating as disruption of the flexor tendons due to the influence these tendons have on the lumbricals and interossei.

Rupture of the flexor digitorum profundus tendon from the distal phalanx may be treated conservatively or with surgery. Splinting is usually in place for 6 weeks and then an active exercise programme is introduced. To minimise the tension on the tendons, flexion exercises are performed with the wrist in extension and extension exercises are performed with the wrist in flexion. Strengthening exercises are not started until there is good active extension of the wrist and the metacarpophalangeal and interphalangeal joints, which usually occurs 8 weeks post-surgery. Strengthening exercises are progressed depending on how well the patient is managing, with the introduction of co-ordination exercises and endurance work.

If the common extensor tendon that inserts into the base of the middle phalanx is damaged, a boutonnière deformity may result. This is a common injury in sport and may be caused by a severe flexion force to the proximal interphalangeal joint (PIP) or direct trauma to the posterior aspect of this joint. A boutonniere injury should be suspected if there is more than 30° extension lag at the PIP joint. Rehabilitation for the common extensor tendon requires immobilisation of the PIP joint in full extension for 6–8 weeks. Gentle mobility exercises can be started after 4 weeks for flexion/extension of the PIP joint with immobilisation between exercise sessions. Strengthening work can be commenced 2–3 months post-injury.

Treatment of the rupture of the distal attachment of extensor digitorum (Mallet's finger) involves splinting for approximately 6 weeks or longer if there is insufficient healing. An avulsion fracture is treated with open reduction and internal fixation of the fracture, usually with 'K-wires', followed by immobilisation. The splint will remain in situ until active extension can be carried out at the distal interphalangeal (DIP) joint. At this point, which is usually around 8 weeks post injury or surgery, active exercises can be commenced with progressive strengthening exercises. The splint is disregarded at approximately 9–10 weeks as long as there is no extensor lag in the DIP joint, and unrestricted use can commence at approximately 12 weeks.

Overuse injuries

Carpal tunnel syndrome is particularly common in individuals working at computer terminals for long periods, where the wrist is held in extension, or in a gymnast who repeatedly weight-bears through the wrist. It can also occur in situations of extended gripping, such as racquet sports or where a person has spent an unusually long period of time gripping a paint brush. Other causes of carpal tunnel syndrome that have been identified include fluid retention, particularly in pregnancy, infection, renal problems, and gout or collagen disorders. It occurs when the median nerve is compressed as it travels through the carpal tunnel and which can lead to ischaemia of the nerve. Other symptoms may include loss of sensation in the hand as well as weakness and pain along the pathway of the median nerve. The pain is particularly apparent at night in people who have a tendency to sleep with the wrist slightly flexed, as this position will also cause nerve compression and consequently pain. If carpal tunnel syndrome is suspected it is important that the cervical spine is thoroughly investigated as the symptoms may be referred from the neck. Various modalities can be used to relieve the symptoms, including a wrist splint that maintains the wrist position in neutral and is useful particularly at night. Exercise is not effective when the patient is

symptomatic (Piazzini *et al.*, 2007), but when the symptoms have reduced, an active exercise programme may be reintroduced. Surgery to relieve the compression on the median nerve may be considered in extreme cases.

Joint diseases

Osteoarthritis is a common disease that can either be a primary condition or follow a pre-existing condition. As a primary condition, the most common area in the hand and wrist for osteoarthritis to manifest is the first carpometacarpal joint of the thumb. Osteoarthritis of this joint is typified by pain at the base of the thumb, especially when gripping an object. Osteoarthritis is more common in women than men, especially over the age of 45–50 years of age. Conservative management includes splinting, gentle moist heat, usually administered by wax baths, and gentle exercises.

Secondary osteoarthritis can develop in any area of the wrist or hand following a previous injury, particularly fractures in which a joint or joint surface is involved. It is a progressive degenerative condition and is exacerbated with use. It is very common following injuries to the scaphoid and in extreme conditions it can lead to degeneration of the joint between the scaphoid and radius, and consequently lunate and capitate, which will ultimately result in a collapse of the wrist. Support may be offered to the joint through splinting, and gentle non-resisted exercises will help maintain some range of movement.

Rheumatoid arthritis and juvenile arthritis are conditions that affect the whole of the body, but can cause particular problems in the upper limb, wrist and hand. Treatment and rehabilitation will help relieve symptoms to a certain degree and help minimise disability. The repeated inflammatory episodes of various joints of the body can cause substantial damage to the soft tissues and extra-articular structures. This can result in pain, stiffness, joint instability and ultimate deformity, including ulnar deviation of the metacarpophalangeal joints, boutonnière deformity and swan-neck deformity. Joint laxity, weakness of the muscles and loss of range of movement will lead to major dysfunction of the hand and wrist, making even the simplest tasks in everyday living almost impossible to perform.

Interventions for this disease include stabilisation, to allow better function of the wrist and hand by utilising the muscles of the forearm, controlling the inflammatory process and protecting the joints. Some patients present with stiff and immobile joints due to scarring following inflammatory episodes or surgery and these patients require sustained exercise therapy. Patients may also present with joint laxity following surgery that may require splinting for long periods.

Active exercises should be used to maintain joint range followed by isometric strengthening exercises. Resisted exercises should be undertaken with extreme caution due to the inflammatory nature of the disease. There are many pieces of adaptive equipment that can be introduced and which will reduce the stresses of everyday living for the patient with rheumatoid arthritis. Avoidance of repetitive actions and patient education are paramount for improvement in symptoms.

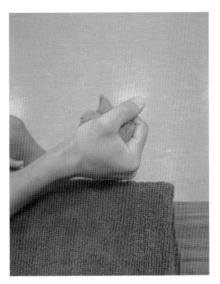

Figure 9.1 The power grip.

SECTION 2: PRACTICAL USE OF EXERCISE

Assessment of the wrist and hand

The most important aspect of any rehabilitation programme involving the wrist and hand is to restore full function to the movements of the fingers and thumb. The ability to manipulate various objects and the application of dexterity and range of uses that humankind is capable of set us aside from all other creatures. Prehensile or gripping activities have been described in various ways over the years but essentially they are all variations of the power grip (Fig. 9.1), precision grip (Fig. 9.2) and the hook grip.

In the power grip all the fingers and thumb are flexed around the object with the thumb controlling the movement if any is required. The purpose of this grip is to hold an object firmly, so that it can be worked on by the other hand or wielded as a tool or weapon. The precision grip uses very fine, small movements of the digits. The object is grasped between the ends of the fingers and thumb or just the thumb and index finger. The manipulation or positioning of the object is carried out at the wrist

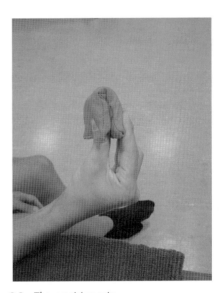

Figure 9.2 The precision grip.

or in particularly fine work the lumbricals and interossei of the hand. The hook grip is used to pull or suspend objects. It may sometimes be used as a power grip when carrying out activities such as climbing, where it is used to suspend or elevate the body. The thumb may or may not be used as the fingers are flexed into the palm as far as the dimensions of the object allow. These movements should be fully assessed by the clinician prior to design of a programme.

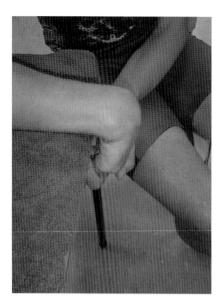

Figure 9.3   Passive wrist flexion.

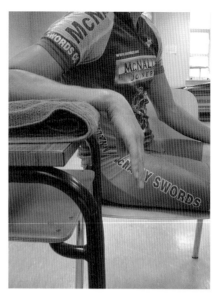

Figure 9.5   Active wrist flexion.

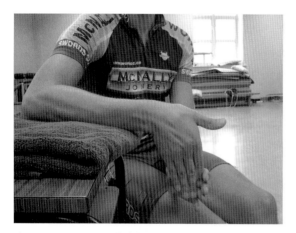

Figure 9.4   Passive radial deviation.

Movements of the hand and wrist in all planes should be tested first actively and then passively. It is important to establish which is the dominant side, as this may have some bearing on the results. It is vital to note the position of the fingers when testing mobility as the long tendons cross over many joints, and if the fingers are flexed movement in the wrist may be restricted.

Exercise management of the wrist and hand

The early phase – passive exercises/mobilisation

Assessment of the strength of the hand and wrist should include both isometric and dynamic tests. These tests should include the lumbricals and interossei and all other movements of the wrist hand and digits. The initial tests should be single joint movements such as flexion, extension radial and ulna deviation of the wrist (Figs 9.3–9.5). The more complex patterns involving multiple joints should follow if the initial tests are comparable with the opposite side.

In the initial stages of rehabilitation of the wrist and hand passive movements can be introduced to re-establish full mobility. Passive movements involve the therapist manipulating specific joints, while the patient tries to relax and takes no active part. With many wrist problems there is a loss of supination and pronation at the distal radioulnar joint. To regain full range of active movement it is essential that these movements are re-established. To mobilise the distal radioulnar joint the forearm can be in either a prone or supine position. The therapist places one hand around the radial head and the other around the head of the ulna.

To make the patient more comfortable when mobilising the wrist joint a pad can be placed under the distal forearm and the hand placed over the edge of the treatment couch or table. With the patients' forearm in pronation and the wrist in neutral, the therapist should secure the lower end of the forearm around the radial and ulnar styloids with one hand and place the other hand over the carpal bones. A longitudinal distraction force should be applied by the second hand; this force can either be sustained or oscillatory.

To increase either radial or ulna deviation the forearm is placed with either the radial or the ulnar side uppermost, depending on the area that needs to be mobilised. For an increase in ulnar deviation the forearm is placed radial side up with the wrist in neutral, with the stabilising hand over the radial and ulna styloids and the mobilising hand over the carpals. A downward force is applied by the mobilising hand. For radial deviation, the ulna is uppermost and the same directional force is applied.

To increase flexion or extension of the wrist, the forearm is placed in pronation with the wrist in neutral. The therapist stabilises the forearm by grasping the radial and ulnar styloids and mobilises the wrist by placing the other hand over the carpal bones. To increase flexion, an antero-posterior (AP) force is applied parallel to the wrist joint. To increase extension, a postero-anterior (PA) force is applied in the same manner.

The carpal joints can be mobilised on an individual basis if required, but it is important to understand the shape of the bones involved and their relationship with their neighbours to ensure that the correct force is applied in the most appropriate direction. To mobilise the individual carpal joints the therapist uses a pinch grasp on a pronated hand; one hand stabilises while the other hand carries out the mobilising technique.

The proximal row of carpal bones has a convex shape that fits in to the radius and ulna, which are both concave. To increase flexion in the radiocarpal joint a posterior force is applied to the radius, and to increase extension an anterior force is applied. The ulnocarpal joint is further complicated by the presence of a articular cartilaginous disc between the distal radioulnar joint and also between the

ulnar medial part of the lunate, and the triquetral if the hand is adducted. The disc can block free movement if disrupted. The ulnocarpal joint can be mobilised by applying an anterior force that will help to mobilise the disc. The scaphoid is convex compared with the concave shape of the trapezium and trapezoid thereby to increase flexion the scaphoid should be fixed and an AP glide of the trapezium and trapezoid should be carried out. To increase extension an AP glide of the scaphoid on the distal carpals is carried out. Mobilisation of other carpal bones is similar, by securing one carpal bone with a stabilising thumb and finger and then mobilising the joint with the other thumb and finger using either an AP or PA glide.

Techniques to mobilise carpometacarpal and metacarpophalangeal joints are similar to those previously described; in addition, traction forces can be applied to the joints and this is particularly effective when treating the first carpometacarpal joint for increasing opposition and rotation movements.

When passive range has been re-established active exercises can be recommenced. It is important that active movements are recommenced as soon as possible as they have advantages over purely passive movements. Exercises to improve active flexion of the wrist and hand are shown in Figure 9.6.

Intermediate stage – strengthening exercises

When normal joint range and function have been restored, progressive strengthening exercises can be gradually introduced. These can be commenced with static or isometric contractions and then progressed to active or dynamic exercises that include concentric eccentric and isotonic contractions. A strengthening programme should commence with specific exercises for particular joints and progress onto exercises that involve the kinetic chain for the whole of the upper limb. If possible, functional patterns of movement should be followed. It is important that both the interossei and the lumbricals (Fig. 9.7) are included in any strengthening protocols particularly following any type of immobilisation.

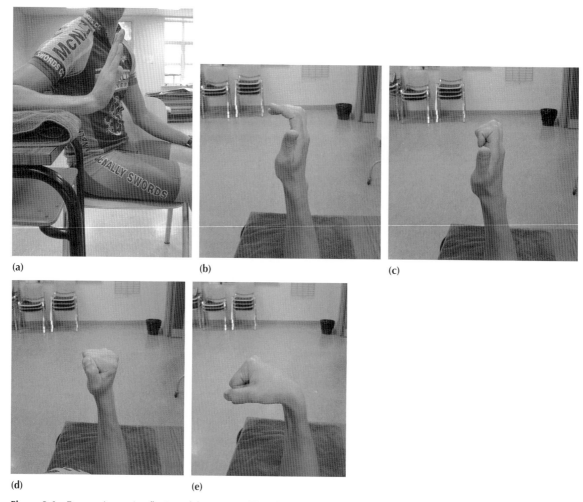

(a)   (b)   (c)

(d)   (e)

Figure 9.6   Progressive active flexion of the wrist and hand.

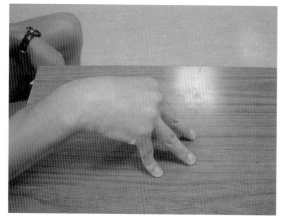

Figure 9.7   Lumbrical strengthening.

Resisted exercises can be performed manually, using the clinician or self administered for a home exercise programme. Pieces of equipment that can be used for resisted work include: therapeutic putty of various densities denoted by a variety of colours, elastic bands and hand springs and small dumbbells. However, it is essential that a full range of movement is completed, which is not always possible with putty, hand springs or dumbbells. Figures 9.8–9.13 illustrate different strengthening exercises using a range of equipment.

Grip strength exercises are essential to restore normal function of the wrist and hand. These exercises can be carried out using ball of various sizes and different densities of therapeutic putty. Elastic bands around the fingers are useful and offer a good

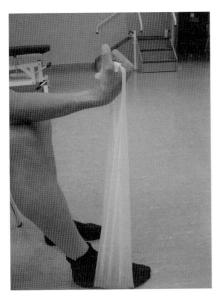

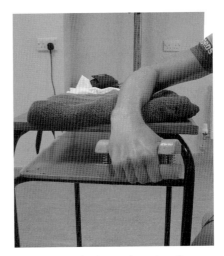

Figure 9.10 Strengthening of wrist flexors against resistance.

Figure 9.8 Concentric strengthening of wrist flexors.

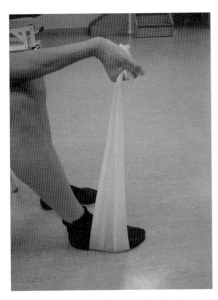

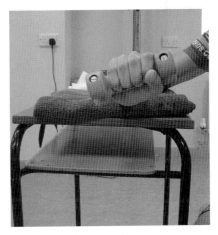

Figure 9.11 Strengthening of wrist extensors against resistance.

Figure 9.9 Eccentric strengthening of wrist flexors.

source of resistance for extension exercises of the digits.

Late or functional stage

Functional exercises for the hand and wrist will differ greatly between patients due to the demands made in normal everyday life, particularly in employment or sporting activities. The functional exercise programme should incorporate as many normal activities as possible to re-establish functional movement patterns at the correct speed and stress levels that will be encountered in normal life.

Plyometric and proprioception exercises for the wrist and hand are the same as those used for the elbow and shoulder. Many other plyometric and proprioceptive exercises can be introduced using a

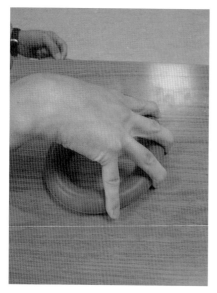

Figure 9.12 Strengthening of the lumbricals and finger flexors.

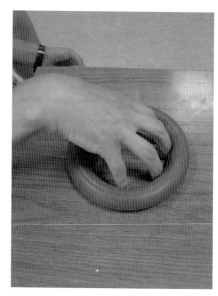

Figure 9.13   Strengthening of the finger extensors.

ball. This can be a normal ball or a medicine ball. The actions used in volley ball when setting or passing the ball are plyometric for the fingers and wrist and can be carried out against a wall. Dropping a ball and catching it before it reaches the floor palm down requires strength dexterity and good reaction time. This can be made more demanding by increasing the weight of the ball. Proprioception exercises include various gripping actions of various sized objects and throwing and catching balls of different weights and sizes. Practising precision grips with different sized objects will also promote an increase in proprioceptive abilities.

SECTION 3: CASE STUDIES AND STUDENT QUESTIONS

Case study 1

A 70-year-old woman fell on her outstretched right hand and sustained a fracture of the distal end of the radius and ulna.

Management

The patient's forearm was immobilised with plaster of Paris and she was encouraged to move her fingers and flex her elbow as much as she could during immobilisation. Following 6 weeks of immobilisation, passive, active and active-assisted exercises were commenced. This included passive movements to mobilise the carpus and first carpometacarpal joint. When full range of movement had been achieved gentle strengthening exercises were introduced using therapeutic putty and elastic bands.

Case study 2

A young cricket player caught a ball, which forced a hyperextension of a distal interphalangeal joint.

Management

On examination it was found that the patient had a 'Mallet finger' deformity, suggesting a rupture of the long extensor tendon and which was confirmed on magnetic resonance imaging (MRI). Open reduction was carried out and a splint applied post-surgery. The hand was kept in the splint for 6 weeks, at which point the splint was removed and the tendon was tested to evaluate whether it could maintain extension of the distal phalanx. This was not the case, therefore the splint was reapplied and checked every 5 days. When the tendon was able to maintain extension, active exercises were commenced. The splint was reapplied between sessions. It was important for the therapist to check for an extensor lag of the distal phalanx at every session. At week 10, gentle progressive exercises were started using therapeutic putty and elastic bands. At this point the splint was disregarded, and at 16 weeks, full sporting activities were recommenced.

Case study 3

A 50-year-old diabetic man noticed a thickening on the palm of the left hand, and his little finger was staring to flex into his palm.

Management

On examination it was found that the patient was developing Dupuytren's contracture. A stretching programme was implemented to try to ease the situation but after a period of time, when the fifth digit was flexing into the palm and the fourth digit was beginning to follow, it was decided that a Z-plasty should be carried out to elongate the palmer fascia and release the contracture. Following surgery, a splint was applied but passive and active exercises were initiated as soon as the patient could tolerate and the wound was checked regularly to ensure that scarring was minimal and scar mobility was maximised, particularly as the patient was a diabetic and wound healing could have been compromised. Success of this surgery may depend on correct splinting and exercise therapy. Hand function was restored as soon as possible but during this time it was noticed that the other hand was developing a thickening and the same procedure had to be repeated on the other hand, which was not unexpected.

Student questions

(1) What are the common complications following fractures of the wrist?
(2) How quickly is an exercise rehabilitation programme reintroduced for flexor tendon ruptures?
(3) What is the most common carpal bone to sustain a fracture and why?
(4) How can plyometric exercises be undertaken for the wrist and hand?
(5) What movements are possible at the first carpometacarpal joint?
(6) Describe an exercise protocol for a patient with rheumatoid arthritis.
(7) Describe a progressive exercise programme for tendinopathy of the wrist.
(8) What is the common cause of carpal tunnel syndrome?
(9) What is the primary site for osteoarthritis in the wrist and hand?
(10) What is the common cause of inter-carpal instabilities.

References

Handoll, H.H., Madhok, R. and Howe, T.E. (2006) In the treatment of fractures of the wrist Rehabilitation for distal radial fractures in adults. *Cochrane Database of Systemic Reviews*, 3, CD003324.

Keogh, J.W., Morrison, S. and Barrett, R. (2007) Strength training improves the tri-digit finger-pinch force control of older adults. *Archives of Physical Medicine and Rehabilitation*, 88, 1055–1063.

Kibler, W.B. (1997) Diagnosis, treatment and rehabilitation principles in complete tendon ruptures in sports. *Scandinavian Journal of Medicine and Science in Sports*, 7, 119–129.

Piazzini, D.B., Aprile, I., Ferrara, P.E., Bertolini, C., Tonali, P., Maggi, L., Rabini, A., Piantelli, S. and Padua, L. (2007) A systematic review of conservative treatment of carpal tunnel syndrome. *Clinical Rehabilitation*, 21, 299–314.

Ronningen, A. and Kjeken, I. (2008) Effect of an intensive hand exercise programme in patients with rheumatoid arthritis. *Scandinavian Journal of Occupational Therapy*, 15, 173–183.

Thien, T. B., Becker, J.H. and Theis, J.C. (2004) Rehabilitation after surgery for flexor tendon injuries in the hand. *Cochrane Database of Systematic Reviews*, 4, CD003979.

Wakefield, A.E. and McQueen, M.M. (2000) The role of physiotherapy and clinical predictors of outcome after fracture of the distal radius. *Journal of Bone and Joint Surgery, British Volume*, 82, 972–976.

10

The Hip and Pelvic Complex

Kevin Sims

SECTION 1: INTRODUCTION AND BACKGROUND

While hip and pelvic girdle pain are not as common as low back pain, the incidence of hip osteoarthritis (OA) or pelvic girdle pain (PGP) does increase with age and in pregnancy (Felson *et al.*, 2000; Van De Pol *et al.*, 2007). The purpose of this chapter is to review exercise approaches to these two closely related regions.

Evidence of exercise efficacy in the management of hip pain

Specific evidence for the role of exercise in hip disorders is surprisingly scarce. Often the hip and knee are considered together with the assumption that if exercise is beneficial for the knee then the same will apply to the hip. As an example, a recent document published by the Osteoarthritis Research Society International group provided evidence-based, consensus-driven recommendations for the management of hip and knee OA (Zhang *et al.*, 2008). The following recommendations specific to exercise were made:

- 'Patients with symptomatic hip and knee OA may benefit from referral to a physical therapist for evaluation and instruction in appropriate exercises to reduce pain and improve functional capacity'.
- 'Patients with hip and knee OA should be encouraged to undertake, and continue to undertake, regular aerobic, muscle strengthening and range of motion exercises. For patients with symptomatic hip OA, exercises in water can be effective'.

Both of these recommendations are primarily based on randomised controlled trials (RCTs) of the knee. Apart from two RCTs (Stener-Victorin *et al.*, 2004; Cochrane *et al.*, 2005) supporting hydrotherapy, the evidence supporting exercise in hip OA is based largely on expert clinical opinion (Roddy *et al.*, 2005).

However, several studies do support the efficacy of exercise in managing hip OA. Both hip (37%) and knee (59%) OA subjects were included in an RCT, which looked at muscle strengthening and stretching, general mobility and co-ordination plus advice on adaptation of activities of daily living (van Baar *et al.*, 1998). The content, intensity and frequency of treatment were tailored to the patient's needs. A medium reduction in pain (a comparison of visual analogue scale (VAS) scores of each week

Exercise Therapy in the Management of Musculoskeletal Disorders, First Edition. Edited by Fiona Wilson, John Gormley and Juliette Hussey.
© 2011 Blackwell Publishing Ltd

with the previous week) and a small reduction in observed disability (composite score of time taken and quality of performance of functional tasks) was found (van Baar *et al.*, 1998). In a later follow-up, these beneficial effects were shown to decline and by 6 months had disappeared, indicating the need for long-term patient compliance with exercise programmes (van Baar *et al.*, 2001).

In another study, exercise therapy was compared with manual therapy (Hoeksma *et al.*, 2004). The exercise therapy was based on the protocols designed by van Baar *et al.* (1998) and the manual therapy included muscle stretching, traction, manipulation and promotion of physical activity including walking, cycling and swimming. The main outcome measure was the patient's perceived improvement on a six-point scale (ranging from 'much worse' to 'complete recovery'). Using this measure, 81% of the manual therapy group and 50% of the exercise therapy group reported an improvement. These improvements persisted at the 29-week follow-up. The authors concluded that there was support for the beneficial effects of manual therapy although both groups improved in the study (Hoeksma *et al.*, 2004).

Most recently a group of community-dwelling patients with hip (11% control group, 5% treatment group) and knee OA were treated with a twice-weekly, 6-week period of hydrotherapy (Hinman *et al.*, 2007). The intervention consisted of progressive exercises in functional weight-bearing tasks under direct supervision from a physiotherapist. The primary outcome measures were subject-perceived changes in pain and physical function rated on a five-point Likert scale (4 or 5 indicating improvement). The treatment group reported a 72% improvement in pain (compared with 17% in the control group) and 75% improvement in physical function (compared with 17% in the control group). These benefits were maintained for 6 weeks after the completion of the programme with 84% of participants continuing to exercise independently. However, as the majority of subjects in both groups had knee OA the results of this study are most applicable to this condition. There is no evidence for conditions other than hip OA.

Aerobic exercise

There is no specific evidence on the effect of aerobic exercise and hip disease. However, an RCT which examined the effects of hydrotherapy on hip and knee OA found a reduction in pain and an increase in physical function utilising a programme which included an aerobic exercise component (Cochrane *et al.*, 2005). Several studies in subjects with knee OA suggest that aerobic walking programmes lead to a reduction in pain and disability (Kovar *et al.*, 1992; Talbot *et al.*, 2003). This would suggest that similar benefits would occur in subjects with hip OA.

Muscle strength and endurance

A large-scale review of exercise and OA bemoans the 'almost complete absence of published data' on the effects of structured exercise and hip OA (Vignon *et al.*, 2006). As strengthening exercises have benefits for subjects with knee OA (see Chapter 11) one is left to extrapolate that similar effects probably occur in subjects with hip OA. One major study investigating the benefits of exercise (including strengthening) in people with hip OA has shown a reduction in pain and disability (van Baar *et al.*, 1998). A recent case series also includes a description of strengthening of the hip abductors and external rotators as routine in all subjects (MacDonald *et al.*, 2006). Although this is encouraging, further evidence is required.

Another alternative is to review published data on muscle weakness associated with hip OA. This provides a rationale for targeting certain muscle groups although the presence of muscle impairment does not imply cause and effect with hip OA. A weakness of the hip abductors, flexors and adductors (tested with a dynamometer) was found in 27 men (average age 56) with hip OA when compared with healthy controls (Arokoski *et al.*, 2002). Hip extension strength was not different between groups but was weaker on the side of the more affected hip in the hip OA group. There was also a reduction in cross-sectional area (measured with magnetic resonance imaging (MRI)) of the pelvic and thigh muscles in the more severely affected hip compared with the better hip.

More recently, a study investigating predominantly older women (mean age 67) with unilateral hip OA identified weakness (compared with the unaffected limb) in the hip extensors, flexors, abductors, adductors and knee extensors (Rasch *et al.*, 2007). This study also identified a reduced cross-sectional area (measured with computed tomography (CT)) of all the major muscle groups except the hip abductors. This somewhat surprising result may be explained by the inability of CT to detect alterations in intra- and extramuscular fat and other non-contractile components. An additional measure, radiological density, which gives an indication of loss of contractile muscle, did show a reduction in the hip abductors (Rasch *et al.*, 2007). Another study of an active, high functioning population of subjects with unilateral hip OA did not show a weakness in hip flexion, extension, abduction and adduction when compared with a control group of similar functional status (Sims *et al.*, 2002).

In summary, it appears all muscle groups may be weakened in hip OA. Clinical observation suggests that around the hip, tightness and overactivity in the hip flexors (tensor fascia lata (TFL) and rectus femoris) and weakness in the hip extensors/abductors (glutei muscles) are common findings. Thus it is recommended that both glutei are likely to benefit from strengthening exercises in subjects with hip pathology.

Range of motion and flexibility

There are no trials that have specifically addressed this aspect of exercise in hip OA. All studies of exercise and the hip have included range of motion and stretching exercises as part of the programme (van Baar *et al.*, 1998; Hoeksma *et al.*, 2004; MacDonald *et al.*, 2006).

Balance and proprioception

There are no studies that have specifically evaluated balance or proprioceptive exercises in hip OA. One study used kinetic postural control measures (centre of pressure) to evaluate a physiotherapy programme including range of motion, strengthening and relaxation exercises in 80 males with hip OA (Giemza *et al.*, 2007). The specific exercises were not stated but the programme also included massage, heat and ice. Subjects were treated five times a week for 6 weeks. It was concluded that the physiotherapy programme improved the subjects' postural control, with a reduction in centre of pressure medio-laterally and in antero-posterior excursion. This suggests balance can be improved in subjects with hip OA but due to the multi-modal treatment it is not possible to identify the relative importance of specific interventions. The lack of a control group makes it impossible to know if the hip OA group had impaired balance at the start of the programme.

Common injuries/conditions

Hip OA

Hip OA is a common disorder characterised by loss of articular cartilage and new bone formation (Sokoloff, 1969). The incidence of hip OA increases with age (Felson *et al.*, 2000) but genetic and systemic factors (e.g. obesity) are also part of its aetiology (Dieppe and Lohmander, 2005). Occupations involving carrying heavy loads, exposure to vibration, repeated stair climbing or jumping (e.g. farmers and miners) increase the risk of developing hip OA (Vignon *et al.*, 2006). Clinically, there is a loss of joint range of motion, with internal rotation loss most closely linked to with radiographic hip OA (Birrell *et al.*, 2001).

Femoro-acetabular impingement

Femoro-acetabular impingement is characterised by a contact between the head and neck of the femur with the acetabular rim and is associated with abnormalities of the proximal femur and the acetabulum (Beck *et al.*, 2005). One commonly described variety of impingement is cam impingement, where an aspherical femoral head is jammed into the acetabulum during normal ranges of flexion, leading to chondral damage and labral tears (Lavigne *et al.*, 2004). The other common variety is pincer impingement, where there is contact between the acetabular rim and the femoral head neck junction due to acetabular over-coverage (Lavigne *et al.*, 2004). It is proposed that femoro-acetabular impingements are a common cause of early hip OA.

Instability/dislocation

Although the hip is considered to be an inherently stable joint, the concept of hip instability is gaining momentum. Several clinical syndromes have been described that have as their basis an excessive anterior translation of the femoral head during hip motion (Sahrmann, 2002). Atraumatic instability is thought to occur as a result of repetitive hip rotation with axial loading (Shindle *et al.*, 2006). This leads to capsular stretching and labral injury with subsequent micro-instability. Such a process may occur in athletes such as figure skaters, soccer players, ballet dancers and gymnasts. The hip may also dislocate (e.g. dash-board injury in motor vehicle accident) or subluxate (e.g. fall on a flexed hip and knee playing football), commonly in a posterior direction (Shindle *et al.*, 2006).

Labral tears

Tears of the acetabular labrum are increasingly recognised with the anterior labrum most commonly affected (McCarthy *et al.*, 2001). The labrum has sensory nerve endings in the superficial layers, making it a source of pain (Kim and Azuma, 1995). It may be damaged by any of the conditions described above as well as trauma. The labrum is continuous with chondral cartilage and thus labral tears are commonly associated with chondral defects (McCarthy *et al.*, 2001).

Trochanteric bursitis

This commonly used term is best renamed 'greater trochanteric pain syndrome' as recent evidence has failed to find bursal inflammation in subjects with lateral trochanteric pain (Silva *et al.*, 2008). Instead this condition is likely to be a combination of gluteus medius and minimus tears or insertional tendinopathy (Kong *et al.*, 2007). It is more common in older females and is more likely in the presence of low back pain and knee OA (Segal *et al.*, 2007).

Evidence of exercise efficacy in the management of pelvic girdle pain

Dysfunctions of the pelvis are common in pregnancy, with PGP a common feature in 7–25% of women (Wu *et al.*, 2004; Van De Pol *et al.*, 2007). There is a body of evidence which has examined exercise in the management of PGP. A systematic

review of physiotherapy treatments for pregnancy-related low back pain and PGP failed to find evidence of positive effect (Stuge *et al.*, 2003). The authors identified two high-quality trials (Nilsson-Wikmar *et al.*, 1998; Mens *et al.*, 2000) which failed to find a difference in pain intensity and functional status between exercise and control groups.

One of these studies (Mens *et al.*, 2000) utilised an exercise approach, based on the concept of diagonal slings linking the gluteus maximus, latissimus dorsi and the oblique abdominals in stabilising the sacroiliac joint. Attachment of these muscles via the posterior layer of thoraco-lumbar fascia provides compressive forces across the sacroiliac joint, which has been termed force closure (Pool-Goudzwaard *et al.*, 1998). This approach was compared with two control groups. One group did not do any exercises and the other exercised the longitudinal muscles (rectus abdominis, erector spinae and quadratus lumborum). All subjects were approximately 4 months post partum and were treated for 8 weeks. While the diagonal sling proposition is attractive, the results of the study did not show a difference between the groups in terms of pain and perceived improvement (Mens *et al.*, 2000). One possible reason was that in the study design the exercises were given to patients on a videotape, which did not allow for individual modification. Approximately 25% of the treatment group experienced an increase in symptoms from the exercises (Mens *et al.*, 2000), particularly longer lever exercises targeting the gluteus maximus.

Stuge *et al.* (2004) published a study on the physiotherapy management of PGP after their systematic review, in which each subject was examined individually and a programme most appropriate to the individual was formulated and supervised throughout. In this study, both groups received other physiotherapy modalities as appropriate (mobilisation, massage, heat, etc.) but the treatment group performed exercises based on the diagonal sling approach and also utilised specific stabilising exercises (Stuge *et al.*, 2004). The control group received instruction on strengthening and stretching exercises but no specific stabilising exercises. The intervention period was 20 weeks with approximately 11 treatments in this time. Both groups commenced treatment approximately 10 weeks post partum. Subjects undergoing the specific stabilising programme had lower pain intensity, disability and a higher quality of life than the control group (Stuge *et al.*, 2004).

The specific stabilising exercises were low load contractions of the transversus abdominis with co-activation of the multifidus. Other authors have demonstrated that muscles such as the erector spinae, gluteus maximus and biceps femoris also increase sacroiliac joint stiffness and help in force closure (van Wingerden *et al.*, 2004). Thus, it would appear that exercise approaches for persons with PGP should include training for the transverse abdominal wall, pelvic floor, multifidus and gluteus maximus.

However, it would be a mistake to assume that stabilisation exercises are a necessary requirement in the management of all PGP disorders. Recently O'Sullivan (O'Sullivan and Beales, 2007b,c) has argued that appropriate management of subjects with PGP is dependent on subclassifying subjects into groups. Mechanical PGP (as opposed to inflammatory) subjects may present with disorders of inadequate or excessive force closure. The two groups can be identified by, among other things, their different responses to compression. Subjects with reduced force closure are helped with external compression (e.g. the active straight leg raise test) whereas in subjects with excessive force closure, their condition is aggravated by these procedures. Thus, in some cases it may be necessary to embark on a muscle relaxation or stretching programme (O'Sullivan and Beales, 2007b).

Aerobic exercise

No trials have examined the specific effects of aerobic exercise on PGP. Given the positive effects in subjects with low back pain (see Chapter 6) one may expect a similarly beneficial effect in PGP.

Muscle strength and endurance

The preceding section on evidence of PGP exercise programmes has reviewed two studies where the diagonal sling and specific stabilising muscles have been targeted. The subjects in both of these studies were post partum.

Several other studies have investigated exercises designed to improve pelvic girdle support in subjects pre partum. One study compared three groups

that received information or home exercise or supervised exercise (Nilsson-Wikmar *et al.*, 2005). The supervised exercises targeted the gluteals, latissimus dorsi and abdominals whereas the home exercise group performed movements of the arms and legs in sitting, standing and four-point kneeling while maintaining the pelvis in a stable position. Pain and function in all groups improved post partum with no evidence that either of the exercise groups were superior to the information group. It was concluded that perhaps exercise needs to be more specific for the transversus abdominis or may not be effective until after delivery (Nilsson-Wikmar *et al.*, 2005). Stabilising exercises (transversus abdominis and pelvic floor contractions) were found to reduce PGP pain in pre-partum women more effectively than standard intervention (education and unsupervised home exercise programme) (Elden *et al.*, 2005).

Two other studies examined the effects of pre-partum exercises on the resolution of PGP post partum. One compared an intervention which included information, advice on posture and activities of daily living, and exercises (stretching and stabilising but not described in the text) with a control group with PGP who did not receive treatment (Haugland *et al.*, 2006). Four sessions were delivered to small groups once per week for four weeks during weeks 18–32 of gestation. At 6 and 12 months post partum there was no difference in pain levels between the groups. These findings were consistent with another study in which the recovery from PGP post partum was not influenced by either specific stabilising exercises or acupuncture as additions to standard treatment administered between gestational weeks 12 and 31 (Elden *et al.*, 2008).

Range of motion and flexibility

None of the studies have specifically addressed the benefits of this type of exercise although several studies have included stretching in the exercise programme (Stuge *et al.*, 2004; Nilsson-Wikmar *et al.*, 2005; Haugland *et al.*, 2006).

Balance and proprioception

Exercises of this type have not been investigated in subjects with PGP.

Common pelvic conditions/injuries

Inflammatory arthritis

The sacroiliac joint may be affected by spondyloarthropathies such as ankylosing spondylitis, which is a progressive inflammatory disorder. Clinical features include back pain and progressive stiffness of the spine (Dakwar *et al.*, 2008).

Mechanically induced PGP disorders

A recent paper attempted to develop a logical pragmatic approach to identifying mechanically induced PGP (O'Sullivan and Beales, 2007b). This was done in order to bypass the often complicated and confusing clinical models that had previously formed the basis for treatment. Using this approach mechanical PGP disorders can be subdivided into two main groups as described below.

- *Reduced force closure*: The underlying dysfunction in this group is increased strain on sensitive and lax ligamentous tissue in the sacroiliac joint in association with a reduced ability of the central nervous system to provide appropriate muscle support, i.e. reduced force closure. This is commonly present post partum (O'Sullivan and Beales, 2007b). This group will typically respond well to stabilising exercises.
- *Increased force closure*: In this group the pain is due to excessive sustained loading of sensitive structures in the sacroiliac joint by the surrounding muscles i.e.: increased force closure. In this group, PGP is often aggravated by performing stabilising exercises (O'Sullivan and Beales, 2007b).

SECTION 2A: PRACTICAL USE OF EXERCISE AROUND THE HIP

Prior to commencing any exercise programme the physiotherapist must have assessed the patient and identified specific dysfunctions in the neuromuscular system. The following exercise approaches are necessarily general and all patients must have a programme tailored to their specific needs.

Aerobic exercise

As has been noted in Section 1, there is limited evidence that aerobic exercise is beneficial in subjects with hip OA. However, the reader should review Chapter 11, which identifies aerobic exercise as of benefit to subjects with knee OA. A simple graded walking or swimming programme may provide good benefits to patients with hip OA.

An example of a walking programme (modified from Ettinger *et al.*, 1997) is given in Table 10.1.

Note: Care should be taken to ensure an optimal gait pattern. This may require use of walking aids such as a stick or walking poles (Fig. 10.1).

Strengthening exercise

As a general rule the exercises should replicate the function which will be required. For example, the gluteals are required to work in their inner range during stance phase of gait. Thus exercises should be performed in this functional range (Sullivan *et al.*, 1982).

Early phase

In order to encourage a beneficial co-activation of the surrounding hip muscles to optimise support of the joint an early-stage exercise is to ask the patient to gently draw the hip into the socket. This may be done in supine crook lying (Fig. 10.2) and may be facilitated by asking the patient to resist a gentle long axis distraction. Once learned, this action may be incorporated prior to the commencement of other exercises.

Gluteus medius is retrained in side lying with an external rotation of the hip (Fig. 10.3). The emphasis is on hip motion without motion in the pelvis and low back. Adjusting the degree of hip flexion may be required to ensure the activation is of gluteus medius rather than TFL. Emphasis is on maintaining an inner range hold for up to 10 seconds, provided the patient has sufficient endurance. The number of repetitions is again determined by the patient's ability.

Both gluteus maximus and gluteus medius contraction may be facilitated by inner range hip exten-

Table 10.1 Walking programme for hip osteoarthritis

Week	Frequency	Duration	Programme
Week 1	2 days per week	25 min	Warm up 5 min (slow walking, arm circles, trunk rotation, shoulder and chest stretches, and side stretch) Walk 15 min (ideally 50% of max heart rate) Warm down (slow walking and three flexibility exercises: a shoulder stretch, hamstring stretch, and lower back stretch)
Week 2	3 days per week	25 min	As per week 1
Week 3	3 days per week	30 min	Increase walk to 20 min
Week 4	3 days per week	40 min	Increase walk to 30 min
Week 5	3 days per week	50 min	Increase walk to 40 min
Week 6+	3 days per week	60 min	Increase walk to 50 min

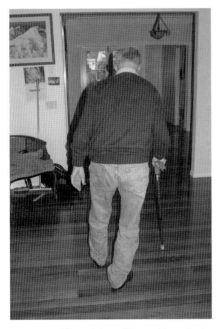

Figure 10.1 An older adult walking with a single stick to minimise limp.

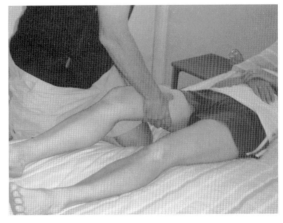

Figure 10.2 Manual facilitation of co-activation of hip muscles to draw the hip into the socket. The therapist is applying a gentle longitudinal distraction along the line of the femur while the patient resists this action.

sion in supine with leg over the side of the bed (Fig. 10.4). This closed kinetic chain exercise has the advantage over open chain exercise such as prone hip extension because the weight-bearing component effectively stimulates mechanoreceptors around the joint, improving muscular contraction (Dee, 1969; Kisner and Colby, 1996).

Open chain hip extension in prone is best performed after the previous exercise when the muscle is likely to be optimally facilitated. Focus initially would be on maintaining an inner range hold (Fig. 10.5).

Hip external rotation may also be retrained in sitting with Thera- Band® resistance (Fig. 10.6). A neutral spine position is essential to the optimal

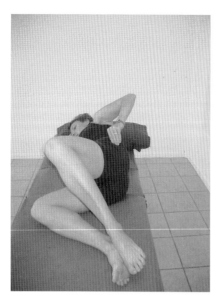

Figure 10.3 Retraining inner range gluteus medius function in side lying. The patient performs hip external rotation without movement in the trunk or pelvis and use their hand to ensure gluteus medius is active.

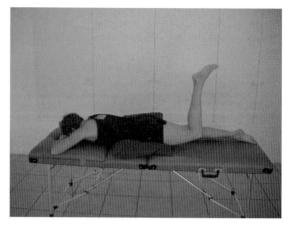

Figure 10.5 Retraining inner range gluteus maximus function in prone. The patient performs hip extension with knee flexion. The pillow helps to maintain the lumbar spine in a neutral position.

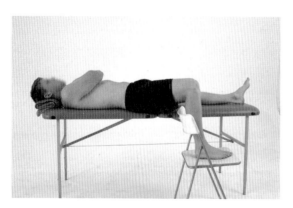

Figure 10.4 Retraining inner range gluteus maximus function in supine lying. The patient performs hip extension with knee flexion to minimise hamstring contribution. The lumbar spine is maintained in a neutral position.

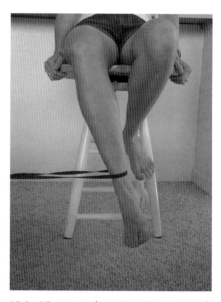

Figure 10.6 Hip external rotation in sitting with Thera-Band® resistance.

performance of this exercise. It is proposed that in addition to gluteus medius, iliopsoas is also active in this exercise (Johnston *et al.*, 1999).

It is important to include retraining of gluteus medius function in standing early in a rehabilitation programme. Initially this may involve optimising the standing posture (specific to the individual patient) and training them to maintain pelvic alignment in the frontal plane while they lift their contralateral limb onto a step (Fig. 10.7). This may

initially require a conscious pre-activation of the stance limb gluteals.

Later phase

Higher-level gluteus medius exercise is done by performing hip abduction with an extended knee (Fig. 10.8). The hip must not drift into flexion or internal

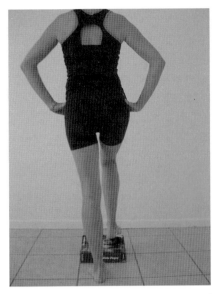

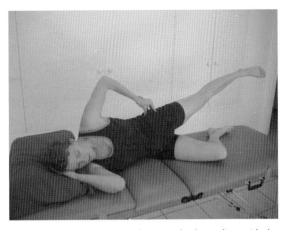

Figure 10.8 Hip abduction keeping the leg in line with the trunk and palpating the gluteus medius to ensure it is active.

Figure 10.7 Stepping while maintaining optimal pelvic alignment of the stance limb.

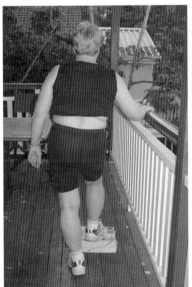

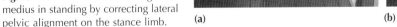

Figure 10.9 Activation of gluteus medius in standing by correcting lateral pelvic alignment on the stance limb.

(a)   (b)

rotation to avoid TFL dominating the abduction synergy. Rehabilitation should target inner range holds initially but may also include through range repetitions.

Standing gluteus medius activity can be progressed by having the patient stand with one foot on a step. The stance limb gluteus medius then eccentrically lowers and concentrically raises the contralateral pelvis (Fig. 10.9). The patient must be aware not to rely on the contralateral trunk lateral flexors (quadratus lumborum) to dominate in this exercise. Use of a mirror may help to reinforce the

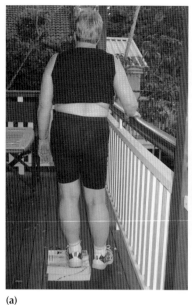 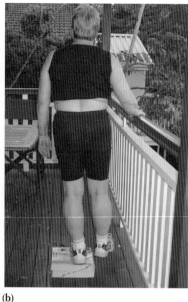

(a)   **(b)**

Figures 10.10 A progression of gluteus medius activation in standing by correcting lateral pelvic alignment on the stance limb as the contralateral pelvis is slowly lowered and raised.

correct movement pattern. This may be progressed by standing on a step with the contralateral limb unsupported. The stance limb abductors then control the lowering and raising of the contralateral pelvis (Fig. 10.10). Depending on the specific dysfunction present in the patient it may be necessary to practise maintaining control of the pelvic position during gait, e.g. stance phase of gait. This may be enhanced by use of a mirror.

Higher-level gluteus maximus function should include double leg squats where instruction of correct technique is important. It is optimal for the patient to keep the anterior knee over the middle of the arch of the foot during the squat (Fig. 10.11). During the return to the upright position the patient must initiate the movement from the pelvis and not the thorax. Bridging exercises are also good to challenge gluteus maximus function to a higher level.

It may also be important to modify standing postures to optimise gluteus medius and maximus function. For example, patients who tend to slouch and stand excessively onto one limb are instructed to limit the amount of hip adduction by maintaining gluteus medius tone (Fig. 10.12). Similarly, people who stand with excessive lumbar extension may need to incorporate gluteus maximus activity to maintain a more neutral position of the pelvis relative to the lumbar spine.

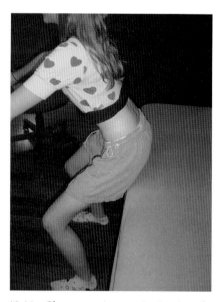

Figure 10.11 Gluteus maximus activation in a functional squat position whilst maintaining good lumbo-pelvic alignment.

Range of motion and flexibility exercises

There is no specific published evidence that stretching exercises are useful when dealing with hip

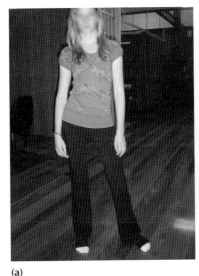
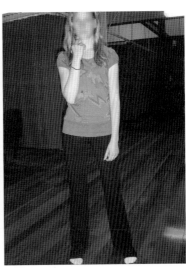

Figure 10.12 Utilising active control to minimise slouch standing on stance limb. (**a**) The patient is standing in excessive lateral pelvic tilt. (**b**) This has been corrected by activation of the gluteus medius.

(a) (b)

pathology. However, two studies which did identify benefits for subjects with hip OA both included stretching in the treatment programme (van Baar *et al.*, 1998; Hoeksma *et al.*, 2004). It is recommended that all patients should be assessed individually to identify specific muscle tightness. However, the hip flexors, hip adductors and hip external rotators will commonly require stretching. Suggested stretches for these regions are shown in Figure 10.13. When stretching the hip external rotators it is important to avoid an increase in groin discomfort.

Proprioceptive and balance training

There is no published evidence on this form of training. It may be that in some cases basic balance training may be a useful means of generally facilitating muscles around the hip prior to strengthening exercises. A progression from maintaining static positions (Fig. 10.14a tandem stance) to more dynamic situations (Fig. 10.14b standing on one leg with contralateral leg swings) to advanced situations (e.g. standing on one leg with contralateral leg swings and eyes closed).

Summary

In order to sustain the beneficial effects of treatment it is important that the patient continues with the programme after a treatment phase. An important way to achieve this is to incorporate exercises into functional tasks that the patient performs regularly. Exercise training should simulate the functional tasks (Pisters *et al.*, 2007) or aim simply to alter movement patterns during the functional tasks so that the appropriate muscles are recruited or stretched.

SECTION 2B: PRACTICAL USE OF EXERCISE AROUND THE PELVIS

This section provides a brief outline of the use of exercise around the pelvis. The specific exercises are outlined elsewhere in this text. Again it is critical to assess each patient to design a programme specifically tailored to their needs.

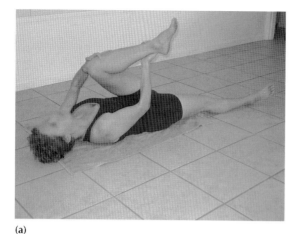

(a)

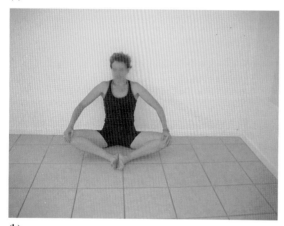

(b)

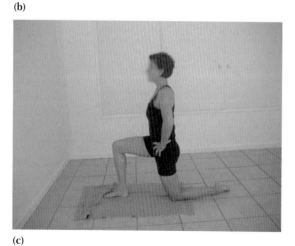

(c)

Figure 10.13 Stretches for the (**a**) buttock, (**b**) hip adductors and (**c**) flexors. Note: (**c**) the neutral lumbo-pelvic position and (**b**) the use of the wall to maintain an upright position of the trunk.

Aerobic exercise

Several studies have indicated that general aerobic activity is beneficial in the management of low back pain (see Chapter 6). There is every reason to believe that a carefully structured aerobic exercise programme would have a similar benefit for patients with PGP.

Any aerobic exercise should take into account the ability to transfer load through the pelvis. Given that in many patients the pain is likely to be aggravated by the excessive impact forces associated with walking and running, the pool may be more appropriate. It is also wise to avoid activities with emphasis on twisting and rapid direction changes (e.g. tennis, squash, netball) until muscle strength and pain are both improved. An example of a low-impact pool session programme is given in Table 10.2.

Strengthening exercise

As seen in Section 1 the evidence suggests that patients with PGP due to reduced force closure will respond well to exercise targeting the transverse abdominal wall, the pelvic floor, multifidus and gluteus maximus. A strengthening programme for the hip musculature would follow the same progressions as outlined in Section 2A. A programme to improve lumbo-pelvic muscle function is described in Chapter 6 on the lumbar spine.

In most cases, the success of any exercise programme hinges on the patient being able to incorporate muscle support into functional situations such as standing and walking. As has been described in Section 2A this may require activation of the gluteals and the transverse abdominal wall muscles to maintain an optimal alignment between the pelvis and the lumbar spine (Fig. 10.15). Neglecting this important aspect of exercise therapy will lead to disappointing results.

Range of motion and stretching exercises

There is no specific evidence regarding stretching and the management of PGP. One study showing

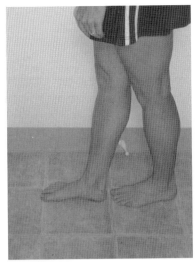 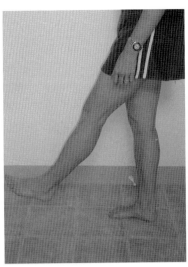

Figure 10.14 (a) Tandem stance and (b) leg swings. This exercise can be progressed by repeating with eyes closed.   (a)   (b)

Table 10.2 A low-impact pool session for patients with PGP

Warm-up	Walk 1 min forward
	Walk 1 min backward
	Walk 1 min side step
	Repeat twice
	Stretch hip flexor/quads/buttock/low back/shoulders overhead
Main set	10 squats
	10 lunges
	10 leg forward leg swings each side (focus on keeping abdominal support)
	Treading water holding onto pool side (1 min)
	Shoulder abduction (bilateral) in squat position 10 ×
	Trunk rotations with arms in 90° flex 10 × each side
	Horizontal shoulder flex/ext in squat 10 × each direction
	Treading water holding onto pool side (1 min)
Cool-down	Walk 3 min
	Gentle bicycling/kicking, holding onto edge of pool (2 min) (focus on relaxation via breathing)

improvement in PGP with exercises included stretching of the buttock, hip flexors and quadriceps in the programme, based on an individual assessment of the patient (Stuge *et al.*, 2004). Stretches of these muscle groups are described in Section 2A. It is likely that patients with PGP related to excessive force closure may respond better to stretching exercises of muscles identified as being overactive.

Proprioception exercises

There is no documented evidence to support this form of training in patients with PGP. However, it may be relevant to re-educate patients and increase their awareness of trunk and pelvis body position to improve sitting and standing postures. The use of a mirror to optimise this is recommended.

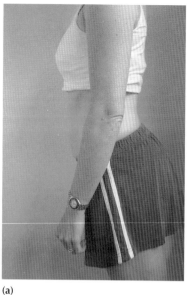
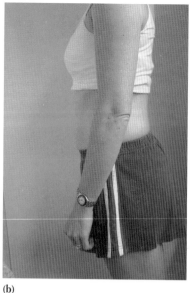

(a)   (b)

Figure 10.15 Correcting lumbo-pelvic position from excessive anterior pelvic tilt (**a**) to a more neutral position (**b**) using activation of the transverse abdominal wall and the gluteals.

SECTION 3: CASE STUDIES AND STUDENT QUESTIONS

Case study 1

A 68-year-old woman presents with 4 years of left groin pain and stiffness gradually becoming more noticeable. An X-ray shows degenerative changes in the hip joint with a loss of superior joint space. Her main functional problems are stiffness after prolonged sitting and in the morning. She also is unable to walk or stand for more than an hour before experiencing significant groin discomfort. Examination reveals a loss of internal rotation, flexion and extension. During left stance phase of gait her left hip is kept in slight adduction the pelvis shifts to the left. She has weakness of the gluteus medius and maximus and an overactive TFL.

Management

This woman has a mild superior form of hip OA. Her functional problems are standing and walking, and treatment is focused on improving these

issues. Manual therapy (a longitudinal distraction) is used early to improve movement, reduce pain and give an associated improvement in muscle activation. Gentle massage and stretching of the left TFL is also done before starting on the exercise approach. Early exercise treatment is based on improving the function of the gluteus medius. This is done in side lying with a pillow between knees and externally rotating the hip. With manual guidance of the motion, the patient is able to activate the gluteus medius without domination of the TFL. She can hold this position for only 2–3 seconds and after four repetitions she is fatigued. Following this, the patient practises standing on the left leg with the right leg on a step. In this position the patient maintains the pelvis in a neutral position in the frontal plane (i.e. avoids stance limb hip adduction) using the gluteus medius and not the TFL. This position does not feel normal to the patient and a mirror is an important tool to improve her awareness of the

Case study 1—cont'd

new position. She is instructed that she must replicate this new position for as long as possible whenever she is standing.

Further treatments involve progressing the gluteus medius into inner range and increasing the length of holding time up to 10 seconds. The standing exercises are progressed to lifting the contralateral limb off the step while maintaining the pelvis in the neutral position. It is important to introduce gait re-education into the programme as her awareness of pelvis neutral improves. Initially this is done using a stick in the opposite hand which allows her to focus (with feedback from therapist and mirror) on minimising the excessive lateral motion of the pelvis. In addition to this she is also given a stretch for the TFL and prone hip extensions to improve gluteus medius activation. From this point the patient is encouraged to walk without the stick as her gait pattern improves. She is also educated about controlling her walking volumes to reduce flare-ups. She also joins a local seniors group for water exercises once a week. Two years later her pain is much reduced and she is able to walk longer distances.

Case study 2

A 28-year-old delivery driver presents with 6 months of right groin pain following an incident in standing when he was forced into lumbar hyperextension with his pelvis fixed. He initially had low back pain, which later settled, and is now troubled by groin pain on walking (as the right hip extends) and prolonged standing. On examination he stands in a sway back posture with increased passive hip extension. He has poor abdominal and gluteal tone bilaterally, worse on the right side and his gluteus maximus activation and strength are poor. His range of hip extension is excessive, psoas is lengthened and weak. Passive accessory glides indicate increased anterior range of motion. An MRI of the hip is normal.

Management

This man has clinical signs of instability which fit in with the mechanism of injury of hip hyperextension. Because his pain is aggravated by standing the initial focus of treatment is to improve the position of passive hip extension in which he habitually stands. This is done by doing posterior pelvic tilts in supine which activate the abdominals and gluteus maximus. This is immediately incorporated into standing with feedback to bring the pelvis back under the trunk. A mirror is required to illustrate this to him and he immediately feels more comfortable in this position. To manage the pain with walking, he is given a squat exercise in standing and a prone hip extension exercise to improve gluteal activation.

Once this programme has been started he is also instructed on maintaining a better neutral spine posture in sitting. He practises moving in and out of this position when driving. This encourages activation of psoas. To further activate this muscle hip external rotation with Thera-Band® resistance in a neutral spine sitting posture is also added. The patient also finds that his pain on walking can be reduced if he tries to keep his pelvis under his trunk. This leads to better recruitment of the abdominals and gluteals (and probably the psoas also). Two months later his pain is absent in standing and his walking is much improved provided that he does not over-stride. He is happy with his progress and elects to self-manage his condition with a continuation of his exercise programme.

Case study 3

A 34-year-old woman presents with right groin pain 6 weeks after the birth of her third child. She noted increased low back discomfort in the last 8 weeks of her pregnancy. This settled but she was anxious to return to activity post partum and as she increased walking volume the groin pain developed 3 weeks post partum. It is also noticeable at night when she rolls over in bed and when she gets out of a chair. On examination she weight-bears more on the right leg and tends to favour this leg on rising from the chair. She has tenderness on palpation through the right adductor longus belly and insertion on the pubic ramus. She has a positive active straight leg raise when lifting the left leg which reproduces her right groin pain. Compression of the sacroiliac joint completely relieves the pain. She has poor gluteal tone and activation bilaterally and stands in a passive sway extension of the lumbar spine and hip.

Management

This patient has adductor pain due to inadequate attempts to provide force closure to the sacroiliac joint. This has been aggravated by attempts to increase activity too soon after birth. She is instructed on transversus abdominis and pelvic floor exercises in supine. She is quickly able to perform this accurately. On the first day she is also given a posterior tilt exercise in supine. In standing she controls her passive lumbar extension by repositioning her pelvis under the trunk. She is quickly able to do this as well. Finally, she is given a squat exercise focusing on equal weight-bearing. She is instructed on pacing her walking so that she is not exceeding her capabilities.

Two weeks later she reports that she is significantly better. The only time she notices any groin pain is if she tries to walk too fast. She has minimal tenderness in the adductor longus and her active straight leg raise is no longer positive. Her abdominal exercises are progressed to include unilateral leg lifts in supine while maintaining a neutral spine position. She is instructed to increase the volume of the squat exercise. She also is asked to include walking up a mild incline near her home as a means of getting good gluteal recruitment. After another 2 weeks she is very happy, with minimal pain, and is able to exercise more without exacerbation of her symptoms.

Student questions

(1) On what is the evidence base for exercise in the management of hip disorders largely based?
(2) Do the beneficial effects of hip exercise in clinical studies persist once the programme has finished?
(3) What is the evidence comparing exercise and manual therapy in managing hip pain and improving function?
(4) Which muscles are most likely to be adversely affected by hip pain and pathology?
(5) What is one possible reason why the study of the effects of exercise of the diagonal sling muscles failed to show a positive effect on the management of PGP?
(6) Which muscles have been identified to play a key role in providing force closure to the sacroiliac joint?
(7) Is there evidence that exercise in pre partum women can influence the recovery from PGP in women?
(8) Do all people with PGP require stability training?
(9) Why is it important to retrain the gluteus medius and maximus in the inner range?
(10) Which group of patients with PGP is likely to respond better to stretching exercises?

References

Arokoski, M., Arkoski, J.P., Haara, M., Kankaapaa, M., Vesterinen, M., Niemitukia, L.H. and Helminen, H.J. (2002) Hip muscle strength and muscle cross sectional area in men with and without hip osteoarthritis. *Journal of Rheumatology*, 29, 2185–2195.

Beck, M., Kalhor, M., Leunig, M. and Ganz, R. (2005) Hip morphology influences the pattern of damage to the acetabular cartilage: femoroacetabular impingement as a cause of early osteoarthritis of the hip. *Journal of Bone and Joint Surgery, British Volume*, 87, 1012–1018.

Birrell, F., Croft, P., Cooper, C., Hosie, G., Macfarlane, G., Silman, A. and PRC Hip Study Group. (2001) Predicting radiographic hip osteoarthritis from range of movement. *Rheumatology*, 40, 506–512.

Cochrane, T., Davey, R.C. and Mattews Edwards, S.M. (2005) Randomised controlled trial of the cost-effectiveness of water-based therapy for lower limb osteoarthritis. *Health Technology Assessment*, 9, 1–114.

Dakwar, E., Reddy, J., Vale, F.L. and Uribe, J.S. (2008) A review of the pathogenesis of ankylosing spondylitis. *Neurosurgical Focus*, 24, E2.

Dee, R. (1969) Structure and function of hip joint innervation. *Annals of the Royal College of Surgeons of England*, 45, 357–374.

Dieppe, P. and Lohmander, L. (2005) Pathogenesis and management of pain in osteoarthritis. *Lancet*, 365, 965–973.

Elden, H., Ladfors, L., Olsen, M.F., Ostgaard, H.C. and Hagberg, H. (2005) Effects of acupuncture and stabilising exercises as adjunct to standard treatment in pregnant women with pelvic girdle pain: randomised single blind controlled trial. *British Medical Journal*, 330, 761.

Elden, H., Hagbreg, H., Olsen, M.F., Ladfors, L. and Ostgaard, H.C. (2008) Regression of pelvic girdle pain after delivery: follow-up of a randomised single blind controlled trial with different treatment modalities. *Acta Obstetricia et Gynecologica Scandinavica*, 87, 201–208.

Ettinger, W.J., Burns, R., Messier, S.P., Applegate, W., Rejeski, W.J., Morgan, T., Shumaker, S., Berry, M.J., O'Toole, M., Monu, J. and Craven, T. (1997) A randomized trial comparing aerobic exercise and resistance exercise with a health education program in older adults with knee osteoarthritis. The Fitness Arthritis and Seniors Trial (FAST). *Journal of the American Medical Association*, 277, 25–31.

Felson, D., Lawerence, R.C., Dieppe, P.A., Hirsch, R., Helmick, C.G., Jordan, J.M., Kington, R.S., Lane, N.E., Nevitt, M.C., Zhang, Y., Sowers, M., McAlindon, T., Spector, T.D., Poole, A.R., Yanovski, S.Z., Ateshian, G., Sharma, L., Buckwalter, J.A., Brandt, K.D. and Fries, J.F. (2000) Osteoarthritis: new insights. Part 1: the disease and its risk factors. *Annals of Internal Medicine*, 133, 635–646.

Giemza, C., Ostrowska, B. and Matczak-Giemza, M. (2007) The effect of physiotherapy training programme on postural stability in men with hip osteoarthritis. *Aging Male*, 10, 67–70.

Haugland, K., Rasmussen, S. and Daltveit, A.K. (2006) Group intervention for women with pelvic pain in pregnancy. A randomized controlled trial. *Acta Obstetrics et Gynecologica Scandanavica*, 85, 1320–1326.

Hinman, R., Heywood, S. and Day, A.R. (2007) Aquatic physical therapy for hip and knee osteoarthritis: Results of a single-blind randomized controlled trial. *Physical Therapy*, 87, 32–43.

Hoeksma, H., Dekker, J., Ronday, H.K., Heering, A., van der Lubbe, N., Vel, C., Breedveld, F.C. and van der Ende, C.H. (2004) Comparison of manual therapy and exercise therapy in osteoarthritis of the hip: a randomized clinical trial. *Arthritis and Rheumatism*, 51, 722–279.

Johnston, C., Lindsay, D.M. and Wiley J.P. (1999) Treatment of iliopsoas syndrome with a hip rotation strengthening program: A retrospective case series. *Journal of Orthopedic and Sports Physical Therapy*, 29, 218–224.

Kim, Y. and Azuma, H. (1995) The nerve endings of the acetabular labrum. *Clinical Orthopedics and Related Research*, 320, 176–181.

Kisner, C. and Colby, L. (1996) *Therapeutic Exercise – Foundations and Techniques*. FA Davis Company, Philadelphia, Pennsylvania.

Kong, A., Van der Vliet, A. and Zadow, S. (2007) MRI and US of gluteal tendinopathy in greater trochanteric pain syndrome. *European Radiology*, 17, 1772–1783.

Kovar, P., Allegrante, J.P., MacKenzie, C.R., Peterson, M.G., Gutin, B. and Charlson, M.E. (1992) Supervised fitness walking in patients with osteoarthritis of the knee. A randomized, controlled trial. *Annals of Internal Medicine*, 116, 529–534.

Lavigne, M., Parvici, J., Beck, M., Siebenrock, K.A., Ganz, R. and Leunig, M. (2004) Anterior femoroacetabular impingement: part 1. Techniques of joint preserving surgery. *Clinical Orthopedics and Related Research*, 418, 61–66.

MacDonald, C., Whitman, J.M., Cleland, J.A., Smith, M. and Hoeksma, H.L. (2006) Clinical outcomes following manual physical therapy and exercise for hip osteoarthritis: A case Series. *Journal of Orthopedic and Sports Physical Therapy*, 36, 588–599.

McCarthy, J., Noble, P.C., Schuck, M.R., Wright, J. and Lee, J. (2001) The role of labral lesions to development of early degenerative hip disease. *Clinical Orthopedics and Related Research*, 393, 25–37.

Mens, J., Snijders, C.J. and Stam, H.J. (2000) Diagonal trunk muscle exercises in peripartum pelvic pain: a randomized clinical trial. *Physical Therapy*, 80, 1164–1173.

Nilsson-Wikmar, L., Holm, K., Oijerstedy, R., and Harms-Ringdahl, K. (1998) Effects of different treatments on pain and on functional activities in pregnant women with pelvic pain [abstract]. *Third Interdisciplinary World Congress On Low Back & Pelvic Pain; 1998 Nov 19–21; Vienna, Austria*, pp. 330–331.

Nilsson-Wikmar, L., Holm, K., Oijerstedt, R. and Harms-Ringdahl, K. (2005) Effect of three different physical therapy treatments on pain and activity in pregnant women with pelvic girdle pain: A randomized clinical trial with 3, 6, and 12 months follow-up postpartum. *Spine*, 30, 850–856.

O'Sullivan, P. and Beales, D. (2007b) Diagnosis and classification of pelvic girdle pain disorders – Part 1: A mechanism based approach within a biopsychosocial framework. *Manual Therapy*, 12, 86–97.

O'Sullivan, P. and Beales, D. (2007c) Diagnosis and classification of pelvic girdle pain disorders, Part 2: Illustration of the utility of a classification system via case studies. *Manual Therapy*, 12, e1–12.

Pisters, M., Veenhof, C., van Meeteren, N.L.U., Ostelo, R.W., de Bakker, D.H., Schellevis, F.G. and Dekker, J. (2007) Long-term effectiveness of exercise therapy in patients with osteoarthritis of the hip or knee: a systematic review. *Arthritis and Rheumatism*, 57, 1245–1253.

Pool-Goudzwaard, A., Vleeming, A., Stoeckart, R., Snijders, C.J. and Mens, J.M. (1998) Insufficient lumbopelvic stability: a clinical, anatomical and biomechanical approach to 'a-specific' low back pain. *Manual Therapy*, 3, 12–20.

Rasch, A., Byström, A., Dalen, N. and Berg, H.E. (2007) Reduced muscle radiological density, cross-sectional area, and strength of major hip and knee muscles in 22 patients with hip osteoarthritis. *Acta Orthopaedica*, 78, 505–510.

Roddy, E., Zhang, W., Doherty, M., Arden, N.K., Barlow, J., Birrell, F., Carr, A., Chakravarty, K., Dickson, J., Hay, E., Hosie, G., Hurley, M., Jordan, K.M., McCarthy, C., McMurdo, M., Mockett, S., O'Reilly, S., Peat, G., Pendleton, A. and Richards, S. (2005) Evidence-based recommendations for the role of exercise in the management of osteoarthritis of the hip or knee – the MOVE consensus. *Rheumatology*, 44, 67–73.

Sahrmann, S. (2002) *Diagnosis and Treatment of Movement Impairment Syndromes*. Mosby, St. Louis.

Segal, N., Felson, D.T., Torner, J.C., Zhu, Y., Curtis, J.R., Niu, J., Nevitt, M.C. and Multicenter Osteoarthritis Study Group (2007) Greater trochanteric pain syndrome: epidemiology and associated factors. *Archives of Physical Medicine and Rehabilitation*, 88, 988–992.

Shindle, M., Ranawat, A.S. and Kelly, B.T. (2006) Diagnosis and management of traumatic and atraumatic instability in the athletic patient. *Clinics in Sports Medicine*, 25, 309–326.

Silva, F., Adams, T., Feinstein, J. and Arroyo, R.A. (2008) Trochanteric bursitis: refuting the myth of inflammation. *Journal of Clinical Rheumatology*, 14, 82–86.

Sims, K., Richardson, C.A. and Brauer S.G. (2002) Investigation of hip abductor activation in subjects with clinical unilateral hip osteoarthritis. *Annals of the Rheumatic Diseases*, 61, 687–692.

Sokoloff, L. (1969). *The Biology of Degenerative Joint Disease*. University of Chicago Press, Chicago, Illinois.

Stener-Victorin, E., Kruse-Smidje, C. and Jung, K. (2004) Comparison between electro-acupuncture and hydrotherapy, both in combination with patient education and patient education alone, on the symptomatic treatment of osteoarthritis of the hip. *Clinical Journal of Pain*, 20, 179–185.

Stuge, B., Hilde, G. and Vollestad, N. (2003) Physical therapy for pregnancy-related low back and pelvic pain: a systematic review. *Acta Obstetrica et Gynecologica Scandanavica*, 82, 983–990.

Stuge, B., Laerum, E., Kirkesola, G. and Volestad, N. (2004) The efficacy of a treatment program focusing on specific stabilizing exercises for pelvic girdle pain after pregnancy. A randomized controlled trial. *Spine*, 29, 351–359.

Sullivan, P., Markos, P. and Minor, M.A.D. (1982) *An Integrated Approach to Therapeutic Exercise – Theory and Clinical Application*. Reston Publishing Company, Reston, Virginia.

Talbot, L., Gaines, J.M., Huynh, T.N. and Metter, E.J. (2003) A home-based pedometer-driven walking program to increase physical activity in older adults with osteoarthritis of the knee: a preliminary study. *Journal of American Geriatrics Society*, 51, 387–392.

van Baar, M., Dekker, J., Oostenorp, R.A., Bijl, D., Voorn, T.B., Lemmens, J.A. and Bijlisma, J.W. (1998) The effectiveness of exercise therapy in patients with osteoarthritis of the hip or knee: A randomized clinical trial. *Journal of Rheumatology*, 25, 2432–2439.

van Baar, M., Dekker, J., Oostenorp, R.A., Bijl, D., Voorn, T.B. and Bijlsma, J.W. (2001) Effectiveness of exercise in patients with osteoarthritis of hip or knee: nine months' follow up. *Annals of the Rheumatic Diseases*, 60, 1123–1130.

Van De Pol, G., Van Brummen, H.J., Bruinse, H.W., Heintz, A.P. and Van Der Vaart, C.H. (2007) Pregnancy-related pelvic girdle pain in the Netherlands. *Acta Obstetrica et Gynecologica Scandanavica*, 86, 416–422.

van Wingerden, J., Vleeming, A., Buyruk, H.M. and Raissadat, K. (2004) Stabilization of the sacroiliac joint in vivo: verification of muscular contribution to force closure of the pelvis. *European Spine Journal*, 13, 199–205.

Vignon, E., Valat, J.P., Rossignol, M., Avouac, B., Rozenberg, S., Thoumie, P., Avouac, J., Nordin, M. and Hilliquin, P. (2006) Osteoarthritis of the knee and hip and activity: a systematic international review and synthesis (OASIS). *Joint, Bone, Spine*, 73, 442–455.

Wu, W., Meijer, O., Uegaki, K. Mens, J.M., van Dieen, D.H., Wuisman, P.I. and Ostgaard, H.C. (2004) Pregnancy-related pelvic girdle pain (PPP), I: Terminology, clinical presentation, and prevalence. *European Spine Journal*, 13, 575–589.

Zhang, W., Moskowitz, R.W., Nuki, G., Abramson, S., Altman, R.D., Arden, N., Bierma-Zeinstra, S., Brandt, K.D., Croft, P., Doherty, M., Dougados, M., Hochberg, M., Hunter, D.J., Kwoh, K., Lohmander, L.S. and Tugwell, P. (2008) OARSI recommendations for the management of hip and knee osteoarthritis, Part II: OARSI evidence-based, expert consensus guidelines. *Osteoarthritis and Cartilage*, 16, 137–162.

Mandy Johnson

SECTION 1: INTRODUCTION AND BACKGROUND

The knee joint is one of the most commonly injured joints in both the working and the sporting environment. It is made susceptible to injury because of the shape of the bony surfaces and the two long lever arms, created by the femur and tibia. Its stability is provided by the soft tissues surrounding the joint. Even though the joint is technically unstable it takes tremendous force, more than three times the body weight (Chen and Black, 1980), to disrupt the surrounding soft tissue. The patellofemoral joint is integral to the correct functioning of the knee joint. It acts as a modified pulley system to lengthen the lever arm of the quadriceps mechanism.

Evidence for the use of exercise in the rehabilitation of knee injuries

The use of exercise for the rehabilitation of knee injuries has been well illustrated in the literature for numerous conditions and injuries, both acute and chronic. Fransen *et al.* (2001) carried out a systematic review of the use of exercise therapy for oste-

oarthritis (OA) of the knee. Seventeen randomised controlled trials (RCTs) were identified, which included 2562 patients. The studies looked at the effectiveness of an exercise programme in relation to self-reported pain and increases in physical function. There was a mixture of exercise protocols on both a group and individual basis. The overall conclusions were that therapeutic exercise demonstrates a beneficial effect on pain and physical function for people with symptomatic OA of the knee joint and that group therapy was as effective as individual therapy. Van Baar *et al.* (1999) also conducted a systematic review examining the effectiveness of exercise therapy in patients with OA of the hip or knee. They concluded that there was evidence to support the use of therapeutic exercise in the management of hip or knee OA. In an RCT of 83 patients with OA of the knee, Deyle *et al.* (2000) demonstrated that manual physiotherapy combined with an exercise programme (which included: stretches and range of motion (ROM) exercises; riding a stationary bike; muscle strengthening exercise) decreased pain and stiffness and increased the distance walked in 6 minutes and was associated with less surgery. A frequent mode of delivery of an exercise programme is through hydrotherapy which has a number of benefits, particularly in the management of the more disabled patient. Silva *et al.*

Exercise Therapy in the Management of Musculoskeletal Disorders, First Edition. Edited by Fiona Wilson, John Gormley and Juliette Hussey.
© 2011 Blackwell Publishing Ltd

(2008) examined the effect of a hydrotherapy exercise programme versus a conventional land-based exercise regimen for management of patients with OA of the knee. This RCT of 64 subjects concluded that although both water- and land-based exercises reduced knee pain and increased knee function, hydrotherapy was superior in relieving pain during and after walking. Further evidence in support of aquatic exercise in the management of knee (and hip) OA came from a systematic review of six trials (800 subjects) by Bartels *et al.* (2007). Although there were methodological limitations in a number of trials, the authors concluded that aquatic exercise has a beneficial effect in the short term for patients with OA of the hip or knee.

There are a number of studies on exercise protocols for anterior cruciate ligament (ACL) rehabilitation, pre and post surgical reconstruction, although some show methodological limitations. Trees *et al.* (2005) carried out a systematic review of treatment of isolated ACL injuries. They reviewed nine trials consisting of 391 participants. Two trials examined conservative treatment and the remainder examined exercise programmes, post surgery. The outcome measures for all these studies were return to work and return to pre-injury activity levels measured at 6 and 12 months. The general conclusions of this review were that even though active exercise is an accepted part of treatment of ACL injuries there were no significant differences between the various exercise routines.

Trees *et al.* (2007) carried out a systematic review of the exercise regimes of ACL injuries in combination with meniscal and collateral ligament injury which is more frequent than isolated injuries. Six studies were identified, involving 343 participants. One study was conservative and all the rest followed reconstruction surgery. The outcome measures were the same as in the previous review. Again all the studies involved exercise of various types from isometric to isotonic work, joint mobility, balance and proprioception. Some of the studies compared supervised with home-based programmes or accelerated versus non-accelerated programmes. The general conclusions were similar to the previous review in that there were no significant differences between exercise regimens. These reviews demonstrate that although exercise shows efficacy in the management of ACL injury, there is a requirement for further research, with well-controlled randomised studies, and consensus on suitable outcome

measures and surveillance periods. More specifically, there is a need to identify the exercise mode that is the most effective.

Compared with the number of studies on rehabilitation of the ACL, there is less evidence regarding the role of exercise in posterior cruciate ligament (PCL) rehabilitation, which probably reflects the number of cases seen in practice. Peccin *et al.* (2005), in a review of treatment of the PCL, identified 286 studies that involved use of exercise in the rehabilitation process but none of these trials were randomised or even quasi-randomised. The problem for researchers when carrying out randomised trials for both ACL and PCL rehabilitation is that exercise therapy is traditionally a fundamental part of any rehabilitation programme for both these injuries. It is therefore unlikely that a trial would compare an exercise versus a non-exercise control group due to ethical considerations. It is also difficult to compare different types of exercise programme because many exercises are multifunctional, particularly as soon as weight-bearing begins, e.g. the squat can be used for strengthening, proprioception, balance and in some circumstances range of movement of the knee.

In summary, there are a number of studies which demonstrate the efficacy of general exercise in the management of knee pain related to specific conditions, notably OA and cruciate ligament injury. However, the lack of clear description of the exercise mode and methodological limitations in published studies warrant further work in this area.

Aerobic exercise

One of the difficulties in examining the effect of aerobic exercise in the management of disorders of the knee is the absence of trials investigating aerobic activity only. Many of the studies outlined above combined aerobic exercise with other activities such as muscle strengthening and ROM exercises. Ettinger *et al.* (1997) stratified patients with knee OA into an aerobic exercise group or resistance exercise group as part of an RCT. They found that both groups had modest improvements in a number of outcome measures including measures of disability, physical performance and pain. This suggests that aerobic exercise is important in the management of OA of the knee. Rogind *et al.* (1998) examined the effects of a 'physical training' programme on patients with OA of the knee, demonstrating beneficial effects, even in those with severe OA.

In a number of joints discussed throughout this book, poor levels of physical activity and thus aerobic fitness have been cited as a risk factor for onset, associated disability and pain in musculoskeletal disorders. A number of studies have produced similar findings in disorders of the knee. Manninen *et al.* (2001) examined the association between physical exercise and the risk of severe knee OA requiring arthroplasty. Their results showed that the risk of severe knee OA decreased with increasing cumulative hours of recreational physical exercise. The effect of exercise on levels of disability associated with knee OA was examined by Pennix *et al.* (2001). The study concluded that aerobic and resistance exercise may reduce levels of disability in older people with knee OA. Similarly, Dias *et al.* (2003) and Evcik and Sonel (2002) also found that an exercise and walking protocol had a positive effect on the quality of life of elderly individuals with knee OA. Thus, while it is unclear how activity levels are related to onset of knee OA, evidence suggests that the inclusion of aerobic exercise is needed for optimal management.

On the contrary, a number of recent studies have noted an increased risk of knee OA and musculoskeletal disorders of the knee in general with high levels of physical activity, particularly in sports such as soccer (Drawer and Fuller, 2001). These studies must be considered with caution as they examine the effects of high-intensity exercise, often with the inclusion of contact injury. Intensity of aerobic exercise in the management of OA of the knee was investigated by Brosseau *et al.* (2003), who analysed a number of trials in the area, and concluded that both high- and low-intensity aerobic exercise are equally effective in improving a number of outcome measures in subjects with OA knee. The analysis also concluded that programmes with higher-intensity exercise components had a greater drop-out rate, indicating that low-intensity aerobic exercise may be the safest and most successful type of programme. The type of exercise prescribed in these studies was primarily stationary cycling, presumably chosen as it loads the knee joint less than a weight-bearing activity. The biomechanics of this activity, however, should be considered with caution. Neptune and Kautz (2000) examined the effects of backward and forward pedalling on a stationary bike to establish the relative loading of the knee joint complex. It was found that backward pedalling offers reduced tibiofemoral compressive loads for knee disorders such as meniscus damage and OA but higher patellofemoral joint loads. The authors recommended that backward pedalling should not be prescribed for patients with disorders of the patellofemoral joint or after ACL injury or reconstruction.

Thus there appears to be clear evidence for the benefits of aerobic exercise in the management of disorders of the knee although there is a requirement for further trials considering aerobic activity as a sole intervention. While evidence suggests that high levels of activity may increase risk of injury, it should be noted that this research was conducted on a specific group of patients who also exposed the knee joint to extreme loading as a result of contact injury. Further, there is evidence to the contrary that low levels of activity may predispose individuals to a higher level of disability associated with OA of the knee.

Balance and proprioception

The role of proprioception in the function of the knee joint complex has received growing attention in recent years. This is a result of studies which have noted proprioceptive deficits following injury or deficits associated with pathology. While it is unclear if the proprioceptive deficits precede or are as a result of disorders of the joint, proprioceptive training has being adopted as an integral part of knee rehabilitation. Baker, V., *et al.* (2002) found abnormal knee joint proprioception in individuals with patellofemoral pain syndrome while Bonfim *et al.* (2003) and Reider *et al.* (2003) noted similar deficits in patients with ACL impairments (lesions and following reconstruction). The role of proprioception in knee OA is less clear with conflicting evidence in the literature. Koralewicz and Engh (2000), Pai *et al.* (1997) and Hassan *et al.* (2001) all found evidence of proprioceptive deficits in individuals with knee OA when compared with controls. However, Bayramoglu *et al.* (2007) found that in 50 patients with bilateral knee OA, repositioning error was not affected in those with a mild-to-moderate form of the disease. Reasons for altered joint position sense, particularly in OA, have not been clearly established yet. Pain has been cited as a factor in proprioceptive deficits although there is no consensus regarding this idea. Erden *et al.* (2003) found a positive correlation between pain and altered joint position sense, while Bennell *et al.* (2003) found no significant correlation between pain and proprioceptive function in patients with OA of the knee.

Sensorimotor or proprioceptive training has been shown to have benefits in improving joint position sense in knee disorders in a number of trials. Tsauo *et al.* (2008) showed that sensorimotor training using a sling suspension system improved proprioception in the knee joints as well as self-reported function in patients with knee OA. In a prospective cohort study of team handball players, Panics *et al.* (2008) showed that proprioceptive training improved knee joint position sense and suggested that this improvement may have reduce the rate of injury.

While there is still a need for further research in the area, particularly to establish if poor proprioception is a risk factor for injury or is a consequence of pathology, the evidence above suggests that proprioceptive training should be an integral part of a knee rehabilitation programme.

Range of movement and flexibility exercises

The rehabilitation of hamstring injuries is well documented in the literature, which reflects the incidence of the injury, especially in the sporting population and particularly the elite athlete population. Mason *et al.* (2007) performed a systematic review of rehabilitation of hamstring injuries. The review compared three RCTs. All the trials investigated used stretching exercises as an integral part of the rehabilitation programme, which reflects the acceptance of this technique in contemporary treatment protocols. All three studies showed an improved rate of recovery with the stretching exercises but other treatment protocols were employed with the stretches, which could have influenced the results, therefore no one protocol seemed to be more successful than the other two.

As with aerobic exercise, there is a paucity of studies examining the role of ROM or stretching exercise in the management of knee pathology. Many of the trials described above include ROM exercise in their protocol but only with the addition of aerobic and strengthening exercise. Deyle *et al.*

(2000) included passive joint movements, muscle stretching and soft-tissue mobilisation as well as 'ROM exercises for the knee' in an 8-week programme for knee OA. However, strengthening exercises for the hip and knee were also included as part of the intervention. While the programme was concluded to be successful with a significant number of subjects reporting a 'decrease in stiffness in the knee', this measure is likely to be a subjective report as measurement of knee joint ROM was not carried out in any part of the trial.

ROM exercises are routinely used by many clinicians, as most knee disorders, particularly those which are degenerative in nature, present with decreased ROM. While many clinicians would support the efficacy of this approach, there is a requirement for more research to endorse this clinical application.

Muscle strength and endurance

Muscle strengthening exercise is a core component of rehabilitation of knee disorders for most practitioners. This is likely to be a reflection of the fact that muscle weakness surrounding the joint, particularly of the quadriceps, has been found to be both a risk factor and a common finding in conditions such as OA (Slemenda *et al.*, 1997; Lewek *et al.*, 2004). A number of studies have focused on this single component of rehabilitation, particularly in the treatment of knee osteoarthritis. Baker, K.R., *et al.* (2001) examined the efficacy of home-based progressive strength training in adults with knee OA. A combination of functional exercises such as squats and resistance exercises with ankle weights were performed by patients three times per week for 4 months. The researchers' findings showed that high-intensity, home-based strength training can produce substantial improvements in strength, pain, physical function and quality of life in patients with knee OA. In a similarly designed trial, O'Reilly *et al.* (1999) showed that a home exercise programme, which consisted of strengthening exercise for the quadriceps, significantly improved self-reported knee pain and function in patients with knee OA.

There is debate regarding the optimal mode of exercise in the management of knee disorders, particularly of OA. Jan *et al.* (2008) examined the relative effects of high versus low load resistance strength training in patients with knee OA resulting in significant improvements in pain, function, walking time and muscle torque for both modes. The effects of high resistance strength training were larger than that of low load training although this finding was not statistically significant. Cheing *et al.* (2002) found that a 4-week programme of simple isometric exercise was effective in reducing knee pain in those with OA. Eyigor (2004) investigated the efficacy of isokinetic and progressive resistance exercise in 40 patients with knee OA, and found that both modes of exercise reduced pain and relieved function, with no statistically significant differences between the two programmes. As a simple progressive resistance programme is cheaper and more easily performed by the patient than isokinetic exercises it presents a viable option in the management of knee OA. This mode of training is supported by the findings of Sevick *et al.* (2000), who examined the cost-effectiveness of aerobic and resistance exercise in seniors with knee OA. In a study including 439 patients with OA of the knee, they found that resistance training was more economically efficient than aerobic exercise in improving physical function.

Research in recent years has been directed at analysis of strengthening protocols for the management of specific pathologies, notably patellar tendinopathy and ACL deficiency. Visnes and Bahr (2007) performed a critical review of the role of eccentric training as treatment for patellar tendinopathy. Following analysis of seven studies, the authors concluded that most studies suggest that eccentric strength training with the inclusion of an incline board provides the best outcome in management of this condition. However, no specific protocol demonstrated superiority over any other. Heintjes *et al.* (2003) performed a systematic review of exercise therapy for patellofemoral pain syndrome (PFPS). Twelve studies were identified (nine RCTs and three concurrent controlled trials). Three studies compared a group receiving exercises against groups that did not. One group underwent a programme of eccentric exercises, another group underwent a programme of static open chain exercises along with isokinetic exercises and the final group used a brace that provided progressive resistive resistance during activities of daily living. All the other studies compared one exercise protocol with another, and of which five studies compared open kinetic chain (OKC) with closed kinetic chain

(CKC) exercises. Of the three studies that compared exercise groups with non-exercise groups, all trials found that there was an improvement in pain levels but little change in functional capacity. Of the studies comparing OKC with CKC exercises both were said to be significantly effective but no method was more successful. This conclusion was supported by Herrington and Al-Sherhi (2007) and Witvrouw *et al.* (2004), who showed significant improvements in clinical outcomes with both open and closed kinetic chain exercises both in the short and in the long term. O'Sullivan (2005) went further, stating that to achieve the most successful recruitment of the vastus medialis obliquus (VMO) during the rehabilitation of PFPS, both open and closed kinetic chain exercises should be carried out. Cowan *et al.* (2002) showed that by applying a specific progressive rehabilitation programme, the motor control of the VMO could be altered in relation to the vastus lateralis, leading to a positive outcome. However, Syme *et al.* (2008) demonstrated similar results with the use of either VMO selective training or general quadriceps strengthening only and suggested that clinicians should not over focus on selective activation before progressing rehabilitation.

However, in a more recent study, Fredberg *et al.* (2008) examined the effect of prophylactic eccentric training in asymptomatic soccer players with ultrasonographic abnormalities in Achilles and patellar tendons. The findings were that a stretching and eccentric programme reduced the risk of abnormal ultrasound findings but had no effect on reducing injury risk. However, it was also shown that in asymptomatic players with abnormal ultrasound findings, the exercise protocol increased injury risk. As this study examined both eccentric exercise and stretching, it was not possible to come to a clear conclusion regarding eccentric exercise and injury risk, suggesting that there is still a requirement for more research in this area.

There has been a great deal of debate about the efficacy of open versus closed kinetic chain work for knee ligament injuries. CKC exercises are considered to be safer as they are thought produce less shear factors across the joint. The major problem with CKC exercises is that even though they are less stressful to the ACL they put more pressure on the patellofemoral joint. It therefore makes it difficult to treat a patient with multiple pathologies. Tagesson *et al.* (2008) examined the role of closed versus open kinetic chain exercise in 42 patients with ACL deficiency, who were randomised into rehabilitation with either a CKC or OKC strengthening programme. Sagittal static and dynamic tibial translation was evaluated as were muscle strength and activation and jump performance. It was found that there were no differences in static or dynamic tibial translation between both groups although the OKC group had significantly greater quadriceps strength following the protocol. The authors concluded that the risks associated with OKC exercise were not confirmed and that it appears that patients with ACL deficiency may need OKC exercise to regain good muscle torque. However, despite this finding, in a review of contemporary literature, Grodski and Marks (2008) suggested that there is still a lack of consensus regarding OKC versus CKC and more high-quality trials are needed.

In summary, while it is clear that resistance training is beneficial in the rehabilitation of knee disorders, there is a lack of clarity regarding the most effective programmes because of the many variables involved.

Disorders of the knee joint complex

Ligament sprains

The ligaments surrounding the knee are considered to be passive stabilisers of the joint and disruption can lead to instability. The ligaments of the knee can be divided into two distinct groups, the intra-articular group or central pivot, consisting of the anterior and posterior cruciate ligaments and the extra-articular or peripheral group. Knee ligaments are commonly injured in the sporting environment but can be easily damaged in a non-sporting incident such as a fall or a road traffic collision. The cruciate ligaments provide joint stability in all planes of movement in collaboration with the peripheral musculoskeletal structures. If the joint is put under a valgus force with external rotation the ACL and medial collateral ligament (MCL) prevent anterior translation of the tibia. The close association of all these soft tissues and their collaboration in providing stability of the knee joint explain why these structures are rarely injured in isolation and also why these relationships need to be considered

in any rehabilitation programme. The ACL is commonly injured in sporting activities which involve rapid twisting and turning. The ligament is most commonly injured when an excessive valgus force is applied to an extended knee joint, when the foot is planted on the floor creating a lateral rotation of the femur on the tibia. This movement regularly occurs in multidirectional sports such as football or rugby where an athlete rapidly changes direction. The injury can occur with or without contact from another person.

An ACL rupture may be partial or complete. Occasionally a patient may present after a number of incidents that result in small tears, which lead on to the final insult that completed the total rupture. An acute total ACL rupture is characterised by severe pain and varying degrees of haemarthrosis, and the patient may complain of instability. There may be a loss of extension and a positive Lachman's and anterior drawer test, but these may be difficult to perform due to spasm in the hamstrings. Management may be conservative or surgical depending on the age of the patient and their degree of activity, sporting or otherwise.

Management following repair of an ACL depends on the method of surgery used. If other structures had been damaged in conjunction with the ACL they would be allowed to heal before a repair was attempted. Rehabilitation can either be delayed or accelerated depending on the type of surgery used, the preferences of the surgeon, other associated injuries and the expectations of the patient. In an accelerated programme if there were no problems, full contact sporting activities may be reintroduced after approximately 6 months.

PCL injuries are far less frequent than ACL injuries and usually occur following forceful hyperextension or a fall on a flexed knee. Following rupture, reconstruction of the PCL is performed far less frequently than for the ACL and usually only if other structures are involved. A PCL-deficient knee is less likely to have problems with instability, and conservative management is most common with an emphasis on quadriceps strengthening and proprioception exercises with introduction of co-contraction exercises when the signs of inflammation have diminished.

The MCL can be damaged if a direct blow occurs to the outside of the joint as in a tackle or indirectly if a player, wearing a studded boot, plants his foot in soft ground and twists, creating a rotational force about the joint. If a direct force is applied to the outside of the joint, with the knee slightly flexed, in a weight-bearing position, it causes an external rotation of the tibia in relation to the femur, which can cause damage to the MCL. This can occur in isolation, or more usually in combination with the medial meniscus and if the force exceeds the physiological limits the ACL may become involved. In extreme situations the PCL may become compromised. This results in global instability of the joint. The lateral collateral ligament is less commonly damaged than the MCL and often in isolation, although if the force is severe enough associated damage may occur to the lateral meniscus or either cruciate ligament. It is usually damaged following a direct varus force to the knee with some hyperextension.

Meniscus injuries

Injuries to the menisci of the knee rarely occur in isolation and are less common than injuries to ligaments and problems with the patellofemoral joint. When isolated tears do occur they are usually degenerative in nature and are sustained by the older rather than the younger generation. Acute meniscal tears usually involve other soft tissue structures. Meniscal injuries can occur following a number of different mechanisms including rotational and translational forces as well as overuse or degeneration.

Damage to the medial meniscus is more common than the lateral meniscus by a ratio of approximately 10:1. Approximately 80% of injuries to the medial meniscus are associated with damage to other soft tissue structures of the knee particularly the MCL and ACL due to their common attachments. Symptoms of meniscal tears are often characterised by 'locking' or 'clicking' of the knee joint, as a portion or flap of meniscus becomes impinged in between the femoral condyles and tibial plateau, when the joint is moved into extension or sometimes flexion. The patient also often reports that the knee 'gives way' and feels unstable. There may be a small effusion and tenderness along the joint line with McMurray's and Appley's compression tests often positive. If the effusion is aspirated and blood is present it would usually indicate ligament involvement. A posterior horn tear would produce pain on full squatting.

Osteoarthritis of the knee

OA of the knee often produces significant pain that worsens on weight-bearing and consequently leads to an increase in functional disability. It is characterised by morning stiffness, diminished joint range and crepitus on movement. If inflammation is present, it is localised to the joint involved. The medial compartment of the knee is more likely to be affected than the lateral compartment, which can ultimately lead to a varus deformity, joint laxity and muscle weakness, particularly of the quadriceps. The cause of the laxity may be multifactorial and can be due to a combination of soft tissue pathology, primary laxity of the ligaments and capsule, previous injury or degeneration of the articular cartilage and bone, which would result in a loss of joint space.

Gait patterns can become compromised with a loss of knee flexion during weight-bearing that increases the load on the articular cartilage. To compensate for the laxity or weakness around the knee joint, the patient will often demonstrate a reflex stiffening of the joint with associated co-contractions of the quadriceps and hamstrings, which increases the pressure inside the joint. A combination of increased internal pressures and increased load on the articular cartilage can increase the risk of cartilage destruction.

Anterior knee pain

Anterior knee pain is an umbrella term for a number of conditions that affect the patellofemoral joint. Sometimes it is difficult to differentiate between the separate conditions and it is not uncommon to have multiple pathologies. These include PFPS, patella tendinopathy, bursitis and plicae syndrome.

Patellofemoral pain syndrome

PFPS is common in all groups within the active and sedentary population with a high incidence in the adolescent population. There are a number of factors which have been attributed to the cause of PFPS, both static and dynamic including biomechanical and muscle weakness/ imbalance factors. The most common are listed in Table 11.1. The differences in symptoms between PFPS and patellar tendinopathy are sometimes very slight and these

Table 11.1   Clinical signs of patellofemoral pain syndrome (PFPS) and patellar tendinopathy (PT)

Clinical signs	PFPS	PT
Painful activity	Running, stairs, eccentric work	Jumping, landing
Site of pain, tenderness	Diffuse at the patella, may not be palpable	Localised, inferior pole patella, length of tendon
Crepitus	In severe cases at patella	In tendon
Giving way	Yes, due to pain, quadriceps weakness	Not usual
Effusion	At patella in severe cases	At tendon in severe cases
Range of motion	↓ in severe cases	normal
Patella mobility	↓ medial glide due to tight lateral retinaculum	normal
Vastus medialis obliquus	Wasted; vastus medialis obliquus/vastus lateralis imbalance	General quads wasting.
Effect of activity	↑ pain with ↑ activity	Initial pain ↓ with activity, ↑ when stopped.
Pseudo locking	Yes	No

Adapted from Houghum (2005).

Table 11.2   Differentiating between intra- and inter-muscular haematomas

Intra-muscular haematoma	Inter-muscular haematoma
Area inflamed	Not noticeably inflamed
Loss of power and stretch	Loss of power but not stretch
No bruising visible due to encapsulation in muscle sheath	Bruising visible below injury site 24–48 hours after injury
Joint range limited and returns slowly due to pain and internal pressure	Joint range returns quickly
Internal pressure high due to blood encapsulated within muscle sheath	Internal pressure low due to blood loss via ruptured sheath

sometimes occur at the same time. The clinical signs are shown in Table 11.1.

Muscle injuries

The muscles around the knee joint that provide dynamic stabilisation of the joint are essentially the hamstrings and quadriceps. Both groups are vulner-able to injury but especially the muscles that cross both the hip and knee, which include the hamstrings and rectus femoris. Sartorius, which even though is not part of the quadriceps group, falls into the same category as rectus femoris. Care must be taken with the diagnosis to differentiate between inter- and intra-muscular haematomas as the treatment protocols are different in the initial stages (Table 11.2). In the case of an intra-muscular haematoma blood is trapped within the sheath and becomes a 'space-occupying lesion'. In severe cases, this may require surgical decompression.

Myositis ossificans is a rare complication which occurs when the haematoma calcifies. This may occur with disruption of the periosteum at the time of the injury or with too aggressive rehabilitation following an intramuscular haematoma. Injuries often result from previous injury if rehabilitation has been inadequate.

Quadriceps

These muscles are commonly injured in sport, particularly in all codes of football. Common causes of strains and tears include fatigue, poor flexibility, and sudden contraction of the muscle, which may occur while jumping or with a sudden change in direction. Other contributory factors may be muscle imbalance; particularly an abnormal quadriceps:hamstring ratio (usually hamstrings have 60–80% power of quadriceps). Tears are characterised by sudden pain in the front of the thigh and signs of inflammation, and a defect may be palpable. Surgery is rarely indicated even in the most severe cases.

The hamstrings

The hamstring muscles are a common site of injury in the active population, not just in sporting activities. The hamstring muscles are important trunk stabilisers in posture and also extend the hip and flex the knee when walking and running. Hamstring tears are usually the result of overload of the muscle fibres, particularly during an eccentric contraction. Symptoms are similar to those of quadriceps tears with pain in the posterior aspect of the thigh. Any posterior thigh pain must be investigated thoroughly as it may be neural rather than muscular in nature. This is particularly important in children who rarely suffer from hamstring tears, even those in elite sports. Posterior thigh pain in children is usually a consequence of a growth spurt and with neural stretches will settle quickly, unlike true hamstring tears, which can take a number of weeks to settle.

SECTION 2: PRACTICAL USE OF EXERCISE

When planning a rehabilitation programme for the knee joint it is helpful to consider both primary and secondary issues. The primary issues deal with the specific problem that has affected the knee joint, such as the damage to the joint or soft tissue surrounding and supporting it, and the secondary factors, which are the areas affected as a consequence of the primary problem and could include increased or decreased stability of the joint, loss of range, decreased muscular power, endurance and strength, reduced proprioception and co-ordination difficulty in activities of daily living. To identify the primary and secondary factors surrounding a knee injury a comprehensive assessment must be carried out.

Rehabilitation protocols of the knee joint have been developed with specific pathologies in mind so the programmes outlined below reflect this. However, it must be noted that the general principles described may be used in management of many presentations of knee pain. Further, it should be considered that knee pain is commonly caused by a number of structures simultaneously and while a working diagnosis may be given, the protocols should be a guideline rather than a generic approach to management.

The pathologies which will be considered here are: OA of the knee, patellar tendinopathy, PFPS, ACL injury, and meniscal and ligament injury.

Osteoarthritis of the knee joint

As osteoarthritis is a degenerative disorder with no known cure other than joint replacement, the management of this condition aims to use exercise to reduce pain and improve joint function.

Aerobic exercise

Early phase

Brosseau *et al.* (2003) confirmed that 'both high and low intensity aerobic exercise were equally effective at improving a patient's functional status, gait, pain and aerobic capacity for people with OA of the knee'. The ultimate aim of the programme should be to allow the patient to reach the activity as recommended in the American College of Sports Medicine (ACSM) guidelines, although early goals will focus on improving general function. The choice of activity will depend on the ability of the patient to perform the activity within limits of pain and the activity should not aggravate the condition. Many patients will find that weight-bearing activity aggravates their symptoms so non- weight-bearing activity should be the exercise of choice in the early stage of rehabilitation. Hydrotherapy is an excellent option in patients with OA of the knee as the lower limb is de-loaded by the buoyancy of the water. Also the water provides resistance that will allow the

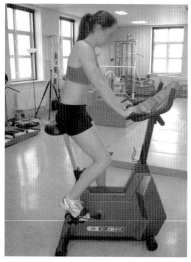
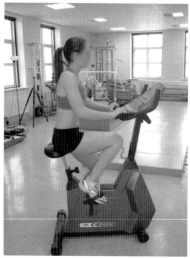

(a)   **(b)**

Figure 11.1 (**a**) Cycling with a high saddle. (**b**) Cycling with a low saddle to encourage knee flexion.

heart rate to be raised more easily in fitter individuals. Use of a buoyancy vest will allow the patient to perform walking and running patterns with the lower limb, which will be the precursor to improving these functions on the land. Use of a static bicycle for cycling is another appropriate option. In the early stage of rehabilitation, the height of the saddle should be set so that the patient's knee is moving through a movement range that is comfortable as this may be limited by pain; this may mean that the saddle is high to begin with but should be gradually lowered throughout rehabilitation to try to improve the range, see Figure 11.1 (a: early phase; and b: late phase). If high-intensity training is chosen, the patient should exercise at 70% heart rate reserve (HRR) and for low intensity, 40% HRR should be selected. Choice of exercise intensity will depend on factors such as the cardio-respiratory health of the patient and will be decided following appropriate assessment of the patient.

Late phase

The choice of late-stage aerobic activity should reflect the specific functional requirements of the patient. A walking programme should be commenced as soon as possible with the ultimate aim to achieve 1 hour of this activity on most days of the week. Simple walking programmes have demonstrated efficacy in management of OA of the knee (Evcik and Sonel, 2002). Patients may benefit from a Nordic walking approach (see Chapter 2), as the walking poles give them extra support. All patients should progress to walking without any support and move from a stable surface (smooth pavements) to less regular surfaces such as a field or sandy beach. The footwear of choice should be training shoes to correct foot biomechanics and attenuate shock. The patient should be told that the walking programme should be continued following discharge and, as far as possible, incorporated into daily life.

Range of motion and flexibility exercises

As mentioned above, the nature of OA of the knee means that exercise therapy is likely to be ineffective in restoring full ROM to the joint. Therefore, the aim of ROM exercises should be to achieve a ROM that facilitates better function according to the demands of the patient's lifestyle.

Early phase

Pain may limit ROM in the early stage of rehabilitation and the aim should be to avoid aggravating the condition. Active-assisted exercise may be beneficial and a good example was outlined above, using a static exercise bicycle. There should be no tension on the wheels and if the therapist manually starts

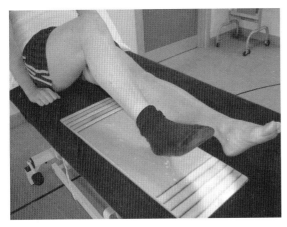

Figure 11.2 Use of a sliding board to ease heel sliding and facilitate knee flexion.

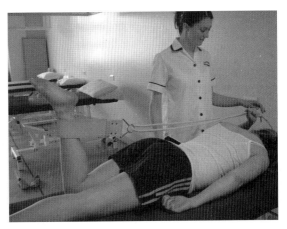

Figure 11.3 Use of a padded rope around the ankle to facilitate knee flexion.

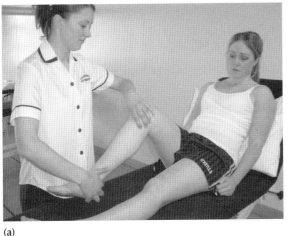

(a)

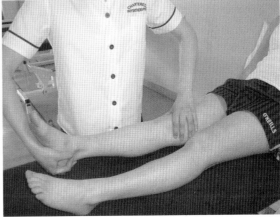

(b)

Figure 11.4 (a) Passive knee flexion. (b) Passive knee extension.

the wheel crank, the natural momentum will help facilitate movement. This exercise may be done at the same time as the aerobic exercise outlined above. A continuous passive motion (CPM) machine is frequently used following surgery to ensure that the joint is moved regularly, although there is no reason why this should not be used in a typical rehabilitation session. Other activities to encourage knee ROM include putting the patient in a long sitting position and encouraging them to slide the heel towards the buttock to flex the knee and sliding outwards into full extension. This activity can be made easier by reducing the friction of the surface by polishing the surface and placing a sock on the heel (Fig. 11.2). It is important not to forget mobil-

ity in the patellofemoral joint and it may be necessary for the clinician or patient to mobilise the patella in all directions while in a relaxed, long sitting position. Use of a padded rope in a prone position may allow the patient to facilitate their own knee flexion (Fig. 11.3).

The addition of passive ROM exercises may be appropriate in the early phase of rehabilitation, particularly to the patellofemoral joint and these may be particularly useful to improve joint range when active and active-assisted exercise are no longer as effective (Fig. 11.4).

Stretches of muscles that cross the knee joint should be incorporated into the ROM programme and will be done most effectively following aerobic exercise. These should include stretches to the hamstrings, quadriceps, adductors, abductors and gastrocnemius (Fig. 11.5).

Late phase

Progression from the early phase of ROM exercise allows the patient to include some active, weight-bearing and functional ROM exercise. Many of these exercises will be naturally part of a strengthening regimen outlined below, particularly functional exercise. Single knee flexion and extension may be performed in standing (Fig. 11.6) and sitting (Fig. 11.7). A standing squat with support (Fig. 11.8a), which is progressed to the same exercise without support (Fig. 11.8b) may be used to improve ROM as well as strength. Exercises such as step-ups on a shallow step, progressing to a deeper step, will increase ROM as well as strength in a functional manner (Fig. 11.9).

Proprioception and balance exercise

Early phase

A number of studies have demonstrated proprioceptive deficits in the knee joint of subjects with OA (Pai *et al.* 1997; Koralewicz and Engh, 2000; Hassan *et al.*, 2001), but other studies have not found repositioning errors in subjects with OA of the knee (Bennell *et al.*, 2003; Bayramoglu *et al.*, 2007). However, optimal management of the patient demands that the knee joint positioning error should be measured at initial assessment and if deficits are found, the exercise used to address such errors should be included in the exercise programme. One of the most effective ways to measure repositioning error is to attach an electrogoniometer to the knee joint, and position the knee at 40°, then 60° and then 90°. The knee is then returned to extension and the patient is asked to reposition the knee in the three positions while the therapist reads the angles on the goniometer (Fig. 11.10). If the patient is unable to re-create the positions he or she may use an electrogoniometer as visual feedback during practice, progressing to checking the display only after repositioning to check the angle. This exercise should be progressed to functional positions such as standing and stride standing.

Late phase

Progression of proprioceptive exercise will take place at the same time as partial weight-bearing (PWB) strengthening exercise. PWB exercises are classified as CKC exercises where multi-joint, multi-muscle actions are reinforced. These exercises enhance proprioception and kinaesthetic awareness, balance, equilibrium and co-ordination and weight-bearing control. Specific movement patterns can be introduced that will replicate patterns of movement which will be used by the patient when the process of rehabilitation is complete. Static balance exercises can be commenced, and there are a number of ways to progress proprioception training of the knee, using various exteroceptors – which are the five senses. Progression of proprioception is affected by the type of base, i.e. whether it is rigid or soft, the height of the base from the floor, which can be altered by lowering the support surface from which the body has to raise, therefore the exercise could be started initially from a high chair to a chair, a stool and then a bench. As the base becomes smaller, the proprioceptive demands are greater. The size of the base can be changed by starting with a wide foot position, gradually bringing the feet together and ultimately standing on the injured leg alone. Adding superimposed movements such as bouncing a ball against a wall while standing on one leg. will challenge balance further.

Muscle strength and endurance exercise

Slemenda *et al.* (1997) found that quadriceps weakness was a significant finding in patients with OA of the knee and for many clinicians, restoring strength in this muscle group is the starting point in any rehabilitation programme. Further, Baker, K.R., *et al.* (2001) emphasised the importance of strength training in the management of OA of the knee by demonstrating that 'high intensity, home based strength training can produce substantial improvements in strength, pain, physical function and quality of life in patients with knee OA'.

Early phase

Exercises to maintain strength in the musculature around the knee joint can be carried out from a

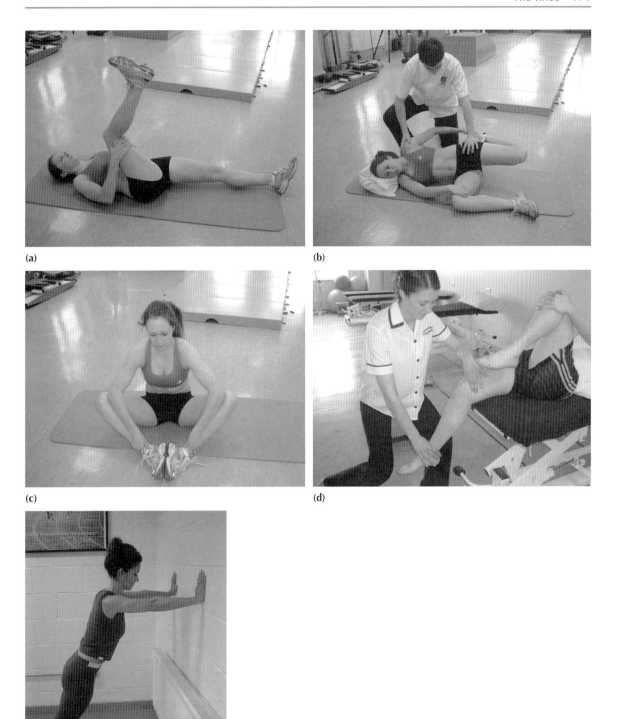

Figure 11.5 (**a**) Hamstring stretches. (**b**) Quadriceps stretches. (**c**) Adductor stretches. (**d**) Abductor stretches. (**e**) Calf stretches.

very early stage in any knee injury in the form of isometric exercises. Isometric exercises can be carried out if the joint is immobilised or if there is insufficient dynamic strength or too much discomfort in the area to allow active joint movement. For OA of the knee, isometric contraction of the quadriceps group in a long-sitting position, followed by

straight leg raises (Fig. 11.11) of various derivatives are the usual starting point in strengthening exercises. A high degree of tension can be produced in the muscle but no active movement is produced at the joint itself. Position of the patient is important to ensure that they do not use trick movements to lift the leg off the surface. The loading of the exercise can be increased by placing an ankle weight *in situ* and repeating the movement.

While Jan *et al.* (2008) demonstrated that both high and low load resistance training improved clinical effects in patients with knee OA, the emphasis in the early stage of rehabilitation is usually to improve the endurance of the muscles to enhance basic function. For this reason, high repetitions with no or minimal load or alternatively, sustained contractions should be carried out at this stage. The patient may then progress to isotonic exercise, loading the knee joint through its movement range with particular emphasis on the quadriceps, and also addressing other muscle groups that demonstrated deficits at initial assessment. Ankle weights, pullies or isokinetic resistance machines may be used to provide resistance. Suggested exercises include knee extension, knee flexion, hip extension, hip adduction and hip abduction. Baker, K.R., *et al.* (2001) suggest that two sets of 12 repetitions should be performed three times a week for each exercise, increasing the weights according to the patient's progress.

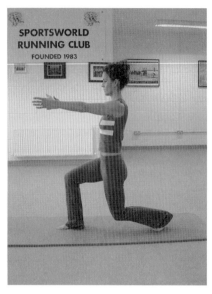

Figure 11.6 Knee flexion in standing.

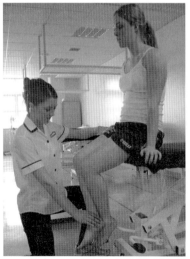

(a)

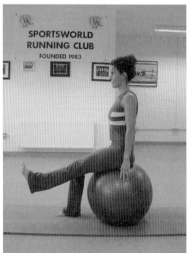

(b)

Figure 11.7 Knee flexion in sitting.

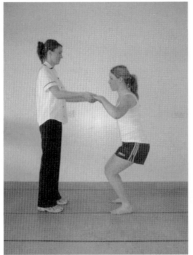
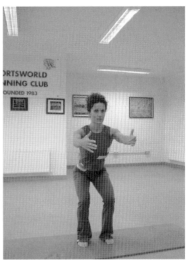

Figure 11.8 (**a**) Standing squat with support. (**b**) Standing squat without support.

(a)   **(b)**

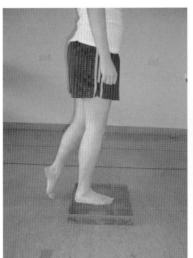
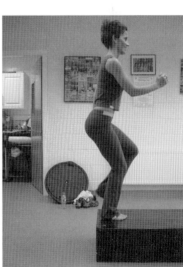

Figure 11.9 (**a**) Step-ups on a shallow step. (**b**) Step-ups on a deep step.

(a)   **(b)**

Late phase

While some of the strengthening exercises outlined above may constitute the late stage by virtue of their progression, the emphasis at this stage should be on functional exercise. Weight-bearing exercise such as lunges and squats allow CKC patterns to be used, which facilitates co-contraction of a number of muscle groups. Exercises such as rising to standing from a sitting position are very functional and resistance may be increased by holding a weight at the chest (Fig. 11.12). Step-ups on to a low bench may be progressed by increasing the height of the bench or placing a weighted back pack on the patient. Lunges may be progressed by asking the patient to hold a weight, although the therapist should observe the patient carefully for biomechanical faults because a high level of proprioception is required in such an exercise.

The components of the late phase of strength training depend on the stage of OA. Patients with moderate and severe disease may only be able to

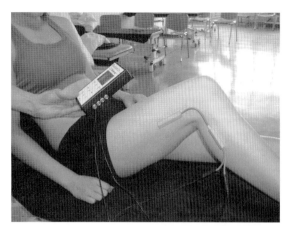

Figure 11.10 Use of an electrogoniometer to train joint repositioning.

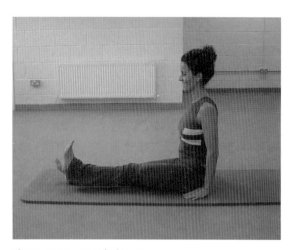

Figure 11.11 Straight leg raise.

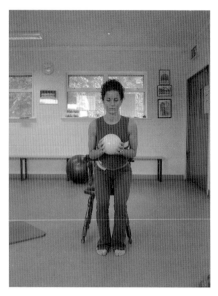

Figure 11.12 Sitting to standing holding a weight.

manage simple exercise such as squats, with minimal loading and the exercise programme should always be aimed at the functional requirements of the patient. It must be noted that although the components of the OA rehabilitation programme are outlined separately above, they should be carried out simultaneously for optimal effect.

Patellar tendinopathy

Great advances in the management of patellar tendinopathy have been seen in recent years with the introduction of eccentric exercise protocols.

Previous treatment focused on the management of the condition as an inflammatory process but recent studies have negated this theory. For the purpose of management of this condition, it will not be divided into the different exercise components as in OA (above) but will be described as a rehabilitation protocol derived from analysis and review of research to date. Visnes and Bahr (2007) concluded from a review of the management of patella tendinopathy that eccentric training has a positive effect on the injury although individual protocols varied, with no clear definition of which was most effective. Further, they suggested that a clinical approach will also use factors such as warm-up and stretching, which are not analysed in many studies. The protocol described below is adapted from Jonsson and Alfredson (2005).

Early phase

While the main component of treatment is the eccentric exercise programme, full assessment of the patient should establish deficits in flexibility, aerobic fitness and proprioception of the knee joint and surrounding structure. While this injury is frequently seen in competitive athletes, aerobic fitness may still be an issue as it must be maintained during a period of rehabilitation. Purdam *et al.* (2004) stated that subjects were not allowed to take part in their normal sporting activity during the first 8

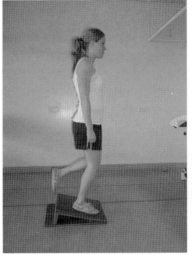 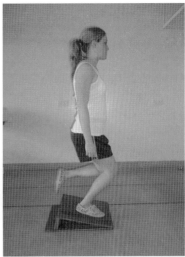

Figure 11.13 (**a**) Standing on 25° incline board. (**b**) Flexion to 70°.   (**a**)   (**b**)

weeks of the eccentric protocol trial. Weight-bearing programmes may not be appropriate in the early stage, so stationary cycling is a good choice of activity, although backwards pedalling should be avoided due to increased load on the patellofemoral joint. Flexibility of the hamstrings (Fig. 11.5a) and quadriceps (Fig. 11.5b) in particular should be addressed with inclusion of stretches to other groups indicated following assessment. The aerobic exercise and stretching component may precede the eccentric training protocol as a warm-up, although the aim should not be to exercise to any level of fatigue, meaning that an aerobic programme may also be carried out separately to a level required by the more competitive athlete. Following the warm-up, the protocol is as follows.

A starting position is standing with the trunk upright on a 25° incline board with the entire body weight on the injured leg (Fig. 11.13a). The knee is then slowly flexed to 70° (Fig. 11.13b). To return to the starting position, the other leg is used to push back up to avoid concentric activity. The patient should be informed that the activity may cause muscle soreness initially and will be painful in the tendon during exercise. The exercise is repeated 15 times, twice a day, 7 days a week.

Late and functional phase

The programme is carried out for a period of 12 weeks. After the first 4 weeks, the patient may progress the aerobic component to slow jogging on flat ground, increase the intensity of cycling or add in swimming (Purdam *et al.*, 2004), provided that these activities do not increase the pain. The eccentric programme should be carried out as above but weight should be added in the form of a loaded backpack on the patient. Weights should be added when the patient no longer finds the exercise painful, to a load that re-creates the pain. The proprioceptive component of the programme will be monitored by the therapist, who must ensure correct biomechanics during all activities of the programme, in particular, ensuring that the patient squats to the correct angle, using an electrogoniometer if necessary.

After 8 weeks, the patient should be allowed to make a graduated return to normal activity while completing the final stage of the programme ensuring that appropriate stretching protocols are adhered to. Functional exercises such as walking can be progressed to fast walking then jogging, half pace running, three-quarters pace running, and then sprinting, forwards, backwards and sideways. This should be done initially in straight lines ,then multi-directional work can be introduced, including rotational work, which will involve shearing and compressive forces. Finally, the joint should be taken through sudden acceleration and deceleration manoeuvres to ensure there is functional stability. Jumping and landing can be introduced, initially with two feet and progressing to one.

There is some emerging evidence that eccentric training and stretching may have a prophylactic effect on recurrence or onset of ultrasonographic changes in the patellar tendon (Fredberg *et al.*, 2008), although further work is required to establish a direct link with injury risk. However, it may be appropriate to include eccentric training as a regular warm-up exercise in patients who are at risk of injury following discharge from treatment.

Patellofemoral pain syndrome

Exercise has been the mainstay of treatment for PFPS, particularly with the introduction by McConnell (1996) of a specific programme that targets patellar tracking and timing of the vastus muscle group. While McConnell placed emphasis on patellar taping to correct tracking in her original research, there is a need for further studies to establish its efficacy (Vagan and Hunt, 2008); and recent research has even suggested that taping may inhibit contraction of the VMO (Ng and Wong, 2009). For this reason, taping is not included in the programme described below but the clinician must make an informed decision on its use according to available evidence as it is still widely used clinically.

The programme outlined below is based on that described by Crossley *et al.*, (2002) and will not be formally separated into components of fitness as for OA.

Early phase

The emphasis of exercise in the early stage of rehabilitation should be correction of timing and intensity of VMO contraction relative to the vastus lateralis (VL). Stretches to appropriate muscle and soft tissues aim to correct the patellar position and allow normal biomechanics of the lower limb. As the position of the whole of the lower kinetic chain will influence patellar position, initial assessment of lower limb biomechanics should be comprehensive, including assessment of dynamic function.

Maintenance or achieving aerobic fitness may be challenging in the management of a patient with PFPS, as many forms of activity will be limited by pain. While there have been no studies examining

cardiovascular fitness and its relationship to PFPS, maintenance of minimal activity levels should be addressed. Activities such as stationary cycling may be chosen. However, the seat should be high so that the knee joint moves through a small ROM, ensuring that the hip does not medially or laterally rotate, and that the patella is directed over the second toe during the cycling motion of the leg. The foot should also face straight ahead in the pedal. There should be no loading on the crank and backwards pedalling should be avoided.

Stretches should be applied to any tissue which is hypomobile at initial assessment. In particular, Crossley *et al.* (2002) recommend:

- Mediolateral (glide and tilt) mobilisation of the patella (stretching of the lateral retinaculum) (Fig. 11.14a)
- Hamstring muscle stretches in sitting (Fig. 11.14b)
- Anterior hip structures stretch with the subject in prone with hip externally rotated and the hip and knee flexed (Fig. 11.14c).

Three repetitions of each stretch with a 30-second hold is recommended. McConnell (1996) suggests that isometric quads exercise should be taught early, placing emphasis on VMO activity. Addition of adduction of the thigh (placing a ball between the patient's knees and asking them to squeeze while contracting the quads) will help facilitate the VMO. Crossley *et al.* then recommend:

- Isometric VMO contractions in sitting with knee at 90° flexion
- Squats to 40° knee flexion combined with isometric gluteal contractions (Fig. 11.15).

(Four sets of 10 repetitions each.)

- Isometric hip abduction against the wall while standing.

(Four sets of 15-second hold.)

All the above exercises should be carried out twice daily.

Late and functional phase

Crossley *et al.* (2002) specify that the above programme should be carried out for 2 weeks. After that, the knee joint may be moved through more

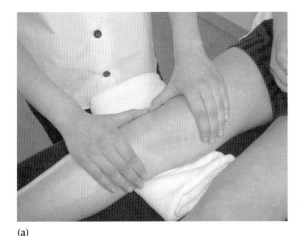

(a)

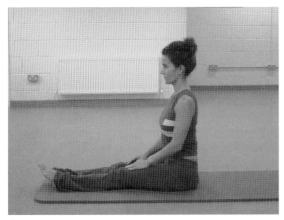

(b)

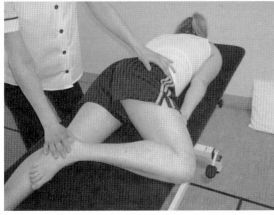

(c)

Figure 11.14 (**a**) Mobilisation of the patella. (**b**) Hamstring stretches in long sitting. (**c**) Stretches of the anterior hip structures.

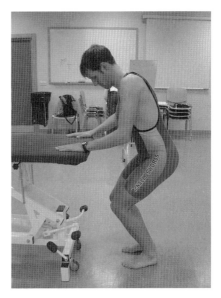

Figure 11.15 Squats to 40° combined with isometric gluteal contraction.

challenging motion patterns with the introduction of gravitational loading. Aerobic exercise should be increased progressing to walking on a flat surface. If orthoses are prescribed by a podiatrist, these should be worn at all times to optimise lower limb biomechanics. Provided that the vastus group is functioning well, this may be progressed to jogging in straight lines. Crossley *et al.* recommend the following exercise for the last 4 weeks of the programme.

- Step-downs – slow lowering of unaffected leg, standing on affected leg with a 10 cm step (three sets of five repetitions progressing to three sets of 10 repetitions) (Fig. 11.16)
- Isometric hip abduction while standing (4 sets of 30 second hold) (Fig. 11.17).

The height of the step may be increased to 20 cm provided that the patient is able to complete the activity correctly and without pain. The stretches described in the early phase should be continued. Proprioceptive work will be done throughout this programme as a high level of control is required to complete the exercises correctly and constant feedback should be given to the patient to reinforce correct movement patterns.

The patient will be allowed a graduated return to activity on completion of the programme but must maintain flexibility of soft tissues. Athletes

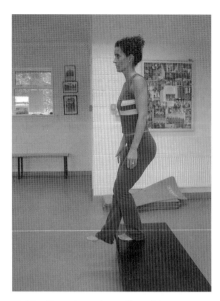

Figure 11.16   'Step-downs' on affected leg.

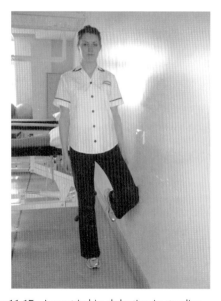

Figure 11.17   Isometric hip abduction in standing.

may want to start loading with exercises such as the weighted squat and the principles of correct biomechanics and muscle activity patterns should be observed while carrying out exercises. Functional activities described above for patellar tendinopathy may be introduced, with sport-appropriate exercises.

It should be noted that some authors suggest that over-emphasis on selective VMO timing may not be necessary and that exercises which simply exercise the quadriceps group in general may be adequate (Syme *et al.*, 2008).

Anterior cruciate ligament injury

It is common for both the medial meniscus and the MCL to be injured at the same time as the ACL, although the rehabilitation programme described below should address deficits noted in both combined and ACL injury only. A systematic review of studies by Trees *et al.* (2007) suggests that while exercise is efficacious in the management of ACL injury (both surgically and post-operative) it was not possible to conclude which mode of exercise or programme produces the best results. However, a review by Wright *et al.* (2008) concluded that early weight-bearing and early ROM exercises are safe and that CKC exercises are beneficial in the first 6 weeks.

The exercise programme outlined below is based on the results of the review by Trees *et al.* (2007) and adaptation of the programme designed by Tagesson *et al.* (2008). Tagesson *et al.* describe the distinct phases of an ACL rehabilitation programme as:

- Phase 1 (weeks 1–4) – *protection.*
- Phase 2 (weeks 5–8) – *early strength training.*
- Phase 3 (weeks 9–12) – *intensive strength training.*
- Phase 4 (weeks 13–16) – *intensive strength training and return to sports.*

Phase 1 (weeks 1–4) – protection

The aims of this phase are to increase ROM of the knee joint, improve gait patterns, improve proprioception of the knee, improve or maintain aerobic fitness and to improve muscle function. This stage may constitute the immediate post-operative phase or the initial stage of a conservative programme. Standard approaches such as anti-inflammatory medication and cryotherapy may be necessary at this stage to reduce swelling.

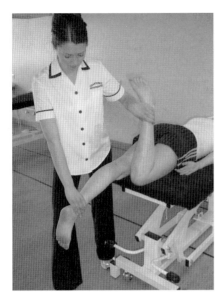

Figure 11.18 Assisted knee extension.

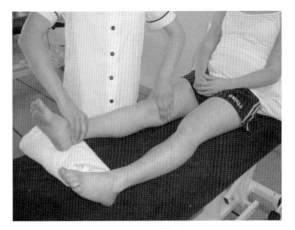

Figure 11.19 Use of a heel block to encourage knee extension.

Aerobic exercise

At this stage, aerobic exercise may be limited by the fact that the patient may be on crutches, non-weight-bearing. The patient should progress to heel walking with a normal walking pattern achieved as soon as possible, partial weight-bearing initially, progressing to full weight-bearing over the first 4 weeks following surgery or injury. The patient may find that walking up stairs or step-ups on a small step may be sufficient to challenge the aerobic system. Once an appropriate ROM is achieved, the patient may start stationary cycling with the seat high up, lowering it as the range of knee flexion increases.

ROM exercise

This stage is particularly important as delays in achieving full range of knee extension at an early stage can delay progression of rehabilitation and can cause long-term problems. A good exercise to improve extension is to place the patient lying prone with the knee and lower leg hanging off the end of the bed, with the therapist assisting extension as required (Fig. 11.18). The patient should also rest with their knee extended and unsupported and a prop underneath the heel to encourage further extension (Fig. 11.19). The range of flexion can be achieved by heel slides (Fig. 11.2).

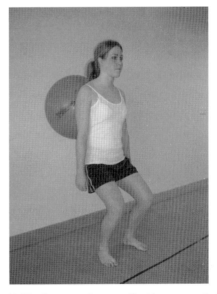

Figure 11.20 Squats against a wall with a gymnastic ball.

Muscle strength and endurance exercise

Static quadriceps contractions should be carried out on an hourly basis at this stage if possible, progressing to a straight leg raise as soon as possible. These exercises are progressed to squatting exercises, which can be combined with proprioceptive function. A two-legged squat leaning back against a gym ball against a wall is a good CKC exercise to improve muscle function of both the hamstring and quadriceps muscles (Fig. 11.20). Slow step-ups on to a low step and small lunges to the front and side are appropriate at this stage.

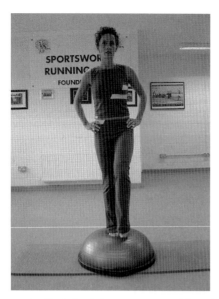

Figure 11.21 Single leg balance on an unstable surface.

Proprioception and balance exercise

All exercises described above incorporate proprioceptive function as the patient must work to ensure correct movement patterns are maintained. However, specific proprioceptive exercise may be introduced, such as standing on an unstable surface, progressing to small squats (Fig. 11.21).

Phase 2 (weeks 5–8) – early strength training

At this stage, the patient should have full ROM and normal gait and the aims of this phase are to increase loading in strength training and to continue to improve function.

Aerobic exercise

The patient may start activities such as a stepper machine or increase the resistance on an exercise bicycle. Walking may be increased in tempo, progressing to very light jogging, particularly if the patient is returning to a sport that involves running.

ROM exercise

As the patient should have full ROM at this stage, the emphasis should be on stretching of appropriate muscle groups to maintain full ROM. These muscle groups will include the hamstring and quadriceps muscle groups in particular. Stretching will be most effective following the aerobic exercise of the programme.

Muscle strength and endurance exercise

This is the most important component of the phase and will see the introduction of a variety of exercise. A combination of both open and closed chain exercise will add variety as both will enhance different functions of the muscle. Lunges may now be loaded with a weight on the shoulders ensuring correct biomechanics at all times. Squats may be progressed by loading in a shoulder press machine and performing on one leg. Other resisted movements which should be included are hip abduction, hip adduction, hip extension, heel raise, leg curl and seated knee extension (avoiding shearing on the tibia). Tagesson *et al.* (2008) suggest that load at this stage should be at 50–60% of 1 RM (repetition maximum), with three sets of 10 repetitions of the exercise performed three times a week. A combination of free weights and machine weights is useful but the additional proprioceptive challenge that free weights provide will be beneficial at this stage.

Proprioception and balance exercise

Once the patient is competent at performing a few of the resisted exercises with free weights, some of them may be performed (with care and reduced loading) on unstable surfaces such as wobble boards. Single leg squats on trampolines and wobble boards are also appropriate exercises.

Phase 3 (weeks 9–12) – intensive strength training

The aim of this phase is to introduce more functional exercise and to increase strength.

Aerobic exercise

The patient may continue with static cycling and the step machine, but may also include exercise that is appropriate to allow them to return to their particular sport. Jogging may now increase and progress to running. Running should initially take place on a flat surface, in straight lines but should quickly proceed to up and down a hill, diagonal patterns and directional changes, and running on uneven surfaces.

ROM exercise

As the patient should have very good ROM, the emphasis of this phase should be as above, to maintain the ROM with a good stretching regimen for appropriate muscle groups.

Muscle strength and endurance exercise

All exercises included in phase 2 should be continued in phase 3 with an increase in loading. Again, the exercises are performed 10 times in three sets and repeated three times a week.

Proprioception and balance exercise

Exercise can be continued in this phase with wobble boards and trampolines as for the previous phase. Running in between cones or hopping over a line on the floor will introduce more dynamic proprioceptive activity.

Phase 4 (weeks 13–16) – intensive strength training and return to sports

The aim of this phase is to increase strength, coordination and to introduce functional activity to allow the patient to return to sport or work.

Aerobic exercise

Running may increase with changes in tempo. Turns and agility drills should be introduced. Acceleration and deceleration activities should be included over various distances. Sports specific activity may be included. For example, if the patient is a footballer, ball skills will be an important component of the programme at this stage. The patient should be reaching optimal fitness by the end of this phase.

ROM exercise

As full ROM should have been achieved in the early phase of the programme, the emphasis is on main-

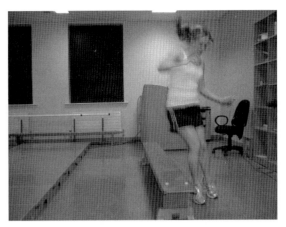

Figure 11.22 Plyometric training jumping over a bench.

tenance. Particular attention should be applied to ROM of the patellofemoral joint, ensuring that movement is normal before discharge, particularly if the graft site was the patella tendon.

Muscle strength and endurance exercise

The exercises shown above (phase 2) may be continued with the load at 80% of 1RM, increasing this load by 10% at week 15. Plyometric activity is an important addition to this stage of the programme. Jump training will fulfil this requirement, to the front and side and over objects to challenge the proprioceptive system as well (Fig. 11.22). Vertical jumps, landing on a soft surface will increase the challenge of the activity. Hopping between the rungs of a ladder placed on the ground will require a high level of control and is suitable for the late stage of activity. Jumping up a small step with both feet, progressing to a higher step on the affected leg will provide a good challenge at the latter stage of the programme.

Proprioception and balance exercise

Exercise carried out in the previous phases should be continued but the greatest proprioceptive challenge in this phase will be seen in the plyometric drills and introduction of agility drills in the late stage of functional rehabilitation.

The emphasis on return to sport should be to maintain the health of the knee and avoid further injury to the same knee (after conservative treatment) or the other knee. Certain sports present considerable risk of injury to the knee, notably soccer.

In recent years, a programme of prophylactic exercise used in soccer has shown efficacy in the reduction of risk of ACL injury (Mandelbaum *et al.* 2005; Gilchrist *et al.* 2008). The 'prevent injury, enhance performance' (PEP) programme is a routine which includes warm up, stretching, strengthening, plyometric and agility exercise. This programme shows promise for the use of exercise in reducing the risk of injury.

SECTION 3: CASE STUDIES AND STUDENT QUESTIONS

Case study 1

A 60-year-old postman presents with diffuse pain in his right knee which is aching in nature, painful on rising in the morning, and aggravated by sitting for more than 20 minutes with the knee flexed. Walking in training shoes at a moderate pace eases the pain within 10 minutes. Investigations show that he has early OA, both in the tibiofemoral and patellofemoral joints.

Management

As this patient has presented with a degenerative disorder, the aim of the treatment will not be to achieve complete resolution of symptoms but rather to improve pain and function. As this patient is already active as part of his occupation, a functional approach should be adopted in his rehabilitation. Aerobic exercise will consist of his daily walking activity, ensuring that he is wearing good footwear to optimise lower limb biomechanics. Limitations in ROM will be addressed with a programme to stretch muscle groups which cross the knee joint and activities such as heel slides and full knee extension exercises in a long sitting position. If the patellofemoral joint is hypomobile, passive mobility exercises may should be performed by the therapist. Specific strengthening exercises may incorporate proprioceptive training, by performing squats in standing, progressing to standing on an unstable surface. Single leg squats will progress the exercise, performed slowly and ensuring that the knee is well positioned over the second toe. Step-ups and step-downs may be performed, gradually increasing the depth of the step. However, as the patellofemoral joint is involved, step-downs may be painful and should be avoided if this is the case. The number of repetitions of the strengthening exercises should be high as they are only loaded by body weight and the aim is to improve the endurance of the musculature. The patient should be discharged with advice to continue daily walking and ROM exercises if possible, and strengthening exercises three times a week if possible. Regular review of this patient is necessary to monitor any progression of the OA.

Case study 2

An 18-year-old man, who is a semi-professional footballer, sustained an injury to his right knee during a game. He went in for a block tackle and felt pain on the medial aspect of his right knee. There was no immediate swelling or locking but there was pain on weight-bearing. There was no evidence of a fracture. The following day the knee was swollen, hot and painful. A diagnosis of a severe grade 2 medial ligament sprain was made.

Management

The knee was iced on a regular basis and placed in a rigid brace for weight-bearing. The brace was

Case study 2—cont'd

left *in situ* for 6 weeks but removed regularly for non-weight-bearing mobility and strengthening exercises. During the period that the brace is *in situ*, it is very important that this patient's aerobic fitness is maintained with non-weight-bearing activity such as cycling, and the uninjured leg may be used to pedal alone in the first phase of rehabilitation. Careful ROM exercises will aim to achieved full flexion and extension from an early stage in an unloaded position with full extension avoided for the first 2–4 weeks. Proprioceptive activity could be carried out in the early stage using an electrogoniometer to practise repositioning of the knee.

Between the second and fourth week, the crutches may be removed and the patient may progress to full weight-bearing. Isometric quadriceps exercise and straight leg raise exercises will aim to restore muscle function. After the fourth week, ROM exercise should aim to achieve full range, and strengthening exercise may now become weight-bearing without loading (squats and lunges) progressing to loaded exercises (leg press, hamstring curls and knee extension). Squats may be performed on an unstable surface to enhance proprioception. At 6 weeks the brace should be removed with care, provided good control of the knee joint is demonstrated. Exercises may be now more functional with the introduction of fast walking, progressing to running, initially in straight lines and then multi-directional. Strengthening exercises should continue as above with loading increased until the patient's injured knee has 80–90% of the strength of the unaffected knee, depending on which is dominant. When the patient can run comfortably, ball work may be commenced and a gradual reintegration of football training undertaken until full fitness had been achieved.

Case study 3

A 45-year-old man, who is training for a marathon, presents with anterior knee pain which is intermittent in nature but is aggravated by descending stairs and sitting at his desk for more than 20 minutes. He is not able to run for more than 10 minutes as he cannot continue because of pain. Examination reveals genu valgum and pes planus and it is noted that his running shoes are deformed and 8 years old.

Management

A working diagnosis of PFPS was given to this patient. A podiatric referral was organised at initial appointment and a pair of orthoses prescribed. The first phase of rehabilitation addressed hypomobility of soft tissue with particular emphasis on stretching the hamstrings, quadriceps, iliotibial band and tensor fascia lata. The patella was mobilised to improve lateral tilt and to improve mobility in the lateral retinaculum. As taping the patella did not change any symptoms, it was not used in this case. Initial strengthening exercise consisted of isometric quads contraction, with particular emphasis on VMO activity. This is progressed to squats to 40° in standing and isometric hip abduction against a wall. Positioning of the knee over the second was monitored and the position of the medial arch of the foot was corrected. Aerobic fitness was maintained with aqua jogging on a daily basis. After 2 weeks, this patient was allowed to start walking, increasing his tempo to a light jog, monitoring position of the knees, hips and feet. He wore his orthoses in a new pair of running shoes which were designed to specifically address his foot pronation. The therapist regularly monitored his VMO activity while walking and jogging to ensure that normal activity was demonstrated. ROM exercises were carried out as above. Squat exercises were progressed to step-downs, introducing some loading at a later stage. At the final stage of the rehabilitation the patient was allowed to increase the distance of a run, progressing to an increased tempo and running on a hilly terrain and changing direction. At discharge, he was advised that all stretches and the VMO programme should be continued and that he should regularly renew his running shoes with specific advice from a podiatrist.

Student questions

(1) A football player has suffered a second-degree tear of his hamstring muscles. Describe the:
- Pre-stretching routine
- Exact stretching routine used
- Post-stretching routine.

(2) Describe your rehabilitation programme for a non-active woman with a sedentary occupation who has OA of the knee.

(3) Discuss an exercise programme for a third-degree MCL sprain of the knee sustained by a young car mechanic, in the intermediate stage of rehabilitation.

(4) Why is proprioception so important in knee rehabilitation?

(5) Demonstrate five non-weight-bearing exercises you might use in the treatment of a repaired medial meniscus.

(6) Discuss the factors that are important in the progression in proprioception training for a knee injury.

(7) What are the differences in a quadriceps muscle with an intra-muscular and an inter-muscular haematoma? How would the treatment approach differ?

(8) Describe the progressions of strength training for a knee ligament injury.

(9) What benefits are there in aerobic training for a retired school teacher who has OA of the knee?

(10) A rugby player is referred to you 8 weeks after an injury to his MCL to his right knee for your opinion on his fitness to resume match play. What are your considerations?

References

Baker, K.R., Nelson, M.E., Felson, D.T., Layne, J.E., Sarno, R. and Roubenoff, R. (2001) The efficacy of home based progressive strength training in older adults with knee osteoarthritis. A randomised controlled trial. *Journal of Rheumatology*, 28, 1655–1665.

Baker, V., Bennell, K., Stillman, B., Cowan, S. and Crossley, K. (2002) Abnormal knee joint position sense in individuals with patellofemoral pain syndrome. *Journal of Orthopaedic Research*, 20, 208–214.

Bartels, E.M., Lund, H., Hagen, K.B., Dagfinrud, H., Christensen, R. and Danneskiold-Samsoe, B. (2007) Aquatic exercise for the treatment of knee and hip oste-

oarthritis. *Cochrane Database of Systematic Reviews*, 4, CD005523.

Bayramoglu, M., Toprak, R. and Sozay, S. (2007) Effects of osteoarthritis and fatigue on proprioception of the knee joint. *Archives of Physical Medicine and Rehabilitation*, 88, 346–350.

Bennell, K.L., Hinman, R.S., Metcalf, B.R., Crossley, K.M., Buchbinder, R., Smith, M. and McColl, G. (2003) Relationship of knee joint proprioception to pain and disability in individuals with knee osteoarthritis. *Journal of Orthopaedic Research*, 21, 792–797.

Bonfim, T.R., Paccola, C.A.J. and Barela, J.A. (2003) Proprioceptive and behaviour impairments in individuals with anterior cruciate ligament reconstructed knees. *Archives of Physical Medicine and Rehabilitation*, 84, 1217–1223.

Brosseau, L., MacLeay, L., Robinson, V.A., Tugwell, P. and Wells, G. (2003). Intensity of exercise for the treatment of osteoarthritis. *Cochrane Database of Systematic Reviews*, 2, CD004259.

Cheing, G.L.Y., Hui-Chan, C.W.Y. and Chan, K.M. (2002) Does four weeks of TENS and/or isometric exercise produce cumulative reduction of osteoarthritic knee pain? *Clinical Rehabilitation*, 16, 749–760.

Chen, E.H. and Black, J. (1980) Materials design analysis of the prosthetic anterior cruciate ligament. *Journal of Biomedical Materials Research*, 14, 567–586.

Cowan, S.M., Bennell, K.L., Crossley, K.M., Hodges, P.W. and McConnell, J. (2002) Physical therapy alters recruitment of the vasti in patellofemoral pain syndrome. *Medicine and Science in Sport and Exercise*, 34, 1879–1885.

Crossley, K., Bennell, K., Green, S., Cowan, S. and McConnell, J. (2002) Physical Therapy for patellofemoral pain: A randomised, double–blinded, placebo controlled trial. *American Journal of Sports Medicine*, 30, 857–865.

Deyle, G.D., Henderson, N.E., Matekel, R.L., Ryder, M.G., Garber, M.B. and Allison, S.C. (2000) Effectiveness of manual physical therapy and exercise in osteoarthritis of the knee. A randomised controlled trial. *Annals of Internal Medicine*, 132, 173–181.

Dias, R.C., Dias, J.M.D. and Ramos, L.R. (2003) Impact of an exercise and walking protocol on quality of life for elderly people with OA of the knee. *Physiotherapy Research International*, 8, 121–130.

Drawer, S. and Fuller, C.W. (2001) Propensity for osteoarthritis and lower limb joint pain in retired and professional soccer players. *British Journal of Sports Medicine*, 35, 402–408.

Erden, Z., Otman, S., Atilla, B. and Tunay, V.B. (2003) Relationship between pain intensity and knee joint position sense in patients with severe osteoarthritis. *Pain Clinic*, 15, 293–297.

Ettinger, W.H., Burns, R., Messier, P., Applegate, W., Rejeski, W.J., Morgan, T., Shumaker, S. and Berry, M.J. (1997) A randomised trial comparing aerobic exercise and resistance exercise with a health education programme in older adults with knee osteoarthritis. The fitness arthritis and seniors trial (FAST). *Journal of the American Medical Association*, 277, 32–37.

Evcik, D. and Sonel, B. (2002) Effectiveness of a home-based exercise therapy and walking programme on osteoarthritis of the knee. *Rheumatology International*, 22, 103–106.

Eyigor, S. (2004) A comparison of muscle training methods in patients with knee osteoarthritis. *Clinical Rheumatology*, 23, 109–115.

Fransen, M., Mc Connell, S. and Bell, M. (2001) Exercise for osteoarthritis of the hip or knee (review). *Cochrane Database of Systematic Reviews*, 2, CD004376.

Fredberg, U., Bolvig, L. and Andersen, N.T. (2008) Prophylactic training in asymptomatic soccer players with ultrasonographic abnormalities in Achilles and patellar tendons: the Danish Super League Study. *American Journal of Sports Medicine*, 36, 451–460.

Gilchrist J., Mandelbaum, B.R., Melancon, H., Ryan, G.W., Silvers, H.J., Griffin, L.Y., Watanabe, D.S., Dick, R.W. and Dvorak, J. (2008) A randomised controlled trial to prevent noncontact anterior cruciate ligament injury in female collegiate soccer players. *American Journal of Sports Medicine*, 36, 1476–1483.

Grodski, M. and Marks, R. (2008) Exercises following anterior cruciate ligament reconstructive surgery: biomechanical considerations and efficacy of current approaches. *Research in Sports Medicine*, 16, 75–96.

Hassan, B.S., Mockett, S. and Doherty, M. (2001). Static postural sway, proprioception and maximal voluntary quadriceps contraction in patients with knee osteoarthritis and normal control subjects. *Annals of Rheumatic Diseases*, 60, 612–618.

Heintjes, E., Berger, M.Y., Bierma-Zeinstra, S.M.A., Bernsen, R.M.D., Verhaar, J.A.N. and Koes, B.W. (2003) Exercise therapy for patellofemoral pain syndrome (review). *Cochrane Database of Systematic Reviews*, 4, CD003472.

Herrington, L. and Al-Sherhi, A. (2007) A controlled trial of weight-bearing versus non-weight-bearing exercises for patellofemoral pain. *Journal of Orthopaedic and Sports Physical Therapy*, 37, 155–60.

Houghum, P. (2005) *Therapeutic Exercises for the Musculoskeletal Injuries*, 2nd edn. Human Kinetics, Champaign, Illinois.

Jan, M.H., Lin, J.J., Liau, J.J., Lin, Y.F. and Lin, D.H. (2008) Investigation of clinical effects of high and low resistance training for patients with knee osteoarthritis: a randomised controlled trial. *Physical Therapy*, 88, 427–436.

Jonsson, P. and Alfredson, H. (2005) Superior results with eccentric compared to concentric quadriceps training in patients with jumper's knee: a prospective randomised study. *British Journal of Sports Medicine*, 39, 847–850.

Koralewicz, L.M. and Engh, G.A. (2000) Comparison of proprioception in arthritic and age-matched normal knees. *Journal of Bone and Joint Surgery, American Volume*, 82, 1582–1588.

Lewek, M.D., Rudolph, K.S. and Snyder-Mackler, L. (2004) Quadriceps femoris muscle weakness and activation failure in patients with symptomatic knee osteoarthritis. *Journal of Orthopaedic Research*, 22, 110–115.

Mandelbaum, B.R., Silvers, H.J., Watanabe, D.S., Knarr, J.F., Thomas, S.D., Griffin, L.Y., Kirkendall, D.T. and Garrett, W. (2005) Effectiveness of a neuromuscular and proprioceptive training program in preventing anterior cruciate ligament injuries in female athletes. *American Journal of Sports Medicine*, 33, 1003–1010.

Manninen, P., Riihimaki, H., Heliovaara, M. and Suomalainen, O. (2001) Physical exercise and the risk of severe knee osteoarthritis requiring arthroplasty. *Rheumatology*, 40, 432–437.

Mason, D. L., Dickens, V. and Vail, A. (2007) Rehabilitation for hamstring injuries (review). *Cochrane Database of Systematic Reviews*, 1, CD004575.

McConnell, J. (1996) Management of patellofemoral problems. *Manual Therapy*, 1, 60–66.

Neptune, R.R. and Kautz, S.A. (2000) Knee joint loading in forward versus backward pedalling: implications for rehabilitation strategies. *Clinical Biomechanics*, 15, 528–535.

Ng, G.Y.F. and Wong, P.Y.K. (2009) Patellar taping affects vastus medialis obliquus activation in subjects with patellofemoral pain before and after quadriceps muscle fatigue. *Clinical Rehabilitation*, 23, 705–713.

O'Reilly, S.C., Muir, K.R. and Doherty, M. (1999) Effectiveness of home exercise on pain and disability from osteoarthritis of the knee: a randomised controlled trial. *Annals of Rheumatic Diseases*, 58, 15–19.

O'Sullivan, S.P. (2005) Activation of vastus medialis obliquus among individuals with patellofemoral pain syndrome. *Journal of Strength and Conditioning Research*, 19, 302–304.

Pai, Y.C., Rymer, W.Z., Chang, R.W. and Sharma, L. (1997) Effect of age and osteoarthritis on knee proprioception. *Arthritis and Rheumatism*, 40, 2260–2265.

Panics, G., Tallay, A., Pavlik, A. and Berkes, I. (2008) Effect of proprioception training on knee joint position sense in female team handball players. *British Journal of Sports Medicine*, 42, 472–476.

Peccin, M.S., Almeida, G.J.M., Amaro, J., Cohen, M., Soares, B.G.O. and Atallah, A.N. (2005) Interventions for treating posterior cruciate ligament injuries of the knee in adults. *Cochrane Database of Systemic Reviews*, 3, CD002939.

Pennix, B.W., Messier, S.P., Rejeski, W.J., Williamson, J.D., DiBari, M., Cavazzini, C., Applegate, W.B. and Pahor, M. (2001) Physical exercise and the prevention of disability in activities of daily living in older persons with osteoarthritis. *Archives of Internal Medicine*, 161, 2309–2316.

Purdam, C., R., Johnsson, P., Alfredson, H., Lorentzon, R., Cook, J.L. and Khan, K.M. (2004) A pilot study of the eccentric decline squat in the management of painful chronic patellar tendinopathy. *British Journal of Sports Medicine*, 38, 395–397.

Reider, B., Arcand, M.A., Diehl, L.H., Mroczek, K., Abulencia, A., Stroud, C.C., Palm, M., Gilbertson, J. and Staszak, P. (2003) Arthroscopy. *Journal of Arthroscopic and Related Surgery*, 19, 2–12.

Rogind, H., Bibow-Nielsen, B., Jensen, B., Moller, H.C., Frimodt-Moller and Bliddal, H. (1998) The effects of a physical training programme on patients with osteoarthritis of the knees. *Archives of Physical Medicine and Rehabilitation*, 79, 1421–1427.

Sevick, M.A., Bradham, D.D., Muender, M., Chen, J., Enarson, C., Dailey, M. and Ettinger, W.H. (2000) Cost effectiveness of aerobic and resistance exercise in seniors with knee osteoarthritis. *Medicine and Science in Sports and Exercise*, 32, 1534–1540.

Silva, L.E., Valim, V., Pessanha, A.P.C., Oliviera, L.M., Myamoto, S., Jones, A. and Natour, J. (2008) Hydrotherapy versus conventional land based exercise for the management of patients with osteoarthritis of the knee: A randomised clinical trial. *Physical Therapy*, 88, 12–21.

Slemenda, C., Brandt, K.D., Heilman, D.K., Mazzuca, S., Braunstein, E.M., Katz, B.P. and Wolinsky, F.D. (1997) Quadriceps weakness and osteoarthritis of the knee. *Annals of Internal Medicine*, 127, 94–104.

Syme, G., Rowe, P., Martin, D. and Daly, G. (2008) Disability in patients with chronic patellofemoral pain syndrome. A randomised controlled trial of VMO training versus general quadriceps strengthening. *Manual Therapy*, 14, 252–263.

Tagesson, S., Oberg, B., Good, L. and Kvist, J. (2008) A comprehensive rehabilitation programme with quadriceps strengthening in closed versus open kinetic chain exercise in patients with anterior cruciate ligament deficiency. *American Journal of Sports Medicine*, 36, 298–307.

Trees, A.H., Howe, T.E., Dixon, J. and White, L. (2005) Exercise for treating isolated anterior cruciate ligament injuries in adults. *Cochrane Database of Systematic Reviews*, 4, CD005316.

Trees, A.H., Howe, T.E., Grant, M. and Gray, H.G. (2007) Exercise for treating anterior cruciate ligament injuries in

combination with collateral ligament and meniscal damage of the knee in adults. Cochrane Database of Systematic Reviews, Issue 3. Art No.: CD005961. DOI:10.1002/14651858.CD005961.

Tsauo, J.Y., Cheung, P-F. and Yang, R.S. (2008) The effects of sensorimotor training on knee proprioception and function for patients with knee osteoarthritis: a preliminary report. *Clinical Rehabilitation*, 22, 448–457.

Vagan, V. and Hunt, E. (2008) Patellofemoral pain syndrome: a review on the associated neuromuscular deficits and current treatment options. *British Journal of Sports Medicine*, 42, 789–795.

Van Baar, M.E., Assendelft, W.J.J., Dekker, J., Oostendorp, R.A.B. and Bijlsma, J.W.J. (1999) Effectiveness of exercise therapy in patients with osteoarthritis of the hip or knee. *Arthritis and Rheumatism*, 42, 1361–1369.

Visnes, H. and Bahr, R. (2007) The evolution of eccentric training as treatment for patellar tendinopathy (jumper's knee): a critical review of exercise programmes. *British Journal of Sports Medicine*, 41, 217–223.

Witvrouw, E., Danneels, L., Van Tiggelen, D., Willems T.M. and Cambier, D. (2004) Open versus closed kinetic chain exercises in patellofemoral pain: a 5-year prospective randomized study. *American Journal of Sports Medicine*, 32, 1122–1130.

Wright, R.W., Preston, E., Fleming, B.C., Amendola, A., Andrish, J.T., Bergfeld, J.A., Dunn, W.R., Kaeding, C., Kuhn, J.E., Marx, R.G., McCarty, E.C., Parker, R.C., Spindler, K.P., Wolcott, M., Wolf, B.R. and Williams, G.N. (2008) A systematic review of anterior cruciate ligament reconstruction rehabilitation: part II: open versus closed kinetic chain exercises, neuromuscular electrical stimulation, accelerated rehabilitation, and miscellaneous topics. *Journal of Knee Surgery*, 21, 225–234.

The Foot and Ankle Complex

12

Ruth Magee

SECTION 1: INTRODUCTION AND BACKGROUND

The treatment of the foot and ankle complex is multifactorial, requiring the clinician to use many treatment approaches for the successful management of both acute and chronic injuries. However, the emphasis in this chapter is on basic exercise rehabilitation of the foot and ankle, although it is important that the therapist considers all the other variables which affect the foot and ankle complex.

Evidence for the use of exercise in the rehabilitation of foot and ankle injuries

Evidence which supports treatment interventions to the foot and ankle is limited overall, and there has been a large emphasis in the research on the ankle and rearfoot complex, with little on the midfoot and forefoot. Much of the research has focused on a small number of conditions, notably anterior talofibular ligament (ATFL) sprain.

Handoll *et al.* (2001) conducted a review of research under the Cochrane Collaboration. Studies which examined various interventions for the prevention of ankle ligament injuries were included. Although a large number of studies that were included in the review had methodological limitations, some conclusions were drawn. Co-ordination training using ankle discs in those with a prior history of ankle sprain demonstrated a decreased risk of ankle sprain in the intervention group compared with controls in a number of studies. Some evidence was also presented indicating that a supervised physiotherapy programme that emphasised balance reduced risk or re-injury when compared with controls. The review found good evidence for the use of external ankle supports to prevent ligament injuries of the ankle but concluded that further research was needed to be conclusive regarding exercise therapy.

A more recent Cochrane review conducted by Kerkhoffs *et al.* (2007) examined surgical versus conservative treatment for acute injuries of the lateral ligament complex of the ankle in adults. Of the 20 trials that were included, the authors suggested that all had methodological flaws that could have affected their results and the overall conclusion was that there was not enough evidence to say if surgery or conservative treatment, including exercise therapy, was the optimal treatment for ankle sprains. De Fries *et al.* (2006) reviewed studies which examined interventions, including exercise therapy, for treating chronic ankle instability. Again, methodological flaws were highlighted in many studies and the authors were unable to conclude if any specific intervention was optimal for

Exercise Therapy in the Management of Musculoskeletal Disorders, First Edition. Edited by Fiona Wilson, John Gormley and Juliette Hussey.
© 2011 Blackwell Publishing Ltd

treating ankle instability. However, it was found that following surgical construction, early functional rehabilitation, or exercise therapy was superior to immobilisation regarding time to return to work and sports. Zoch *et al.* (2003) reviewed studies that examined rehabilitation of ligamentous ankle injuries, concluding that a combination of isokinetic strength training with proprioceptive training shortens rehabilitation and serves as a secondary prophylaxis.

Karatosun *et al.* (2008) compared intra-articular injection therapy to exercise therapy in the management of osteoarthritis of the ankle and found that both provided functional improvement, although the authors concluded that larger trials were necessary to compare individual efficacies more accurately. Van der Wees *et al.* (2006) conducted a review of trials which examined the effectiveness of exercise therapy and manual mobilisation in acute ankle sprain and found that exercise therapy was effective in reducing the risk of recurrent sprains and functional instability although the effects of manual mobilisation were limited to having an (initial) effect on dorsiflexion range of motion (ROM).

More recently, Loudon *et al.* (2008) reviewed studies which examined the effectiveness of active exercise as an intervention for functional ankle instability. Results were positive for the inclusion of exercise therapy in management of ankle instability and the authors concluded that conservative treatment interventions including balance, proprioceptive and muscle strengthening exercise were effective in decreasing 'giving way' episodes, improving balance stability and improving function. Thus, while there is some clear evidence for the positive benefits of exercise in the management of ankle ligament sprain and some evidence in the management of ankle OA, there is a demand for further trials which are of robust methodology to support this approach.

Aerobic exercise

There is little evidence to support the use of aerobic exercise in the treatment of foot and ankle dysfunctions and the author was unable to source any trials which examined the role of an aerobic exercise programme specifically for foot and ankle disorders. However, Willems *et al.* (2005a) showed that poor cardio-respiratory endurance was a risk factor for inversion ankle sprain in a study of male subjects

and Tyler *et al.* (2006) showed that a high body mass index, which is frequently related to poor cardio-respiratory endurance, was also a risk factor for the same injury. Valderrabano *et al.* (2006) showed that patients who were more 'sports active' showed better functional results following total ankle replacement compared with patients who were inactive. Although Xu *et al.* (2004) showed that tai chi had a significant effect on improving proprioception in the ankle, it is unclear if such exercise involves aerobic conditioning. Hubley-Kozey *et al.* (1995) evaluated the effects of a general exercise programme on the passive ROM of the lower limb joints including the ankle in elderly women. The programme included aerobic exercise, stretching and muscular strength and endurance exercise and the authors found that ROM improved in all joints lower limb joints following the programme. As there was a stretching component to the programme it is therefore unclear if the aerobic exercise contributed to the improvements.

Part of the reason for lack of research may be related to the difficulties of loading the cardio-respiratory system when the foot and ankle are dysfunctional, leaving limited options such as swimming and non-weight-bearing programmes for aerobic exercise. However, those studies which examined the role of aerobic exercise in the management of multi-joint osteoarthritis should be considered at this point and have been discussed in earlier chapters.

Muscle strength and endurance

For many clinicians, the early focus of rehabilitation of any foot or ankle disorders will be muscle strengthening exercise. Hartsell and Spaulding (1999) showed that chronic ankle instability and muscle weakness do co-exist and Willems *et al.* (2005a) identified decreased dorsiflexion strength as a risk factor for ankle inversion sprain. Konradsen *et al.* (1998) showed that eversion strength is reduced (compared with the non-injured joint) 3 weeks following acute ankle inversion injuries and Munn *et al.* (2003) found that eccentric inversion strength was reduced in ankle instability. Despite these findings, there is a paucity of research into strengthening exercise as rehabilitation following ankle joint injury.

Much of the focus of strengthening exercise in the management of foot and ankle disorders has been on rehabilitation of Achilles tendinopathy. Alfredson *et al.* (1998) were one of the first groups to prospectively study the effect of a 12-week, heavy load, eccentric calf muscle training programme on individuals with chronic Achilles tendinopathy compared with a control group that received conventional treatment during the same period of time (rest, non-steroidal anti-inflammatory drugs (NSAIDs), orthoses, physiotherapy and 'ordinary' training programmes). While the control group showed no improvement in symptoms, the subjects in the intervention group were all able to return to full function (running) following the programme. While this was a moderately small study with some methodological flaws, similar findings were presented by Mafi *et al.* (2001) with a similar intervention and the overall clinical outcome was much better for eccentric calf training that a concentric programme (Niesen-Vertommen *et al.*, 1992; Mafi *et al.*, 2001). Alfredson *et al.* (2008) suggested that eccentric exercise involves muscle activation combined with muscle-tendon unit lengthening and it is likely to affect the dampening characteristics of the calf muscle and change the type 1 collagen production and tendon volume, which will increase the tendon tensile strength over time.

In further support of an eccentric strengthening protocol, Kingma *et al.* (2007) conducted a systematic review of studies with such a programme in management of Achilles tendinopathy. The authors concluded that although further studies are warranted, results to date are promising and support eccentric overload training in the management of Achilles tendinopathy. More recently, similar findings were presented in a systematic review by Magnussen *et al.* (2009), who analysed 16 quality trials, which concluded that eccentric exercises have the most evidence of effectiveness in the management of mid-portion Achilles tendinopathy.

Many of the studies on strengthening exercise and the foot and ankle have also looked at proprioceptive training and will be discussed in the following sections.

Range of motion and flexibility

Restoring full range of movement to the ankle and foot is essential for the correct movement patterns and biomechanical alignment of the foot and ankle. This can be done using joint mobilisation techniques, tissue massage and stretching or ROM exer-

cises. Willems *et al.* (2005a) found that lack of ankle dorsiflexion was a strong predictor of ankle injury, stating that poor dorsiflexion is associated with 2.5 times the risk of injury. If there was excessive dorsiflexion, and a hypermobile ankle, the risk increased to eight times. However, Willems *et al.* (2005b) found that a greater ROM, in this case in the first metatarsophalangeal (MTP) joint, was a risk factor for ankle inversion sprain in females. Beedle and Mann (2007) determined that the optimal stretch to increase ROM at the ankle joint was a static stretch following a warm-up, which was superior to ballistic stretching following a warm-up.

There is a lack of consensus regarding the immobilisation of acute ankle inversion injuries. Boyce *et al.* (2005) advocated a return to immobilisation, but on a temporary basis and recommended the use of an ankle brace for grade 2 and 3 lateral ligament sprains. Immobilisation was shown to result in significant improvement in ankle joint range of movement at both 10 days and 1 month, when compared with an elastic support.

Flanigan *et al.* (2007) examined the effect of plantar fascia stretching on plantar fascia pain. Previous studies had demonstrated that specific stretching of the plantar fascia was superior to standard weight-bearing Achilles tendon stretching exercises and had a significant effect in reducing pain and functional limitations in subjects with chronic plantar fasciitis (Digiovanni *et al.* 2006). Flanigan *et al.* (2007) concluded that a stretch which included both MTP and ankle joint dorsiflexion was superior to ankle joint or MTP joint alone, having positive effects in the management of plantar fasciitis.

Balance and proprioception

Recent research has placed great emphasis on functional control of the foot and ankle in rehabilitation and the influence of proprioceptive exercise has received focus in a number of studies. The single leg stand test is probably the most useful clinical test in identifying proprioceptive and/or balance dysfunction following foot and ankle disorders.

Trojian and McKeag (2006) state that the single leg balance test is a reliable and valid test for predicting ankle sprains and that the association between a poor single leg stand test and ankle sprain is significant. Javed *et al.* (1999) demonstrated longer reaction time in the peroneus longus muscles of patients who presented with chronic or acute functional instability when compared with controls. Further, they examined the effects of either surgical stabilisation or proprioceptive exercise on peroneal reaction time and found that only the exercise group showed improvement.

Evidence from a number of studies supports the use of wobble boards to improve proprioception in the ankle following inversion injuries (Clark and Burden, 2005). Clark and Burden (2005) noted a significant decrease in muscle onset latency and a significant improvement of their perception of functional instability when a group followed a 4-week wobble board training programme for 10 minutes, three times per week. However, there has been a recent trend among clinicians not to use wobble boards as they are not considered a functional exercise, and it is thought that it is better to focus on a land-based functional programme instead. Delahunt (2007) noted that subjects who have functional instability in the ankle, exhibit feed-forward control deficits to the peroneus longus during dynamic activities. Delahunt suggests that rehabilitation strategies should include exercises that produce sudden unexpected changes in joint movement, as this will facilitate unconscious joint stabilization. The need to rehabilitate the feed-forward mechanism suggests that the use of wobble boards, foam blocks, foam rollers and trampolines will all aid in the rehabilitation of the functionally unstable ankle, as it will produce sudden unexpected change.

A number of studies have noted that introduction of a balance training programme is effective in reducing the risk of ankle sprains. McHugh *et al.* (2007) showed that including a balance training intervention in training for high school football players reduced the incidence of non-contact ankle sprains; Mohammadi (2007) found similar results with the same kind of intervention in soccer players. McGuine and Keene (2006) showed that a balance training programme reduced the risk of ankle sprains in high school athletes. Schweizer *et al.* (2005) attempted to include variation in balance and co-ordination demands by examining stability and co-ordination in the ankles of rock climbers compared with soccer players. The authors suggested that rock climbing demands slow, well-controlled movements of the foot and ankle with the tibiotalar and subtalar joints in varying positions. The study found that the rock climbers exhibited significantly better results in stabilometry testing and greater maximum strength in the ankle

when compared with the soccer players. It was concluded that a rock climbing type of exercise may be of value in the treatment of ankle instability.

Thus although the evidence supporting the use of exercise in the management of foot and ankle disorders is limited in some areas, there is clear support for the use of certain protocols, particularly in the areas of strengthening and proprioception. Such exercises will be discussed practically in Section 2.

Common conditions

Ankle inversion injury

Often an ankle inversion injury is thought to be the same as a lateral ligament sprain; however, this is not always the case. An ankle inversion injury may affect multiple structures beyond the lateral ligament and can cause problems such as a fracture at the fibular head, an osteochondral fracture of the dome of the talus or subluxation of the peroneal tendons – all of which can be very subtle and difficult to diagnose. The patient may present with symptoms very similar to a straightforward lateral ligament sprain. It is essential that the therapist diagnoses the ankle dysfunction correctly and bears in mind the other possible diagnoses. For the purposes of this chapter, a lateral ligament sprain will be discussed, and it is important to remember that an inadequately rehabilitated ankle will lead to prolonged symptoms, a high risk of recurrence and reduced function.

A lateral ligament injury is usually caused by a plantar flexion/inversion movement, and the most commonly injured portion is the ATFL. Depending on the severity of the injury (grades 1–3 ligament sprain), the person may need to stop their activity immediately, or can continue with limitations. The swelling may be immediate or may develop within a few hours. In a grade 1 tear, there is no ligament laxity; in a grade 2 tear there is some ligament laxity but a firm end point and in a grade 3, there is gross laxity with a complete ligament rupture and no end point when testing. Often grade 3 injuries are the least painful, but it is important to get the diagnosis correct as this will dictate the rate of recovery and also the rate of rehabilitation. The management principles for all three grades are the same: control swelling; reduce pain ± immobilisation with a brace, taping or crutches; restore range of movement; restore muscle strength; proprioceptive exercises, and implement a functional sports or work specific programme.

Ankle sprains account for 20% of all sports injuries (Price *et al.*, 2004). Disability from ankle sprains can be severe with 40% of the population having dysfunction that persists for as long as 6 months after the injury (Gerber *et al.*, 1998) and athletes with multiple ankle sprains have significantly reduced proprioception and kinaesthetic awareness (Garn and Newton, 1998). Ankle sprains are the most common injury with an incidence rate of 80% in athletic populations and a recurrence rate of 73% (Yeung *et al.*, 1994). The successful rehabilitation of ankle injuries is crucial in preventing high recurrence rates. Those at risk of an ankle inversion injury include those with a mobile foot type, a more pronated foot, a longer total foot contact time, lateral pressure in the forefoot at push off phase in the gait cycle and those with delayed knee flexion (Willems *et al.*, 2005a). Willems *et al.* (2005b) advocate that the therapist attends to gait patterns and addresses foot biomechanics to prevent inversion injuries. Proprioception is disturbed after an ankle sprain (Hartsell, 2000), thus highlighting the importance of adequate rehabilitation. Often rehabilitation is combined with ankle bracing or taping, as this has been shown to reduce the incidence of re-spraining (Surve *et al.*, 1994).

Chronic pain following an ankle inversion injury may be due to a number of factors including: lateral or deltoid ligament instability; impingement lesion; osteochondral lesion of the talus; syndesmotic instability; or fracture.

Pes Planus, plantar fasciosis and hallux valgus

Pes planus (flat feet) and pain in the region of the plantar fascia (plantar fasciitis or fasciosis) are often seen together, so are being discussed together rather than as separate entities for the purposes of this chapter. Clinically, it is very common to see one condition with the other. The plantar fascia is the major stabiliser of the longitudinal arch, particularly during the mid stance phase of the gait cycle. Pes planus, whether rigid or flexible can lead to injury. The navicular is dropped and the longitudinal arch remains pronated during the gait cycle,

which can cause torsion of the plantar fascia and the Achilles' tendon. The author's experience is that planus must be treated if there is a varus or valgus dysfunction at the subtalar joint causing poor biomechanics; this is particularly important in the childhood/adolescent population. If the patient has a stable subtalar joint, but is genetically flat footed, they would appear to have a low risk or predisposition to injury. Overuse injuries are associated with excessive pronation and it is important to fully rehabilitate not only the long and short intrinsic foot muscles, but also soleus, gastrocnemius and tibialis posterior, as these are likely to absorb shock and reduce the impact on the plantar fascia and midfoot region (O'Connor and Hamill, 2003).

Plantar fasciitis is thought to be due to irritation of the proximal plantar fascia with or without a history of trauma. Pain typically presents under the plantar heel and is worse on weight-bearing although may ease with exercise. There is usually tenderness at the proximal plantar fascia. Magnetic resonance imaging (MRI) may be useful in distinguishing from a stress fracture. Optimal treatment requires a stretching programme for the gastrocnemius, soleus, plantar fascia, orthoses, NSAIDs and in worse cases, surgery (Berkson *et al.*, 2007).

Hallux valgus of the first MTP joint is also known as a bunion, and can have a genetic or biomechanical cause or a combination of both. A hallux valgus diagnosis is given when there is 10° valgus or greater at the first MTP joint, and it is usually associated with a pes planus. This causes the forces at the toe off phase of the gait cycle to pass through the medial aspect of the first ray, thus pushing the ray even further across. Rehabilitation of the foot and ankle may prevent the progression of this condition, but there is a need for further research in this area, particularly in the adolescent population.

Achilles' tendinopathy

Achilles' tendinopathies involve pain in the region of the Achilles' tendon. They can be extremely chronic and difficult to treat and can be very frustrating for the patient, both athlete and non-athlete alike. Until recently it was assumed that overuse of the tendon caused inflammation and thus pain, requiring regular use of NSAIDs. However, more recent research has demonstrated that the pain of tendinopathy may be due to unidentified biochemical factors that activate peritendinous nociceptors without inflammation. Pathological studies have shown that Achilles' tendinopathy is a degenerative process with an absence of inflammatory cells (Smith and Sands, 2007).

Achilles' tendon functions eccentrically to lower the heel to the ground when landing from a jump and it works hard when walking and running uphill. It is usually a chronic overuse injury, of insidious onset, with no specific event to trigger it. However, on further questioning of the patient, it generally becomes obvious that it is associated with excessive stress and either slow or sudden overload on the Achilles' tendon, which can be caused by poor and excessive training methods, poor biomechanics of the lower limb and in particular foot pronation, a change in footwear or training programmes, poor balance within the training programme, which can lead to joint and muscle imbalances causing weakness and lack of flexibility not only of the calf but also of the lumbo-pelvic region and leg. The pain can be both in the mid section of the Achilles tendon and can also be at its insertion into the calcaneum. The latter is much harder to treat and takes a lot longer to settle, so the patient should be aware of the different prognosis, and it is important that the therapist diagnoses it correctly. Tendinopathy frequently occurs in the mid-substance of the tendon in the area of hypovascularity. Patients will complain of pain when rising from a resting position. Examination reveals thickening of the mid-substance of the tendon with local tenderness.

Optimal rehabilitation requires exercise therapy and biomechanical considerations. As it is now known that this disorder is not defined by inflammation, traditional anti-inflammatories approaches, such as NSAIDs, should be avoided. The greatest advance in the management of this condition over the past 20 years has been in the use of eccentric exercise therapy with a number of quality trials demonstrating its efficacy (Rees *et al.*, 2009). The evidence for use of eccentric exercise is strong for the management of mid portion Achilles' tendinopathy but less robust in the management of insertional Achilles' tendinopathy although recent work has demonstrated increased efficacy of eccentric exercise in insertional pathology when the exercise does not move beyond plantigrade (Jonsson *et al.*, 2008). Section 2 outlines practical implementation of the eccentric exercise programme.

SECTION 2: PRACTICAL USE OF EXERCISE

The evidence supporting the use of exercise therapy in the management of foot and ankle disorders is very condition specific and so this chapter will discuss rehabilitation with reference to chosen pathologies or disorders.

Ankle inversion injury

Early rehabilitation

Aerobic exercise

The primary concern when prescribing aerobic exercise following an inversion injury is the stability of the ankle. In the acute stage, single leg cycling with the unaffected leg will allow the cardiovascular system to be challenged without compromising the affected joint. The patient may then progress to cycling with the affected leg with the clinician ensuring that the ankle is maintained in a close packed, dorsiflexed position by keeping the heel rather than the toe at the front of the pedal. Swimming is also suitable, particularly front and back crawl. Breast stroke may be tried with the ankle in dorsiflexion, although avoid the 'whip kick' in as this can be painful. If the ankle is too painful with any leg kicking movement, the patient may put a float between the legs and concentrate on arm movement only.

ROM and flexibility

A programme that includes range of movement exercises and alphabet drawing with the foot is suitable to rehabilitate ROM. Progress the programme to weight transfer and knee bending in standing with support, and gait re-education focusing on heel strike, foot flat and toe off. The patient may not be able to weight-bear more than 25% of their body weight at this stage onto the affected leg, but they should slowly try to progress their percentage body weight onto this leg until they can do a single leg stand with comfort.

See Figures 12.1 and 12.2 for progression of dorsiflexion from non-weight-bearing to weight-bearing. See Figure 12.3 for plantar flexion home

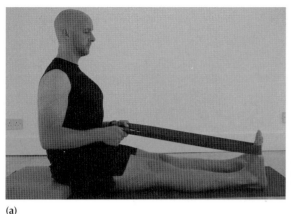

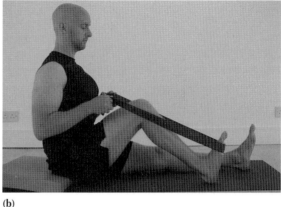

(a)   (b)

Figure 12.1   (**a**) Long-sitting, straight leg dorsiflexion, targeting gastrocnemius. (**b**) Long sitting, bent knee dorsiflexion, targeting soleus.

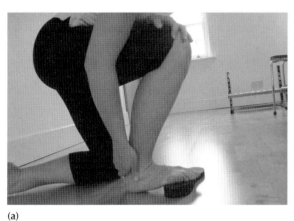

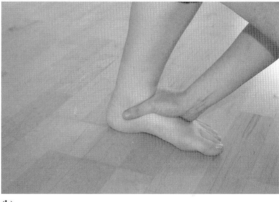

(a)   (b)

Figure 12.2   (**a**) Dorsiflexion. (**b**) Dorsiflexion in weight-bearing.

exercise progression in standing and sitting. It is important that full ROM in all directions are restored to the ankle, particularly dorsiflexion, as this is the movement required not only for gait, but also for the stairs and landing from jumps.

After an ankle inversion injury, the patient often loses the ability to dorsiflex the ankle, and with that, the gastrocnemius and soleus muscles tighten. It is very important to start a flexibility programme early for the calf muscles and to identify the other muscle groups that may also be tight, particularly the peroneals, as these are often overstretched during the injury and subsequently have increased tone and spasm at rest.

It is possible to start the calf stretches in long sitting using a belt, if the patient is unable to weight-bear, if there is too much pain or if there are positive neurodynamics in the form of a straight leg raise. Maintain a straight leg for the gastrocnemius, and

a bent knee for the soleus, while using the belt to dorsiflex the foot and try the exercise in both long sitting (Fig. 12.1) or in a straight leg raise position with knee extension or flexion in supine (Fig. 12.4). It is important that a clinical reasoning approach is used in prescription of every exercise. There is no point in prioritising the exercise in the straight leg raise position if neurodynamic tests are abnormal.

There are many different ways to stretch the calf muscles but the most common way to stretch the gastrocnemius is to start on a flat surface and then progress to a book or a slope (Fig. 12.5) and note the different foot positions available. Starting with the foot in a central position will give a general calf stretch; turning the foot medially can give a more lateral gastrocnemius stretch (Fig. 12.6) and turning the foot laterally (Fig. 12.7) can give a more medial head stretch. It is important to 'chase' the

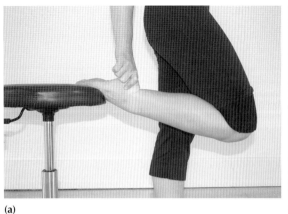

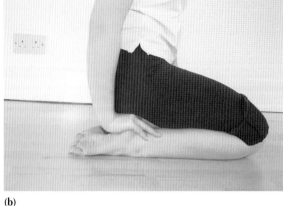

(a)   (b)

Figure 12.3   Plantar flexion in: (**a**) standing and (**b**) sitting.

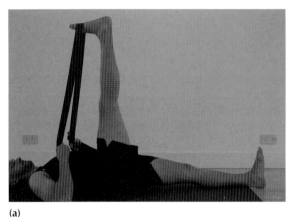

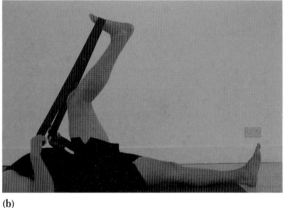

(a)   (b)

Figure 12.4   (**a**) Gastrocnemius stretch. (**b**) Soleus stretch.

stretch – the patient focuses on the tightest and most restricting position. It is also important that the patient does not roll the foot in, and maintains an optimal arch profile by keeping the knee moving over the third metatarsal. If the patient cannot do this, the clinician can place a book along the longitudinal arch to stop it collapsing inwards. They can progress the stretch in standing by asking the patient to stand with both feet on an incline board, aiming to keep the legs straight while moving the pelvis forwards (Fig. 12.8).

To focus the stretch on soleus, perform the stretch as for gastrocnemius (above), but flex the knee, ensuring that the knee moves over the third metatarsal. This can be progressed to a bilateral soleus squat ensuring that both heels remain on the ground and that the knees move forward over the feet ensuring ankle dorsiflexion (Fig. 12.9).

Muscle strength and endurance

There is much crossover between the exercises for muscle strengthening and proprioception/co-ordination. The outline and divisions of this chapter are more for academic reasons, but it is important to bear in mind, that if a patient is doing a single leg stand on toes for balance, they are also doing a concentric strengthening exercise for the gastrocnemius/soleus complex. To turn the same exercise into a strengthening exercise will mean that the patient repeats a heel lift and lower 20–30 times rather than a sustained hold of 30–60 seconds for balance.

Start with the basic isotonic exercises using Thera-Band® or free weights and do the entire ankle movements with both knee flexion and knee extension (Fig. 12.10). If isotonic exercises are too

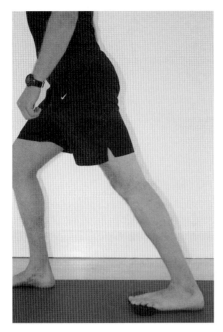

Figure 12.5 Stretch to the gastrocnemius using a block.

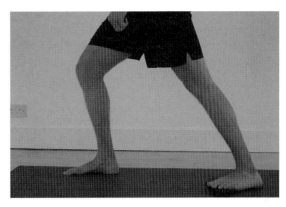

Figure 12.7 Medial gastrocnemius stretch with the foot turned laterally.

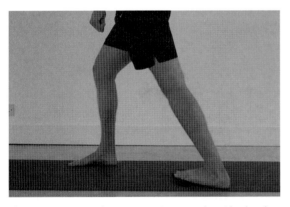

Figure 12.6 Lateral gastrocnemius stretch with the foot turned medially.

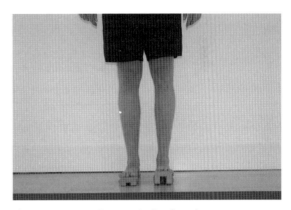

Figure 12.8 Stretch on an incline board.

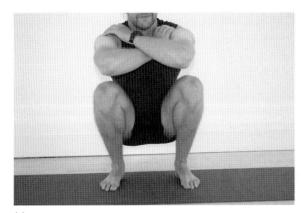

(a)

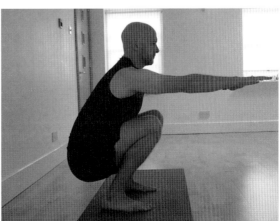

(b)

Figure 12.9 Bilateral soleus squat.

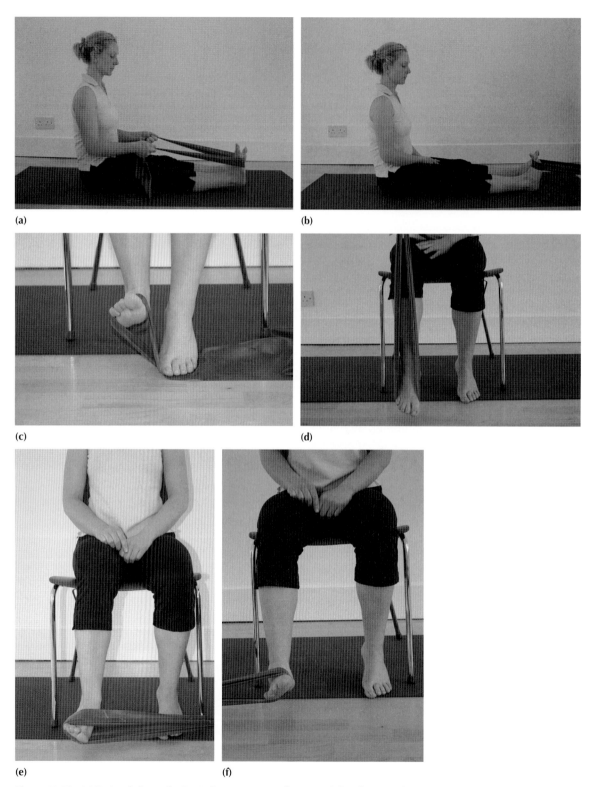

Figure 12.10 (**a**) Resisted plantar flexion in knee extension. (**b**) Resisted dorsiflexion in knee extension. (**c**) Resisted dorsiflexion in knee flexion. (**d**) Resisted plantar flexion in knee flexion. (**e**) Resisted eversion in knee flexion. (**f**) Resisted inversion in knee flexion.

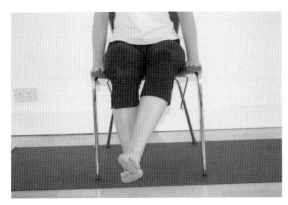

Figure 12.11 Dorsiflexion against resistance of the other foot.

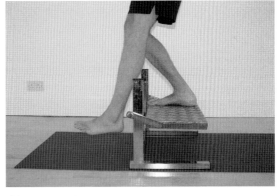

Figure 12.13 Step-over.

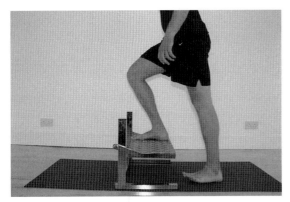

Figure 12.12 Step-up, emphasising dorsiflexion and push up with the right foot. The patient stands on the ball of the left foot to prevent pushing with this side.

painful, start with basic isometrics, where the patient pushes against their other foot for resistance (Fig. 12.11).

Progress the subject to a weight-bearing programme as quickly as possible, and always consider the kinetic chain when doing these exercises. Ensure that there is excellent control around the hip and trunk, and that the patient is not compensating by dipping the pelvis/hip or flexing the trunk forwards. The progression of the rehabilitation will depend on the presenting patient and their functional demands or sport.

Start with the basic step-up and step-down (Fig. 12.12) or step-over (Fig. 12.13). This exercise covers many issues. It helps regain dorsiflexion, but more importantly, it works the gluteus medius and pelvic stabilisers. Ensure that the patient can start to hop, and include multi-directional tasks and add resist-

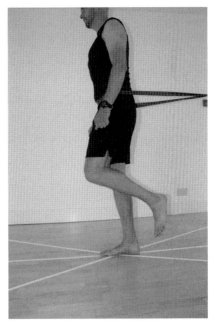

Figure 12.14 Multi-directional task with resistance. The patient jumps forwards and backwards and left and right. The height and distance are gradually increased.

ance as needed (Fig. 12.14). As the patient progresses, start to increase both the distance and the height. Adapt the hopping patterns to suit the patient's needs and design as many hopping patterns as possible. This may include focusing on sideways or backwards hopping more than forwards. Include the trampette – double foot jump, single foot jump, and jumping on and off (Fig. 12.15).

Progress the jumping activity, by asking the patient to jump forwards, backwards and sideways

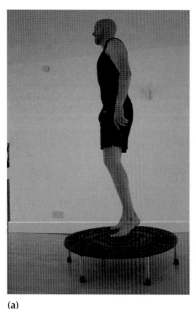

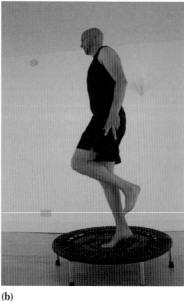

(a)   (b)

Figure 12.15 (**a**) Trampette jumps. (**b**) Single foot trampette jumps.

over an object of varying heights on two feet and one foot (Figs 12.16 and 12.17). Include skipping, shuttle runs (forwards, backwards, and sideways) and figure-of-eights forwards and backwards.

Proprioception

The basic approach to restoring balance is to start the patient standing on one leg. (See Fig. 12.18 for the correct technique.) Refer to Figure 12.19 for a poor technique and excessive weight transference. Although this may be difficult to see in the figure, 'Trendelenburg's' or 'compensatory Trendelenburg's' are very common clinical presentations. If the patient is having difficulties with weight transference and has a large pelvic shift, start in standing, with a narrow base of support, and start with a heel lift, progressing on to a heel and toe lift. Progress the exercise by widening the stance.

Progress the single leg stand exercise with knee flexion on the standing leg. Ensure that, again the patient does not cheat by dipping the pelvis/hip and the only body part to change position is the knee, and that continues to track out over the third metatarsal. If the knee rolls inwards and falls over the first, this will have a pronatory effect on the longitudinal arch and will reduce the work of the intrinsic muscles.

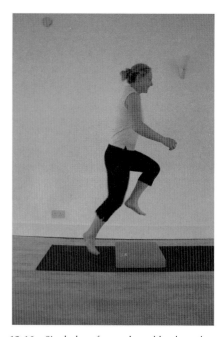

Figure 12.16 Single hop forwards and backwards.

Progress the single leg stand in flat foot position to standing on toes on two feet and one foot with straight legs and then onto toes on two feet and one foot with a bent knee (Fig. 12.20). It is important that the patient keeps the heels high as they bend

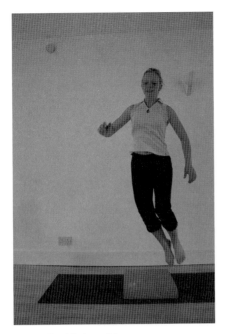

Figure 12.17 Double hop sideways.

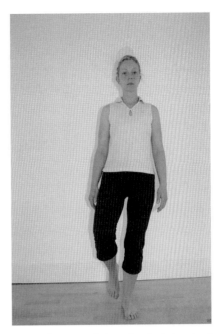

Figure 12.18 Correct technique for single leg stand.

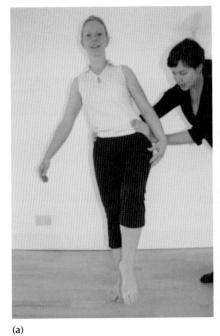

(a)

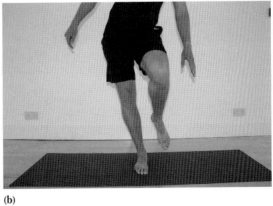

(b)

Figure 12.19 (a) Poor one leg standing technique with (b) 'compensatory Trendelenburg'.

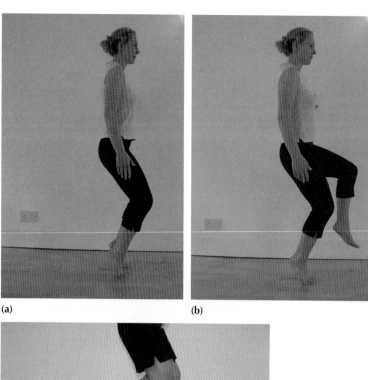

(a) (b)

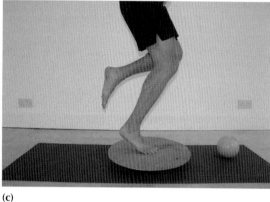

(c)

Figure 12.20 (**a**) Heel lift exercise, two feet. (**b**) Heel lift on one foot. (**c**) Balance exercise on wobble board.

the knee and that the knee continues to move out over the third metatarsal. If the patient can comfortably do these exercises, they can then try to perform them with their eyes closed, and then throwing a ball. The clinician can then progress all the above exercises to the wobble board, foam block and foam roller (Fig. 12.20c). The progression of the patient will depend on many things including their motivation to continue with exercise, their functional ability and prognosis, and also their sporting level.

Functional and late rehabilitation

Functional exercises as outlined above (hopping, jumping, shuttle runs) should be applied when the patient is pain free, has full ROM and good muscle strength and proprioception. It is important to remember that inadequate rehabilitation and early return to sport will increase the chances of re-injury, so it is essential that the patient completes a functional programme and the sooner the clinician can commence this, the more successful will be the rehabilitation. Re-train the movement patterns rather than just focusing on the individual muscles at this stage, and ensure that all the variables of functional training are considered, including load progression, range of movement, base of support, speed and, most importantly, multi-directional activity, by including exercises that challenge the sagittal, transverse and frontal planes. Include squats, dips and plyometric exercises that use different arm positions and different directions to not

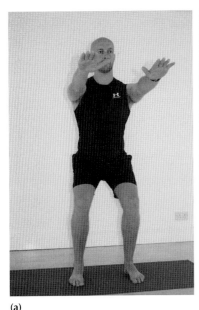 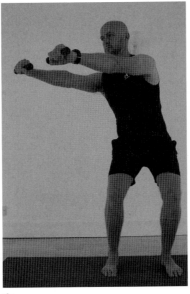 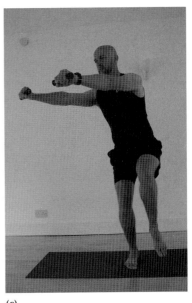

(a)   **(b)**   **(c)**

Figure 12.21   (**a**) Squat with arm raise. (**b**) Double leg squat with trunk rotation. (**c**) Single leg squat with trunk rotation.

only challenge the ankle joint but also the whole kinetic chain (Fig. 12.21).

Planus and plantar fasciosis and hallux valgus

Rehabilitation

Aerobic exercise

All the aerobic exercises described above for ankle inversion injury are appropriate for the management of plantar fasciosis. Activities which are not fully weight-bearing such as rowing are suitable and weight-bearing activities which do not promote constant pronation may be tried. In general, pain is a good indicator of an inappropriate exercise. If the patient has been prescribed orthoses they should be worn during the activity and the prescribing clinician should constantly monitor biomechanics of the foot and ankle, correcting as appropriate.

ROM and flexibility

Start by reducing the pain in the plantar fascia region; this can be done by massaging the sole of the foot and the calf muscles, and also by giving a home exercise of massage or trigger pointing on a

spiky ball and progress to a golf ball as able. Progress the massage treatment to massage of the calf muscles in standing, which will create a wind-up effect of the myofascia and can give very good release of the muscles restricting the normal movement. The therapist must restore full range of movement to the ankle (as outlined earlier), but must also correct the hallux valgus and restore full MTP extension. This can be done in standing (Fig. 12.22a) as well as in sitting (Fig. 12.22b), but the patient must ensure that they abduct the toe before extending it, and ensure that they fixate the MTP joint before extending the hallux.

It is also very important to restore normal movement and function to the toes. Toes, when challenged, can be almost as dexterous as fingers. The effect of a rigid foot, may not only lead to pain, but it may also reduce the shock absorbing capabilities of both the foot and the lower leg. The foot strengthening programme, for both the foot intrinsics and extrinsics can be trained quite easily with the following exercises.

The toe spread (Fig. 12.23)

See if the patient is able to spread their toes (in the same way as they can spread their fingers) and use the interossei muscles without moving the heel or lifting the foot. A progression of this exercise is to

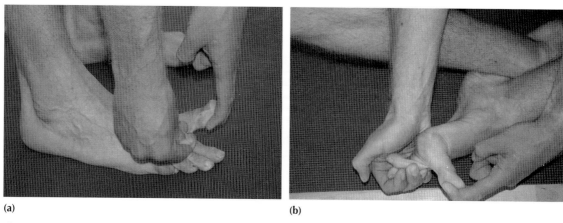

(a)   (b)

Figure 12.22   (**a**) Hallux extension stretch in standing. (**b**) Hallux extension stretch in sitting.

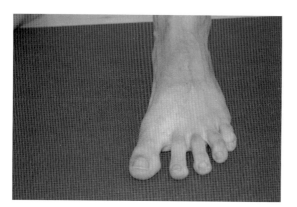

Figure 12.23   Toe spread.

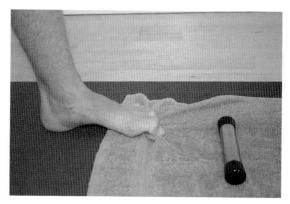

Figure 12.24   Towel exercise.

then 'toe spread and dome'. In this exercise, the patient uses the short intrinsics muscles, and it is important that they do not curl the toes, but still have a slight 'doming effect' where the arch lifts up.

The towel exercise (Fig. 12.24)

This exercise involves the long toe flexors and also helps with the arch lift and requires the patient to spread the toes, placing them on the towel and then scrunching the towel up, until they have managed to pull the whole towel in without moving the heel. A progression of this exercise is to place the towel on a carpet rather than a wooden floor to add more resistance, or place a weight on the towel. Finally, the patient should pick up objects using all the toe flexors, e.g. pencils, markers, buttons, marbles. Ensure that they do not cheat by just using their big toe.

It is also important to include some stretches of not only the calf muscles, as previously demonstrated, but also of the plantar fascia. This can be difficult for the individual who cannot get enough MTP extension, and if that is the case, they may need to do the stretch while keeping the first MTP free. Ensure that the arch profile is maintained throughout the stretch.

Muscle strength and endurance

There are also some specific foot strengthening exercises that should be included. Include walking on toes with the heels kept high and a straight leg to work the gastrocnemius. Repeat with a bent knee, 'the soleus walk', both of which will help to control the rearfoot. Walking on the heels (Fig. 12.25) will help use the tibialis anterior to control the arch position. With this exercise, ensure that the

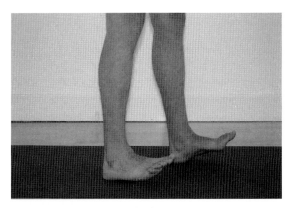

Figure 12.25 Walking on heels.

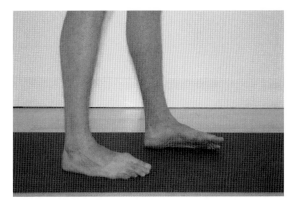

Figure 12.26 Walking on outside of feet.

patient does not cheat by using their toe extensors or by failing to lift their foot up enough into dorsiflexion. Walking on the outsides of the feet (Fig. 12.26) encourages use of tibialis anterior again and the arch drop and lift off the edge of a step works the tibialis posterior tendon eccentrically. The tibialis posterior tendon is the main dynamic stabiliser of the foot and works to invert the subtalar joint and stabilise the arch.

Proprioception

This part of rehabilitation should include the proprioception programme as outlined earlier with specific attention to maintaining the arch profile throughout the exercises without losing rear- or midfoot control. The clinician must also ensure that the patient uses the correct movement patterns and is not overusing the long toe extensors or flexors. They must also avoid toe clawing or extending.

Achilles' tendinopathy

The main aim of treatment is to restore the ankle range of movement, particularly dorsiflexion, lengthen the calf muscles as outlined previously, and start the patient on an eccentric training programme for the gastrocnemius and soleus. Management of this condition should be based on a symptom-related approach.

Aerobic exercise

Aerobic exercise will generally be non-weight-bearing in the acute phase of Achilles tendinopathy. Aerobic exercise described in the management of ankle inversion injury is appropriate. Progression to weight-bearing activities should be with caution and as pain allows and low impact exercise should be prescribed. Late stage of rehabilitation should encourage activities such as plyometrics, skipping and bouncing on a trampette to challenge the tissues of the Achilles' tendon.

Range of motion and flexibility

The exercise programme described to address ROM in the management of plantar fasciosis, as described above, should be applied in the rehabilitation of Achilles' tendinopathy.

Muscle strength and endurance

The programme should commence with the patient performing heel drops over the edge of a step, with both a straight leg and a bent knee (Fig. 12.27). Start without any weight and then gradually increase the patient's load by performing the heel drops with a backpack filled with weights on their shoulders. Again the weight can be gradually increased, as can the repetitions. Alfredson *et al.* (1998) recommend three sets of 15 repetitions, performed twice a day, 7 days a week. This programme should be maintained for 12 weeks. The patient must ensure that they do not load the affected calf concentrically as they move into plantar flexion but must use their non-affected leg to push themselves back up. The patient should be

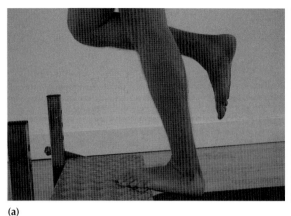
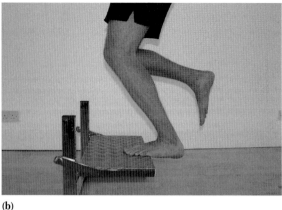

(a)   (b)

Figure 12.27   Heel drop with (**a**) knee extension and (**b**) knee flexion.

warned that the exercises may cause discomfort, particularly in the early stages of the programme, but must stop if the pain becomes disabling. If the patient can do the exercises in the early stages of the programme in bare feet, this allows them to not only focus on their alignment and foot position, particularly of the longitudinal arch, but it also ensures that the foot intrinsic muscles have to work harder. However, if the patient has very poor foot and ankle alignment/biomechanics, or if the step has no carpet on it, this can be too uncomfortable on the sole of the foot and will place too much of a valgus stress on the ankle and midfoot, and will require the patient to wear training shoes.

Proprioception

As discussed previously, it is important to include a good proprioceptive programme, see the above exercises, including Figure 12.20, and ensure that the end-range rehabilitation plan includes functional exercises such as uphill walking and walking downstairs. Step-down exercise will work the calf muscles eccentrically and will also work the hip and leg muscles.

It is very important to address the orthoses issue, ensuring that the patient not only has orthoses that they will wear, but that will also give enough rear- and midfoot control and will act as good shock absorbers. Advice on footwear is essential; ensure that the footwear has a good heel counter, which helps control the calcaneum and also has good shock absorbency. Often clinicians recommend excellent training shoes, with good shock attenuation, and then suggest that the patient wear a rigid orthotic device, which will counteract any shock absorbency benefits of the shoes. It is important that the clinician understands the kind of shoe and device required and for what effect.

SECTION 3: CASE STUDIES AND STUDENT QUESTIONS

Case study 1

A 32-year-old female presents to the clinician with an acute right ankle inversion injury 3 days after inverting her ankle while wearing high heels. She attended the accident and emergency room, was X-rayed and was given a Tubigrip and crutches

and told that she had no fracture but to weight-bear as able. She has been applying the PRICEM (protection, rest, ice compression, elevation, medication) principles since injury, and complains of lateral ankle pain, 'tightness' in the forefoot and

Case study 1—cont'd

marked spasm/pain in the peroneus muscles and, just today, a feeling of tightness in the calf. Assessment reveals marked swelling and discolouration of the lateral ankle and forefoot; marked pain with palpation over the fibula head, all the lateral ankle structures, particularly the ATFL, and muscle spasm and pain in the peroneus muscles. ROM is reduced and painful in all directions – 30° plantar flexion,–10° dorsiflexion, 5° inversion, 5° eversion. Ankle strength cannot be assessed accurately due to pain and lack of movement. Instability tests suggest a grade 2 ATFL sprain. She is afraid to weight-bear on the ankle not only because of pain but also because of the fear that her ankle may 'give way'.

Management

The emphasis in the early stage of management of this patient should be to reduce swelling and pain to allow an increase in function. If the pain is severe, the ankle should be initially immobilised in a brace and the patient should use crutches. At this stage, gait should be re-educated progressing from partial weight-bearing with the crutches to fully weight-bearing as pain allows. Early exercise will include a balance programme comprising weight transference with or without crutches. Soft tissue work on the peroneus muscles, gastrocnemius and soleus muscles may enhance recovery. Active ROM exercise of the ankle may be performed and repeated in a straight leg raise position if neurodynamic tests are positive. ROM exercise may be performed passively with accessory movements added with particular attention to the inferior tibiofibular joint. Aerobic exercise at this stage could include swimming with a kickboard or one leg cycling. Strengthening exercise at this stage would be fulfilled by the performance of the balance programme.

The middle to late phase of rehabilitation requires a progression to functional activities. Single leg stand with knee flexion and extension should be performed as well as 'toe stands' to enhance proprioceptive and build strength. Stair climbing and gait activities with an emphasis on good pelvis control are good functional activities. The patient should perform ROM exercises in functional positions such as squatting in standing. The final stage of rehabilitation should include a full functional programme such as plyometrics and trampette work which includes all components of fitness. The emphasis at this stage is to include multi-directional activities. Taping may provide a psychological and proprioceptive aid in the final stage of management.

Case study 2

A 14-year-old girl, who is a competitive dancer, complains of right heel and arch pain since 8 weeks. Her dance teacher tells her that she has flat feet and that she is not lifting her heels high enough when she dances. The dancer feels that her dancing has deteriorated over the past several months, as she cannot jump as high as she used to, and she now has to really use her arms when she jumps to achieve height. Her mother states that she dances four times a week and that she has noticed that her daughter has become 'heavier on her feet' and has had quite a significant recent growth spurt.

Clinical examination reveals a right early hallux valgus, approximately 10°, bilateral rearfoot varus and compensatory pronation bilaterally. She also has very weak foot intrinsic muscles and is unable to toe spread or dorsiflex in standing (heel walk). The dancer is able to stand on one foot with the eyes open, but is poor with the eyes closed and is unable to stand on her toes on two feet or one foot without significant pronation and heel drop. She has a very poor jump, with little power coming from her calf muscles or her core.

There is a loss of end-range ankle dorsiflexion, MTP 1 extension is 40° with a poor movement

Case study 2—cont'd

pattern and the right hip has lost end of range external rotation. Palpation shows marked tenderness of the right plantar fascia at the calcaneum and also along the longitudinal arch with multiple trigger points in the deep intrinsics.

Management

The aim of management of this patient is to take a global approach, i.e. to address foot dysfunction as well as performance issues. The working diagnosis of this patient is plantar fasciosis. Rehabilitation should commence with ROM activities to include intensive stretching of the plantar fascia, gastrocnemius and soleus, as well as mobilisation of the first MTP joint. Soft tissue work such as massage with the muscle in a

stretched position may aid progress. The intrinsic foot programme (described in text above) should commence early and other issues to correct biomechanics should be addressed at an early stage. Proprioception work in the early stage for this patient should include toe standing on one leg demonstrating good control of the whole limb and the ability to prevent the rearfoot from dropping. The middle to late stage of rehabilitation should progress to jumping and trampette work, teaching the patient to jump correctly by controlling from the hip. This patient should be encouraged to jump with hands behind her back to facilitate lift with the lower limb and good 'core' activity. Jumping and trampette work will challenge the proprioceptive, aerobic and strengthening systems. The patient may be further helped by prescription of correct functional foot orthoses or corrective taping.

Case study 3

A 40-year-old male office worker, who plays tennis once per week and likes to walk daily to and from work, complains of pain in the midportion of his right Achilles' tendon. The pain has been gradually worsening over the past 3 months, and it is particularly stiff first thing in the morning getting out of bed. This stiffness tends to last 10–15 minutes and eases as the patient gets moving. He likes to walk, and has pain at the beginning of the walk, which eases as the walk progresses, but if he overdoes it, the pain will return and he will start to limp. The pain can then last the rest of the day and evening, although eases with the application of a heat pack. He also notices pain walking downstairs. The patient states that he always wears soft slip on leather shoes, and has not changed his running shoes for about 5 years. He also used to wear orthoses, but found that they were too cumbersome and did not fit into his work footwear, so he stopped wearing them about 3 years ago.

Clinical findings show marked tightness in the right soleus and gastrocnemius, with the patient

unable to dorsiflex the right ankle more than 5° in standing, without marked compensatory pronation. The patient is able to do a single leg heel raise without pain, but five single leg hops on the spot provoke his pain, while two hops forwards provoke the pain. There is marked tenderness of Achilles', both with the squeeze test of the tendon and with direct postero-anterior pressure on the tendon.

Management

In the early stage of rehabilitation of this patient, aerobic activities may be continued within the confines of pain. If weight-bearing exercise is painful then non-weight-bearing exercise such as swimming may be acceptable. ROM exercise early in management should emphasise recovery of full ankle dorsiflexion and first MTP ROM. Gait re-education should emphasis, in particular, good heel strike and mid stance. The eccentric

---

Case study 3—cont'd

programme described in the text above should be started as soon as possible, noting that discomfort is likely to be experienced during these exercises. Proprioception such as single leg stands should also be commenced as early as possible. The middle to late stage requires progression of activities described above with increased duration and loading. The eccentric exercise programme should see increased repetitions and the addition of loading with the use of backpack weights by the patient. Ballistic activity should be introduced and exercises which work the Achilles' in a lengthened

position such as uphill lunges should be performed. Multidirectional activities such as 'figure-of-eights' and stop/start exercise should challenge the patient more at this stage. At all times it should be ensured that the patient has good foot and ankle positioning during exercise, particularly in dorsiflexion. As this patient has been prescribed orthoses that are not used, this should be investigated. It is better to compromise with a softer, slimmer device that will be worn continually than to have no orthoses when poor biomechanics are compromising recovery.

Student questions

(1) Design three functional exercises for a painter who complains of Achilles' pain each time he goes up and down the ladder.

(2) What are your goals for the first three days after an acute ankle inversion?

(3) Describe three different ways to stretch the gastrocnemius.

(4) Develop two new proprioceptive exercises for the elite level gymnast.

(5) Why would you give a patient a concentric Achilles' programme as against the recommended eccentric programme?

(6) List the benefits of good footwear.

(7) Why do therapists use wobble boards to train proprioception, a wobble board is not considered a functional exercise? What is the neurophysiological benefit to training on unstable surfaces?

(8) Develop a strengthening programme for the foot with a tibialis posterior tendinopathy.

(9) When would it be appropriate to select a rigid orthotic device for a patient?

(10) Design two new home exercises to improve ankle plantar flexion.

References

Alfredson, H., Pietila, T., Jonsson, P. and Lorentzon, R. (1998) Heavy-load eccentric calf muscle training for the treatment of chronic Achilles tendinosis. *American Journal of Sports Medicine*, 26(3), 360–366.

Beedle, B.B. and Mann, C.L. (2007) A comparison of two warm-ups on joint range of motion. *Journal of Strength and Conditioning Research*, 21, 776–779.

Berkson, E.M., Greisberg, J. and Theodore, G.H. (2007) Heel pain. In: Di Giovanni, C. and Greisberg, J. (eds) *Foot & Ankle, Core Knowledge of Orthopaedics*, pp. 195–199. Elsevier/Mosby, New York, USA.

Boyce, S.H., Quigley, M.A. and Campbell, S. (2005) Management of ankle sprains: a randomised controlled trial of the treatment of inversion injuries using an elastic support bandage or an Aircast ankle brace. *British Journal of Sport Medicine*, 39, 91–96.

Clark, V.M. and Burden, A.M. (2005) A 4-week wobble board exercise programme improved muscle onset latency and perceived stability in individuals with a functionally unstable ankle. *Physical Therapy in Sport*, 6, 181–187.

De Fries, J.S., Krips, R., Sierevelt, I.N., Blankevoort, L. and Van Dijk, C.N. (2006) Interventions for treating chronic ankle instability. *Cochrane Database of Systematic Reviews*, 4, CD004124.

Delahunt, E. (2007) Peroneal reflex contribution to the development of functional instability of the ankle joint. *Physical Therapy in Sport*, 8, 98–104.

Digiovanni, B.F., Nawoczenski, D.A., Malay, D.P., Graci, P.A., Williams, T.T., Wilding, G.E. and Baumhauer, J.F. (2006) Plantar fascia specific stretching exercise improves outcomes in patients with chronic plantar fasciitis. A prospective clinical trial with two year follow up. *Journal of Bone and Joint Surgery, American Volume*, 88, 1775–1781.

Flanigan, R.M., Nawoczenski, D.A., Chen, L., Wu, H. and Digiovanni, B.F. (2007) The influence of foot position on stretching of the plantar fascia. *Foot and Ankle International*, 28, 815–822.

Garn, S. and Newton, R. (1998) Kinaesthetic awareness in subjects with multiple ankle sprains. *Physical Therapy*, 68, 166–171.

Gerber, J.P., Williams G.N., Scoville, C.R., Arciero, R.A. and Taylor, D.C. (1998) Persistent disability associated with ankle sprains: a prospective examination of an athletic population. *Foot and Ankle International*, 19, 653–660.

Handoll, H.H.G., Rowe, B.H., Quinn, K.M. and de Bie R. (2001) Interventions for preventing ankle ligament injuries (Review). *Cochrane Database of Systematic Reviews*, 3, CD000018.

Hartsell, H.D. (2000) The effects of external bracing on joint position sense awareness for the chronically unstable ankle. *Journal of Sports Rehabilitation*, 9, 279–289.

Hartsell, H.D. and Spaulding, S.J. (1999) Eccentric/concentric ratios at selected velocities for the invertor and evertor muscles of the chronically unstable ankle. *British Journal of Sports Medicine*, 33, 255–258.

Hubley-Kozey, C.L., Wall, J.C. and Hogan, D.B. (1995) Effects of a general exercise programme on passive hip, knee and ankle range of motion of older women. *Topics in Geriatric Rehabilitation*, 10, 33–44.

Javed, A., Walsh, H.P.J. and Lees, A. (1999) Peroneal reaction time in treated functional instability of the ankle. *Foot and Ankle Surgery*, 5, 159–166.

Jonsson, P., Alfredson, H., Sunding, K., Fahlstrom, M. and Cook, J., (2008) New regimen for eccentric calf muscle training in patients with chronic insertional Achilles tendinopathy: results of a pilot study. *British Journal of Sports Medicine*, 42, 746–749.

Karatosun, V., Unver, B., Ozden, A., Ozay, Z. and Gunal, I. (2008) Intra-articular hyaluronic acid compared to exercise therapy on osteoarthritis of the ankle. A prospective randomised trial with long term follow up. *Clinical Experimental Rheumatology*, 26, 288–294.

Kerkhoffs, G.M.M.J., Struijs, P.A.A., Marti R.K., Assendelft W.J.J., Blankevoort, L., Dijk Van, C.N. and The Cochrane Collaboration. (2007) *Different functional treatment strategies for acute lateral ankle ligament injuries in adults (review)*. John Wiley and Sons Ltd., Chichester.

Kingma, J.J., de Knikker, R., Wittink, H.M. and Takken, T. (2007) Eccentric overload training in patients with chronic Achilles tendinopathy: a systematic review. *British Journal of Sports Medicine*, 41, e3.

Konradsen, L., Olesen, S. and Hansen, H.M. (1998) Ankle sensorimotor control and eversion strength after acute ankle inversion injuries. *American Journal of Sports Medicine*, 26, 72–77.

Loudon, J.K., Santos, M.J., Franks, L. and Liu, W. (2008) The effectiveness of active exercise as an intervention for functional ankle instability: a systematic review. *Sports Medicine*, 38, 553–563.

Mafi, N., Lorentzon, R. and Alfredson, H. (2001) Superior short-term results with eccentric calf-muscle training compared to concentric training in a randomized prospective multicenter study on patients with chronic Achilles tendinosis. *Knee Surgery, Sports Traumatology, Arthroscopy*, 9, 42–47.

Magnussen, R.A., Dunn, W.R. and Thomson, A.B. (2009) Nonoperative treatment of midportion Achilles Tendinopathy: a systematic review. *Clinical Journal of Sports Medicine*, 19, 54–64.

McGuine, T.A. and Keene, J.S. (2006) The effect of a balance training program on the risk of ankle sprains in high school athletes. *American Journal of Sports Medicine*, 34, 1103–1111.

McHugh, M., Tyler, T., Mirabella, M.R., Mullaney, M.J. and Nicholas, S.J. (2007) The effectiveness of a balance training intervention in reducing the incidence of non-contact ankle sprains in high school football players. *American Journal of Sports Medicine*, 8, 1289–1294.

Mohammadi, F. (2007) Comparison of 3 preventive methods to reduce the recurrence of ankle inversion sprains in male soccer players. *American Journal of Sports Medicine*, 35, 922–926.

Munn, J., Beard, D.J, Refshauge, K. and Raymond, Y.W. (2003) Eccentric muscle strength in functional instability. *Medicine and Science in Sports and Exercise*, 35, 245–250.

Niesen-Vertommen, S.L., Taunton, J.E., Clement, D.B. and Mosher, R.E. (1992) The effect of eccentric versus concentric exercise in the management of Achilles tendonitis. *Clinical Journal of Sport Medicine*, 2, 109–113.

O'Connor, K. and Hamill, J. (2003) The role of selected extrinsic foot muscles during running. *Clinical Biomechanics*, 19, 71–77.

Price, R.J., Hawkins R.D., Hulse, M.A. and Hodson, A. (2004) The Football Association medical research programme: an audit of injuries in academy youth football. *British Journal of Sports Medicine*, 38, 466–471.

Rees, J.D., Maffulli, N. and Cook, J. (2009) Management of tendinopathy. *American Journal of Sports Medicine*, 37, 1855–1867.

Schweizer, A., Bircher, H.P., Kaelin, X. and Ochsner, P.E. (2005) Functional ankle control of rock climbers. *British Journal of Sports Medicine*, 39, 429–431.

Smith, A. and Sands, A. (2007) Achilles tendon problems. In: Di Giovanni, C. and Greisberg, J. (eds) *Foot & Ankle, Core Knowledge of Orthopaedics*, pp. 200–208. Elsevier/ Mosby, New York, USA.

Surve, I., Schwellnus, M.P., Noakes, T. and Lombard, C. (1994) A fivefold reduction in the incidence of recurrent ankle sprains in soccer players using the Sport-Stirrup orthosis. *American Journal of Sports Medicine*, 22, 601–606.

Trojian, T.H. and McKeag, D.B. (2006) Single leg balance test to identify risk of ankle sprains. *British Journal of Sports Medicine*, 40, 610–613.

Tyler, T.F., McHugh, M.P., Mirabella, M.R., Mullaney, M.J. and Nicholas, S.J. (2006) Risk factors for noncontact ankle sprains in High School football players. *American Journal of Sports Medicine*, 34, 471–475.

Valderrabano, V., Pagenstert, G., Horisberger, M., Knupp, M. and Hintermann, B. (2006) Sports and recreation activity of ankle arthritis patients before and after total ankle replacement. *American Journal of Sports Medicine*, 34, 993–999.

Van der Wees, P.J., Lenssen, A.F., Hendriks, E., Stomp, D., Dekker, J. and de Bie, R.A. (2006) Effectiveness of exercise therapy and manual mobilisation in acute ankle sprain and functional instability: A systematic review. *Australian Journal of Physiotherapy*, 52, 27–37.

Willems, T., Witvrouw, E., Delbaere, K., DeCock, A. and DeClercq, D. (2005a) Relationship between gait biomechanics and inversion sprains: a prospective study of risk factors. *Gait Posture*, 21, 379–387.

Willems, T.M., Witvrouw, E., Delbaere, K., Mahieu, N., De Bourdeaudhuij, I. and De Clercq, D. (2005b) Intrinsic risk factors for inversion ankle sprains in male subjects. *American Journal of Sports Medicine*, 33, 415–423.

Xu, D., Hong, Y., Li, J. and Chan, K. (2004) Effect of tai chi exercise on proprioception of ankle and knee joints in old people. *British Journal of Sports Medicine*, 38, 50–54.

Yeung, M.S., Chan, K.M., So, C.H. and Yuan, W.Y. (1994) An epidemiological survey on ankle sprain. *British Journal of Sports Medicine*, 28, 112–116.

Zoch, C., Fialka-Moser, V. and Quittan, M. (2003) Rehabilitation of ligamentous ankle injuries: a review of recent studies. *British Journal of Sports Medicine*, 37, 291–295.

3

Exercise Therapy in Special Populations

Musculoskeletal Disorders in the Developing Child

Juliette Hussey and Mandy Johnson

Physical activity in children – health benefits and guidelines

Health benefits of physical activity in childhood

There are a number of health benefits of physical activity, many of which have been discussed in previous chapters. The benefits of regular activity in early adulthood were first investigated in the Harvard Alumni Health Study where activity levels in 16 396 men aged 35–74 years were investigated. An inverse dose relationship between physical activity and all-cause mortality was found (Paffenbarger et al., 1986).

Other studies (Morris et al., 1966; Lee et al., 1999; Bucksch, 2005) have added further to the evidence for the health benefits of regular activity in adults. The evidence for the effects of physical activity on morbidity and mortality in children is not available at present. The paucity of evidence may in part be due to a lack of studies that have reached a conclusion, or studies that have not been of sufficient length to examine such a relationship. Currently there are a number of population studies investigating the prevalence of cardiovascular

disease risk factors in children and adolescents; these include the Bogalusa Heart Study, the Amsterdam Growth and Health Longitudinal Study, the Northern Ireland Young Hearts Project, the Cardiovascular Risk in Young Finns Study and the European Youth Heart Study (EYHS). While end points have not been reached in these studies they have highlighted the importance of physical activity and fitness in the prevention of cardiovascular risk factors. These and other related studies have produced considerable evidence for the benefits of activity and fitness on insulin sensitivity (Raitakari et al., 1994b; Schmitz et al., 2002), blood lipid profiles (Suter and Hawes, 1993; Raitakari et al., 1994a), flow mediated dilation of the brachial artery (Abbott, 2002) and multiple risk factors including the metabolic syndrome (Bouziotas et al., 2004; Brage et al., 2004; Ribeiro et al., 2004).

Physical activity guidelines in children

Young children tend to be active if given sufficient opportunity and space. The activity they engage in tends to be short bursts of intense activity interspersed with less intense periods. Unlike adults, children tend not to engage in long periods of sus-

Exercise Therapy in the Management of Musculoskeletal Disorders, First Edition. Edited by Fiona Wilson, John Gormley and Juliette Hussey.
© 2011 Blackwell Publishing Ltd

tained activity. As the child gets older he or she commences engaging in more sustained periods of activity generally associated with sport or walking/cycling as a means of transport.

Activity guidelines for children have changed over the last number of years. Physical activity guidelines for children were first presented by the American College of Sports Medicine (ACSM) in 1998. The guidelines were based on those of adults and the recommendation was that children should achieve 20–30 minutes of vigorous activity per day. The general ACSM guidelines for physical activity were that adults should accumulate at least 30 minutes of moderate intensity activity on most, and preferably all days of the week (ACSM, 1990). In 1994 the International Consensus Conference on Physical Activity Guidelines for Adolescents recommended that 'all adolescents are physically active daily, or nearly every day, as part of play, games, sports, work, transportation, recreation, physical education, or planned exercise, in the context of family, school and community activities' and that 'adolescents engage in three or more sessions per week of activities that last 20 minutes or more at a time that require moderate to vigorous levels of exertion (Sallis and Patrick, 1994). More recently in the USA, an expert panel was set up by the Divisions of Nutrition and Physical Activity and Adolescent and School Health of the Centers for Disease Control and Prevention to review and evaluate the evidence on the influence of physical activity on several health and behavioural outcomes in children aged 6–18 years, and to develop evidence-based recommendations (Strong *et al.*, 2005). A total of 850 articles were reviewed, and the areas included adiposity, cardiovascular health, asthma, mental health, injury associated with physical activity and musculoskeletal health. Most of the intervention studies reviewed included supervised programmes of 30–45 minutes of moderate to vigorous activity on 3–5 days per week. The panel recommended that 'school aged youth should participate in 60 minutes or more of moderate to vigorous physical activity that is developmentally appropriate, enjoyable, and involves a variety of activities'.

The strength of the evidence base for the exercise recommendations by Strong *et al.* (2005) could be questioned. It could be argued that a minimum of 60 minutes of moderate to vigorous activity per day is too low, given that, in a study on 7–10 year old

children, while almost all achieved such a level, yet a percentage were overweight (20.7% of boys and 20.2% of girls) (Hussey *et al.*, 2007). Similar findings were those of a EYHS study where among children aged 9 years, 97.4% of boys and 97.6% of girls were meeting the recommendations, and again a number were overweight (Riddoch *et al.*, 2004). The idea that there is a need for both genders to have a higher level of physical activity is supported by Andersen *et al.* (2006), who found a higher level of activity was needed to prevent clustering of cardiovascular disease risk factors. In addition to a higher level of activity required for children it has also been proposed that boys need to do more activity for a given level of body composition. Tudor-Locke *et al.* (2004) recommended different amounts of activity for boys and girls based on data on activity levels collected by pedometer and cut off points for normal weight and overweight/obesity. The selected cut-off points for 6–12 year old children would equate to approximately 120 minutes of activity per day for girls and 150 minutes per day for boys. Therefore it may be that requirements for boys and girls not only need to be higher but need to be different, due to inherent physiological or behavioural differences in the genders.

To the authors' knowledge, there are no long-term longitudinal studies on activity and bone health in children, but there have been a number of studies that have investigated activity over a few years and retrospective studies that have compared adult bone health with activity performed as a child. Both exercise and nutrition are independently recognised as factors essential for optimal bone health during growth. Regular weight-bearing exercise is well recognised as important in bone mineral content and bone mineral density during childhood and growth.

The ASCM recommends that to augment bone mineral accrual in children and adolescents they should engage in impact activities (gymnastics, plyometrics and jumping) and moderate intensity resistance training. Participation in sports that involve running and jumping (soccer, basketball) is likely to be of benefit. The intensity should be high in terms of bone loading forces but resistance training should be <60% of 1 RM (repetition maximum). The frequency should be at least 3 days per week and the duration 10–20 minutes.

In a review on the evidence in this area Daly (2007) concludes that the structural response of bone to exercise during growth is maturity dependent and gender specific. Before puberty exercise appears to increase apposition in both genders but during puberty and late in puberty, exercise appears to result in periosteal expansion in boys but endocortical contraction in girls. While it is accepted that the nature of exercise programmes should be predominately weight-bearing and variable in nature the optimal dose range has yet to emerge. This is echoed by Macdonald *et al.* (2007) who examined the effect of a daily program of physical activity on tibial bone strength in pre or early pubertal children at baseline. The programme included daily jumping and 15 minutes of physical activity in addition to the normal physical education classes. Pre-pubertal boys had a significant increase in bone strength index but there was no difference in girls between the intervention and control subjects. The authors concluded by suggesting the need for a dose response trial for those past the pre-pubertal stage.

Growth and maturation

During childhood and adolescence there is considerable growth in terms of height and weight, and growth spurts can result in changes in the ratios of muscle strength to limb length and in stress on the related soft tissues. Limb growth affects the muscle forces that are required for movement and growth also affects the strength of the tendon, apophysis, ligaments and bone (Hawkins and Metheny, 2001). Muscles and tendons have to lengthen with a growth spurt but if they do not hypertrophy until after the growth spurt, then the increased mass of the limb will require the muscle to generate a greater percentage of their maximum force to produce a movement. This increased force may lead to increased stress on the tendons.

Different types of tissues grow at different rates and at some point go through a process of hyperplasia (an increase in cell number), hypertrophy (an increase in cell size) and accretion (an increase in intercellular substance). Hyperplasia usually occurs before birth whereas hypertrophy occurs after birth, but this does depend on the tissue type (Malina *et al.*, 2004a; Stratton *et al.*, 2004). Neural tissue is essentially defined at the pre-natal stage of development but the amount of muscle tissue is not

defined until after birth. Bone tissue is different again as all three processes of hyperplasia, hypertrophy and accretion occur in bone growth, which can continue into late teens or early twenties.

Maturation occurs in all the various body systems, skeletal, sexual, physiological, neurological, and morphological, etc., but the timing of the process differs with each body system (Malina *et al.*, 2004a). The maturation of the neurological system occurs around the age of 7 years, sexual maturation or the ability to reproduce usually occurs in early teenage years, with girls approximately 2 years ahead of boys. Skeletal maturation is said to have occurred when full skeletal ossification has taken place, and also occurs earlier in girls.

Monitoring and measuring growth

The measurement of growth is termed anthropometry and is used in various ways in both clinical practice and the sporting environment to monitor the development of children. The monitoring of children's growth is well established in paediatric health care, as poor or slow growth can be due to, among other things, poor nutrition, social or economic status or various genetic and/or hormonal deficiencies (Hall, 2000; Hermanussen *et al.*, 2001; Cole *et al.*, 2002). Regular monitoring of growth can often pre-empt problems and can be carried out at a specific chronological age and compared with population reference standards usually in the form of growth charts. Measurements can be taken at one moment in time and compared with the charts but that will only give the information of whether the child at that particular time is small or tall, which if only taken once is clinically meaningless (Zeferino *et al.*, 2003). Usually, measurements are taken at set points over a period of time giving longitudinal data and growth velocity or tempo (Cole *et al.*, 2002). It is accepted that children grow at irregular rates at different chronological ages, which can lead to difficulties in interpreting the results in a meaningful way. Height and weight are the two most commonly used measures to monitor growth, with weight more relevant in infancy and height more relevant after infancy (Cole *et al.*, 2002).

Growth charts are used to monitor the changes that take place longitudinally in a child and were first developed for British children in the early sixties by J.M. Tanner and R.H. Whitehouse, and these charts (in a modified form) are still used along with Freeman charts and the Buckler-Tanner charts (Wright *et al.*, 2002). Different countries use reference data collected from their own national populations which makes it very difficult to compare studies across countries due to the differences in ethnic groups. These differences in ethnicity are beginning to create problems in countries with growing ethnic minorities as the growth charts used for a specific population are not representative of these different groups (Cole *et al.*, 2002). In most sporting environments growth is monitored usually by regular measurements of height and weight.

The adolescent growth spurt

During adolescence there is a sudden increase in the velocity of growth, which is called 'the adolescent growth spurt'. During this time there is an increase in the growth rate that peaks and then gradually slows down until full maturity is reached. The adolescent growth spurt is used in sport to identify the stage of maturation that has been reached by the athlete and whether they are early, normal or late developers as compared with others in the same age group. The onset of the adolescent growth spurt is highly individual and occurs at different chronological and skeletal ages. The adolescent growth spurt in girls occurs at approximately 9–10 years of age and can continue until 14–16 years of age; in boys it commences approximately 2 years later and does not finish until 18 years of age and in some cases even later (Malina *et al.*, 2004a). The adolescent growth spurt has been identified as a particularly vulnerable stage in a young athlete's development. There appears to be an increase in the rate of injury during this time including the risk of fracture. This is thought to be due to the rapid skeletal growth with a delay in bone mineralisation in the cortical bone (Blimkie *et al.*, 1993).

The age of onset of puberty can occur between 8 and 19 years (Baxter-Jones *et al.*, 1995). The assessment of the biological status of young elite performers is becoming more critical as the demands for success grow. Chronological age is a poor indicator of biological status (Mirwald *et al.*, 2002) and it has been shown that physical performance can depend on the stage of biological maturity and development that has been reached (Katzmarzyk *et*

al., 1997; Jones *et al.*, 2000). This information is needed by coaches so they may plan sessions to apply the correct training loads in boys of the same chronological age who are at various levels of physiological development and therefore have different performance abilities. Differences in maturity and development can be as much as 3–4 years for boys of the same chronological age (Hägg and Taranger, 1991; Beunen *et al.*, 1992; Iuliano-Burns *et al.*, 2001). This difference often results in the early maturing boys being in an advantageous position for performance purposes (Malina *et al.*, 2000, 2004b) and often means that late-maturing boys are deselected, even though research has shown that ultimately the late-maturing boys will catch up in all dimensions when they reach adulthood (Philippaerts *et al.*, 2006).

Peak height velocity

When the adolescent growth spurt occurs the rate of the change in height accelerates and then gradually decelerates. Peak height velocity (PHV) is a somatic biological maturity indicator and records the moment of maximum velocity of growth during adolescence. PHV has been used in number of studies as a non-invasive method of assessing the maturation status of players and athletes (Hägg and Taranger, 1991; Beunen *et al.*, 1992; Malina, 1994; Philippaerts *et al.*, 2006). PHV normally precedes all other peak velocities for other tissue growth and the point of time at which this occurs is highly individual and there can be considerable variation among children (Iuliano-Burns *et al.*, 2001). PHV will occur on average between 11.3 and 12.2 years of age in girls and 13.3 and 14.1 years of age in boys (Malina, 1994) with the average PHV occurring up to 2 years earlier in girls than it does in boys (Hägg *et al.*, 1991; Iuliano-Burns *et al.*, 2001). PHV can only be determined in a longitudinal study in which regular height measures are taken and then plotted to determine the growth velocity over time.

Methods of establishing maturity

There are a number of non-invasive methods used to assess maturation. Various maturity indicators can be used including the development of sexual characteristics or morphological age although some critics would argue that maturity cannot be measured by anthropometrical data as body size in itself is not a maturity indicator (Malina *et al.*, 2004a). Age of menarche is used for the maturity assessment of girls as is the age at PHV for both girls and boys; but both these methods can only be used towards full maturity and not prior to the onset of puberty. PHV is limited due to the fact that serial data needs to be taken for at least 4 years (Roche *et al.*, 1988) at least twice a year (Stratton *et al.*, 2004), rendering accuracy and availability of the child over a length of time questionable.

Assessing secondary sexual characteristics is probably the most commonly used method in clinical practice to evaluate maturity status. Criteria have been established for each change in sexual characteristics such as the development of pubic hair, breasts and genitalia, but this system is obviously limited to the pubertal stage of growth.

The only measure of biological maturity from birth to full maturity is the measurement of skeletal age. Skeletal age has been described as being the single best maturational index (Mirwald *et al.*, 2002). Skeletal age can be assessed using a number of techniques ranging from plain X-rays to ultrasound, magnetic resonance imaging and dual energy X-ray absorptiometry (DXA). The hand/wrist is the most commonly used area for assessment of skeletal maturity for a number of reasons. There is minimal exposure to radiation, approximately 0.0017 mSv, which is the equivalent to approximately 1 hour of background radiation in a city centre such as in Manchester. The wrist/hand is easily positioned and there are a large number of bones in a small area that can be assessed.

Musculoskeletal disorders in children

Movement is an essential part of learning for the child. The most common musculoskeletal problems in children are due to trauma, and fractures of the upper limbs are more common than those of the lower limbs. Children engaged in sporting activities are susceptible to overuse injuries for a number of reasons. At a competitive level, children will be engaged in regular competitive training as well as weekly competition. Many of these injuries can be prevented by incorporating specific techniques into training sessions, and many injuries are of a minor nature which may not be reported.

Generally, overuse injuries in children include tendon injury and traction apophysitis, stress fractures, bursitis, and joint disorders. They arise due to highly repetitive activities. Children are vulnerable as their apophyseal growth plates are active and even minor injuries to tendons or growth plates should lead to restriction in activity until the symptoms resolve. Many studies have described the important part that growth and development play in overuse injuries in youth athletes (Krivickas and Feinberg, 1996; Marsh and Daigneault, 1999; Oeppen and Jaramillo, 2003). All these studies acknowledge the fact that longitudinal growth of bone is the primary event and the surrounding soft tissue of joint tendons, ligaments, tendons and muscles elongate as a secondary response. In the short term, this results in an increased tension in the surrounding soft tissues which leads to relative inflexibility and muscle imbalance and consequently weakness. This leaves the athlete vulnerable to injury particularly during repetitive overload which occurs during regular training (Micheli and Klein 1991; Krivickas, 1997; Di Fiori, 1999; Oeppen and Jaramillo, 2003). Biomechanical imbalances are due to the speed of growth in the skeletal tissue compared with the period of time it takes for the surrounding soft tissues to adapt (Marsh and Daigneault, 1999; Hawkins and Metheny, 2001; Oeppen and Jaramillo, 2003).

Prevention strategies include improving flexibility, strength and general fitness in addition to matching children by size rather than chronological age, adherence to the rules, improved playing conditions and the compulsory wearing of protective clothing implements such as shin pads (Schmidt-Olsen *et al.*, 1985; Drawer and Fuller, 2002; Olsen *et al.*, 2004).

In the immature athlete, muscle and tendon strains and ligament sprains are not as common as in fully mature athletes because the soft tissue tends to be stronger than the bone to which it is attached. The resulting injury therefore, is usually an avulsion of the muscle, ligament or tendon from its bony attachment (Bruns and Maffulli, 2000). Overuse injuries, in youth athletes are usually reported by the player when he or she is no longer able to train comfortably rather than when the symptoms are first felt. All types of injury, if incorrectly treated, can have ramifications in the future with regards to the players' balance and proprioception abilities being affected (Emery, 2003).

Specific musculoskeletal disorders in children

The conditions described below are specific to children although management of these conditions should involve application of the same exercise principles described for each joint in the appropriate preceding chapters.

Traction apophysitis conditions

Osgood–Schlatter's syndrome is a traction apophysitis of the tibial tubercle due to repeated stress on the secondary ossification centre of the tibial tuberosity. This condition presents in growing children usually between 8 and 12 years in girls and between 12 and 15 years in boys. The symptoms include pain, swelling and tenderness over the tibial tuberosity. On X-ray, changes seen include irregularity of the apophysis with separation from the tibial tuberosity in the early stages and fragmentation in the later stages (Gholve *et al.*, 2007). The tibial tubercle is the site of insertion of the quadriceps tendon and activities involving strong contractions of the quadriceps, e.g. football, running and basketball are associated with this injury. In adolescents this area is a growth plate and repeated vigorous activity causes traction on the growth plate, which leads to the inflammation and pain. As the tubercle is pulled forward by the quadriceps, contracting bone forms behind and the tubercle can become very prominent. This may in turn lead to pain when kneeling. The condition settles once the growth plate fuses to the tibia. Treatment is aimed at reducing the pain and swelling. Ice packs will provide pain relief, and non-steroidal anti-inflammatories may be recommended. A knee brace may help to reduce strain on the tibial tubercle. Generally symptoms disappear after the growth spurt is complete and only in rare cases is there a need for surgical management such tibial tubercleplasty (Weiss *et al.*, 2007).

Sever's disease affects the calcaneal attachment of the gastrocnemius/soleus musculature (Kaeding and Whitehead, 1998). Other traction apophysitis include the elbow region which may be seen in baseball players or more rarely in those playing racquet sports (Blohm *et al.*, 1999). For both of these conditions, maintenance of joint range of motion (ROM), strength and proprioception should be emphasised, within limits of pain, for the patient. The preceding chapters on the knee and ankle should be reviewed for specific detail.

Scheuermann's disease

Scheuermann's disease is an osteochondrosis of the spine that mainly occurs in adolescents, usually boys, in their last 2–3 years of growth. It is a disturbance in the normal growth of the vertebral epiphyseal ring (Williams, 1979). If the compressive forces in the spine are sufficient it may cause a wedge deformity in the vertebral body causing a kyphosis of the thoracic spine and an associated increase in lumbar lordosis. Small disc herniations in the vertebral end plate called Schmorl's nodes are sometimes identified on X-ray. The condition often remains asymptomatic but can become painful after activity. Treatment would usually consist of moderation of activities to minimise repetitive flexion and extension movements of the spine but with an active exercise programme. See Chapters 5 and 6, which discuss exercise in the thoracic and lumbar spine areas, for specific details of appropriate exercise.

Spondylolysis and spondylolisthesis

The conditions of spondylolysis and spondylolisthesis are commonly found in adolescent athletes (Standaert *et al.*, 2000; Gregory *et al.*, 2004; Iwamoto *et al.*, 2004). Both conditions are described as stress fractures of the pars interarticularis of the lumbar spine. Spondylolysis is when there is a fracture on only one side of the spine; spondylolisthesis is when the stress fractures are bilateral (Standaert *et al.*, 2000; Gregory *et al.*, 2004; Iwamoto *et al.*, 2004). The most common cause of spondylolysis in the immature athlete seems to be repetitive loading of the lumbar spine which creates a stress reaction (Gregory *et al.*, 2004). It can be both symptomatic and asymptomatic, which is only established on routine radiographs (Standaert *et al.*, 2000). The treatment is more commonly conservative, with spontaneous healing occurring in 87.5% of all cases of spondylolysis. (Iwamoto *et al.*, 2004). Spondylolisthesis is more complex because with a bilateral fracture there may be some spinal instability and spinal fusion surgery is not uncommon (Iwamoto *et al.*, 2004). Soler and Calderón (2000) state that spondylolysis is as common in adolescent athletes as a 'lumbar sprain' and that it is said to be 3–4 times more common in athletes than in the general adolescent population. Low back sprains and strains are said to be very common in athletes (Keene, 1983). Rehabilitation would include a stability programme discussed in Chapter 6 on the lumbar spine.

Stress fractures can be commonly experienced in other areas in the adolescent athlete including the foot, tibia and fibula (Oeppen and Jaramillo, 2003), and less commonly – but not unusual – in the tarsal bones and clavicle.

Slipped upper femoral epiphysis

A slipped upper femoral epiphysis (SUFE) is where the growth plate at the upper end of the femur is weakened and the head of the femur moves downwards and backwards, thus affecting the movements at the hip joint. The exact cause is unknown and early diagnosis is important. The child complains of pain in the groin, hip, thigh or knee and has limited movement in the hip joint. The child may walk with a limp and there may be slight shortening of the affected leg. Treatment depends on the severity and is guided by X-rays and scans. Surgery may be required to stabilise the hip. Metal screws are inserted into the head of the femur and removed once the growth plate has closed. Post operatively the child will be non-weight-bearing for about 6 weeks.

Perthes' disease

Perthes' disease is a condition characterised by a loss (temporary) of blood supply to the hip. The area around the head of the femur becomes inflamed. It is usually seen in children between 4 and 10 years of age and is five times more common in boys. Symptoms generally commence with a limp and pain, which may be intermittent over a few months. Pain is brought on by movements of the hip and relieved by rest. Diagnosis is confirmed with X-rays. Treatment may be conservative or surgical. Anti-inflammatory medication is used to reduce the inflammation around the joint. Stretching exercises are prescribed to increase range of movement and the particular focus is on hip abduction

and rotation. The child may require crutches for mobilisation. Casts may be used to maintain the hip in a good position (abduction). Surgical treatment realigns the head of the femur within the acetabulum and the alignment is maintained with screws and plates. The child is kept in a plaster cast for 6–8 weeks post operatively.

In both these conditions, when surgery is required, the general principles of exercise therapy in management of hip pathologies should be applied in post-operative rehabilitation. The reader is referred to Chapter 10 for details.

Scoliosis

Scoliosis is a curvature of the spine in the lateral plane accompanied by rotation. The muscles on the side of the convexity are at a mechanical disadvantage. Scoliosis can be idiopathic or as the result of a neuromuscular condition such as Duchenne's muscular dystrophy, spina bifida or cerebral palsy. Treatment aims at reducing or halting the progression of the deformity by splinting or surgery. In terms of exercise the focus should be on maintaining mobility in the spine and overall musculoskeletal system and a level of fitness. Swimming is recommended to maintain fitness, muscle strength and respiratory function. Prescription of exercise should refer to the principles discussed in Chapters 4–6, which discuss the spine.

General considerations in the exercise management of children

The ability to physically perform at any stage is reflected in a child's progress in growth, maturity and development. A potential exists in all children that follow normal developmental pathways, to learn basic performance skills and movement patterns, which become refined with practice and repetition to form a basic movement framework used in any sport.

The peak bone mass that develops during childhood is an important risk factor in osteoporosis. In children who are physically active higher bone mass is seen (Slemendra *et al.*, 1991). Therefore it is important that clinicians encourage and promote health-enhancing physical activity from an early age. As clinicians are involved in the ongoing management of children with disorders affecting mobility it is essential that weight-bearing activities are encouraged to optimise bone mass. In children with specific paediatric conditions, exercise management may need to be modified to meet particular requirements associated with their overall management. In children with cystic fibrosis, exercise will improve mucociliary clearance, strengthen respiratory muscles and improve bone density, whereas for children with muscular dystrophy the aim may be to increase muscle strength and endurance and thereby prolong the time the child is ambulant. In those with spina bifida the primary aim will be upper limb strength and control of body mass and maximising aerobic power. Specific exercise programmes may need to be devised taking into account the limitations associated with movement in the child with neuromuscular disorders.

References

Abbott, R. (2002) Correlation of habitual physical activity levels with flow-mediated dilation of the brachial artery in 5–10 year old children. *Atherosclerosis*, 160(1), 233–239

American College of Sports Medicine (ACSM). (1990) The recommended quantity and quality of exercise for developing and maintaining cardiorespiratory and muscular fitness in healthy adults. *Medicine and Science in Sports and Exercise*, 22, 265–274.

American College of Sports Medicine (ACSM). (1998) American College of Sports Medicine Position Stand. The recommended quantity and quality of exercise for developing and maintaining cardiorespiratory and muscular fitness and flexibility in healthy adults. *Medicine and Science in Sports and Exercise*, 30, 975–991.

Andersen, L., Harro, M., Sardinha, L., Froberg, K., Ekelund, U., Brage, S. and Anderssen, S. (2006) Physical activity and clustered cardiovascular risk in children: a cross-sectional study (The European Youth Heart Study). *Lancet*, 368, 299–304.

Baxter-Jones, A.D., Helms, P., Maffulli, N., Baines-Preece, J.C. and Preece, M. (1995) Growth and development of male gymnasts, swimmers, soccer and tennis players: a longitudinal study. *Annals of Human Biology*, 22, 381–394.

Beunen, G.P., Malina, R.M., Renson, R., Simons, J., Ostyn, M. and Lefevre, J. (1992) Physical activity and growth, maturation and performance: a longitudinal study. *Medicine and Science in Sports and Exercise*, 24, 576–585.

Blimkie, C., Lefevre, J., Beunen, G.P., Renson, R., Dequeker, J. and Van Damme, P. (1993) Fractures, physical activity, and growth velocity in adolescent Belgian boys. *Medicine and Science in Sports and Exercise*, 25, 801–808.

Blohm, D., Kaalund, S. and Jakobsen, B.W. (1999) 'Little league elbow' – acute traction apophysitis in an adolescent badminton player. *Scandinavian Journal of Medicine and Science in Sports*, 9, 245–247.

Bouziotas, C., Koutedakis, Y., Nevill, A., Ageli, E., Tsigilis, N., Nikolaou, A. and Nakou, A. (2004) Greek adolescents, fitness, fatness, fat intake, activity, and coronary heart disease risk. *Archives of Disease in Childhood*, 89, 41–44.

Brage, S., Wedderkopp, N., Ekelund, U., Franks, P.W, Wareham, N.J., Andersen, L.B. and Froberg, K. (2004) Features of the metabolic syndrome are associated with objectively measured physical activity and fitness in Danish children. *Diabetes Care*, 27, 2141–2148.

Bruns, W. and Maffulli, N. (2000) Lower limb injuries in children in sports. *Clinics in Sports Medicine*, 19, 637–662.

Bucksch, J. (2005) Physical activity of moderate intensity in leisure time and the risk of all cause mortality. *British Journal of Sports Medicine*, 39, 632–638.

Cole, D.A., Tram, J.M., Martin, J.M., Hoffman, K.B., Ruiz, M.D., Jacquez, F.M. and Maschman, T.L. (2002) Individual differences in the emergence of depressive symptoms in children and adolescents: a longitudinal investigation of parent and child reports. *Journal of Abnormal Psychology*, 111, 156–165.

Daly, R.M. (2007) The effect of exercise on bone mass and structural geometry during growth. *Medicine and Sports Science*, 51, 33–49.

Di Fiori, J.P. (1999) Stress fracture of the proximal fibula in a young soccer player: a case report and a review of the literature. *Medicine and Science in Sports and Exercise*, 31, 925–928.

Drawer, S. and Fuller, C.W. (2002) Evaluating the level of injury in English professional football using a risk based assessment process. *British Journal of Sports Medicine*, 36, 446–451.

Emery, C.A. (2003) Risk factors for injury in child and adolescent sport: a systematic review of the literature. *Clinical Journal of Sports Medicine*, 13, 256–268.

Gholve, P.A., Scher, D.M., Khakharia, S., Widermann, R.F. and Green, D.W. (2007) Osgood Schlatter syndrome. *Current Opinion in Paediatrics*, 19, 44–50.

Gregory, P.L., Batt, M.E. and Kerslake, R.W. (2004) Comparing spondylolysis in cricketers and soccer players. *British Journal of Sports Medicine*, 38, 737–742.

Hägg, U. and Taranger, J. (1991) Height and height velocity in early, average and late maturers followed to the age of 25: a prospective longitudinal study of Swedish urban children from birth to adulthood. *Annals of Human Biology*, 18, 47–56.

Hall, D. (2000) Growth monitoring. *Archives of Disease in Childhood*, 82, 10–15.

Hawkins, D. and Metheny, J. (2001) Overuse injuries in youth sports: biomechanical considerations. *Medicine and Science in Sports and Exercise*, 33, 1701–1707.

Hermanussen, M., Lange, S. and Grasedyck, L. (2001). Growth tracks in early childhood. *Acta Paediatrica*, 90, 381–386.

Hussey, J., Bell, C., Bennett, K., O'Dwyer, J. and Gormley, J. (2007) Relationship between the intensity of physical activity, inactivity, cardiorespiratory fitness and body composition in 7–10-year-old Dublin children. *British Journal of Sports Medicine*, 41, 311–316.

Iuliano-Burns, S., Mirwald, R.L. and Bailey, D.A. (2001) Timing and magnitude of peak height velocity and peak tissue velocities for early, average, and late maturing boys and girls. *American Journal of Human Biology*, 13, 1–8.

Iwamoto, J., Takeda, T. and Wakano, K. (2004) Returning athletes with severe low back pain and spondylolysis to original sporting activities with conservative treatment. *Scandinavian Journal of Medicine and Science in Sports*, 14, 346–351.

Jones, M.A., Hitchen, P.J. and Stratton, G. (2000) The importance of considering biological maturity when assessing physical fitness measures in girls and boys aged 10 to 16 years. *Annals of Human Biology*, 27, 57–65.

Kaeding, C.C., Whitehead, R. (1998) Musculoskeletal injuries in adolescents. *Journal of Primary Care*, 25, 211–23.

Katzmarzyk, P.T., Malina, R.M. and Beunen, G.P. (1997) The contribution of biological maturation to the strength and motor fitness of children. *Annals of Human Biology*, 24, 493–505.

Keene, J.S. (1983) Low back pain in the athlete. From spondylogenic injury during recreation or competition. *Postgraduate Medicine*, 74, 209–217.

Krivickas, L.S. (1997) Anatomical factors associated with overuse sports injuries. *Sports Medicine*, 24, 132–146.

Krivickas, L.S. and Feinberg, J.H. (1996) Lower extremity injuries in college athletes: relation between ligamentous laxity and lower extremity muscle tightness. *Archives of Physical Medicine and Rehabilitation*, 77, 1139–1143.

Lee, C.D., Blair, S.N. and Jackson, A.S. (1999) Cardiorespiratory fitness, body composition, and all cause mortality in men. *American Journal of Clinical Nutrition*, 69, 373–80.

Macdonald, H.M., Kontulainen, S.A., Khan, K.M. and McKay, H.A. (2007) Is a school-based physical activity intervention effective for increasing tibial bone strength in boys and girls? *Journal of Bone and Mineral Research*, 22, 434–446.

Malina, R.M. (1994) Physical growth and biological maturation of young athletes. *Exercise and Sports Sciences Reviews*, 22, 389–433.

Malina, R.M., Bouchard, C. and Bar-Or, O. (2004a) *Growth, Maturation, and Physical Activity*, 2nd edn. Human Kinetics, Champaign.

Malina, R.M., Eisenmann, J.C., Cumming, S.P., Ribeiro, B. and Aroso, J. (2004b) Maturity-associated variation in the growth and functional capacities of youth football (soccer) players 13–15 years. *European Journal of Applied Physiology*, 91, 555–562.

Malina, R.M., Reyes, M.E.P., Eisenmann, J.C., Horta, L., Rodrigues, J. and Miller, R. (2000) Height, mass and skeletal maturity of elite Portuguese soccer players aged 11–16 years. *Journal of Sports Sciences*, 18, 685–693.

Marsh, J.S. and Daigneault, J.P. (1999) The young athlete. *Current Opinions in Pediatrics*, 11, 84–88.

Micheli, L.J. and Klein, J.D. (1991) Sporting injuries in children and adolescents. *British Journal of Sports Medicine*, 25, 6–9.

Mirwald, R.L., Baxter-Jones, A.D., Bailey, D.A. and Beunen, G.P. (2002) An assessment of maturity form anthropometric measurements. *Medicine and Science in Sports and Exercise*, 34, 689–694.

Morris, J.N., Kagan, A., Pattison, D.C. and Gardner, M.J. (1966) Incidence and prediction of ischaemic heart disease in London busmen. *Lancet*, 2, 533–539.

Oeppen, R.S. and Jaramillo, D. (2003) Sports injuries in the young athlete. *Topics in Magnetic Resonance Imaging*, 14, 199–208.

Olsen, L., Scanlan, A., MacKay, M., Babul, S., Reid, D., Clark, M. and Raina, P. (2004) Strategies for prevention of soccer related injuries: a systematic review. *British Journal of Sports Medicine*, 38, 89–94.

Paffenbarger, R.S., Hyde, R.T., Wing, A.L. and Hsieh, C.C. (1986) Physical activity, all-cause mortality, and longevity of college alumni. *New England Journal of Medicine*, 314, 605–613.

Philippaerts, R.M., Vaeyens, R., Janssens, M., Van Renterghem, B., Matthys, D., Craen, R., Bourgois, J., Vrijens, J., Beunen, G. and Malina, R.M. (2006) The relationship between peak height velocity and physical performance in youth soccer players. *Journal of Sports Science*, 24, 221–230.

Raitakari, O.T., Porkka, K.V., Räsänen, L., Rönnemaa, T. and Viikari, J.S. (1994a) Clustering and six year cluster-tracking of serum total cholesterol, HDL-cholesterol and diastolic blood pressure in children and young adults. The Cardiovascular Risk in Young Finns Study. *Journal of Clinical Epidemiology*, 47, 1085–1093.

Raitakari, O.T., Porkka, K.V., Räsänen, L. and Viikari, J.S. (1994b) Relations of life-style with lipids, blood pressure and insulin in adolescents and young adults. The Cardiovascular Risk in Young Finns Study. *Atherosclerosis*, 111, 237–246.

Ribeiro, J.C., Guerra, S., Oliveira, J., Andersen, L.B., Duarte, J.A. and Mota, J. (2004) Body fatness and clustering of cardiovascular disease risk factors in portuguese children and adolescents. *American Journal of Human Biology*, 15, 556–562.

Riddoch, C., Andersen, L.B., Wedderkopp, N., Harro, M., Klasson-Heggebo, L., Sardinha, L., Cooper, A. and Ekelund, U. (2004) Physical activity levels and patterns of 9- and 15-yr-old european children. *Medicine and Science in Sports and Exercise*, 36, 86–92.

Roche, A.F., Guo, S.M., Baumgartner, R.N. and Falls, R.A. (1988) The measurement of stature. *American Journal of Clinical Nutrition*, 47, 922.

Sallis, J.F. and Patrick, K. (1994) Overview of the international consensus conference on physical activity guidelines for adolescents. *Pediatric Exercise Science*, 6, 299–301.

Schmidt-Olsen, S., Bünemann, L.K., Lade, V. and Brassøe, J.O. (1985) Soccer injuries of youth. *British Journal of Sports Medicine*, 19, 161–164.

Schmitz, K.H., Jacobs, D.R., Hong C.P., Steinberger, J., Moran, A. and Sinaiko, A.R. (2002) Association of physical activity with insulin sensitivity in children. *International Journal of Obesity*, 26, 1310–1316.

Slemendra, C.W., Miller, J.Z., Hui, S.L., Reister, T.K. and Johnston, C.C. (1991) Role of physical activity in the development of skeletal mass in children. *Journal of Bone and Mineral Research*, 6, 1227–1233.

Soler, T. and Calderón, C. (2000) The prevalence of spondylolysis in the Spanish elite athlete. *American Journal of Sports Medicine*, 28, 57–62.

Standaert, C.J., Herring, S.A., Halpern, B. and King, O. (2000) Spondylolysis. *Physical Medicine and Rehabilitation Clinics of North America*, 11, 785–803.

Stratton, G., Jones, M., Fox, K.R., Tolfrey, K., Harris, J., Maffulli, N., Lee, M. and Frostick, S.P. (2004) BASES position statement on guidelines for resistance exercise in young people. *Journal of Sports Sciences*, 22, 383–390.

Strong, W., Malina, R., Blimkie, C., Daniels, S., Dishman, R., Gutin, B., Hergenroeder, A., Must, A., Nixon, P. and Pivarnik, J. (2005) Evidence based physical activity for school-age youth. *Journal of Pediatrics*, 146, 732–737.

Suter, E. and Hawes, M.R. (1993) Relationship of physical activity, body fat, diet, and blood lipid profile in youths 10–15 yr. *Medicine and Science in Sports and Exercise*, 25, 748–754.

Tudor-Locke, C., Pangrazi, R.P., Corbin, C.B., Rutherford, W.J., Vincent, S.D., Anders Raustorp, A., Tomson, L.M. and Cuddihy, T.F. (2004) BMI-referenced standards for recommended pedometer-determined steps/day in children. *Preventive Medicine*, 38, 857–864.

Weiss, J.M., Jordan, S.S., Andersen, J.S., Lee, B.M. and Kocher, M. (2007). Surgical treatment of unresolved Osgood Schlatter disease: ossicle resection with tibial tubercleplasty. *Journal of Pediatric Orthopedics*, 27, 844–847.

Williams, J.G. (1979) Sports injuries. *Nursing (London)*, 4, 158–162.

Wright, C.M., Booth, I.W., Buckler, J.M., Cameron, N., Cole, T.J., Healy, M.J., Hulse, J.A., Preece, M.A., Reilly, J.J. and Williams, A.F. (2002) Growth reference charts for use in the United Kingdom. *Archives of Disease in Childhood*, 86, 11–14.

Zeferino, A., Filho, A.A.B., Bettiol, H. and Barbieri, M.A. (2003) Monitoring growth. *Journal of Pediatrics*, 79 (Suppl. 1), S23–S32.

Musculoskeletal Disorders in the Cardiac and Respiratory Patient

14

Juliette Hussey

Introduction

The aim of this chapter is to highlight the range of musculoskeletal disorders associated with respiratory and cardiac disease, so the musculoskeletal abnormalities associated with conditions such as chronic obstructive pulmonary disease (COPD), asthma, cystic fibrosis and heart failure will be considered. In addition, the musculoskeletal changes that the patient may experience after cardiac or thoracic surgery will be presented. The evidence for the management of these conditions with exercise therapy will be discussed. Comprehensive details of both cardiac and pulmonary rehabilitation may be found in a previous publication by the authors (Gormley and Hussey, 2005) and will not be discussed in detail in this chapter.

COPD is characterised by airflow limitation. It is progressive and is associated with cough, sputum production and shortness of breath (Global Strategy for the Diagnosis, Management and Prevention of COPD, Global Initiative for Chronic Obstructive Lung Disease (GOLD), 2007) and diagnosis is confirmed by spirometry. Exercise capacity is gradually decreased in these patients due the associated dyspnoea. One of the goals of pulmonary rehabilitation is to address this limitation. Asthma is an inflammatory disorder of the airways with airway obstruction that is reversible either spontaneously or with treatment (British Thoracic Society (BTS), 2001). Symptoms include wheeze, shortness of breath and cough. The symptoms may be provoked by a number of triggers including exercise. The paradoxical relationship with exercise is that exercise induces broncho-constriction in many asthmatic people, but exercise is recommended as part of the overall management of the condition. Cystic fibrosis is a disorder of the exocrine glands and is characterised by excessive mucus secretion. Exercise is recognised as an important part of the management of this condition due to its beneficial effects on mucociliary clearance, lung function, aerobic capacity and bone health.

Musculoskeletal disorders in respiratory disease

Limitations in physical functioning in patient with respiratory disease

Patients with respiratory disease face a number of musculoskeletal problems. These include: postural abnormalities, muscle wasting and dysfunction,

---

osteoporosis, and reduced range of movement in the thoracic cage due to airflow limitation and hyperinflation. These changes are probably due to a number of factors in addition to the disease process and these include: physical inactivity, malnutrition, systemic inflammation, corticosteroid treatment and hypoxaemia.

Exercise tolerance is limited in patients with COPD due to hyperinflation and respiratory muscle fatigue (Roussos *et al.*, 1976). Maximal inspiratory pressure has been found to be a predictor of exercise capacity (Dillard *et al.*, 1989) and in patients with COPD maximal inspiratory and expiratory pressures have been found to be 50% and 39% of predicted (Montes de Oca *et al.*, 1996). In these patients the diaphragm may be already carrying an extra load at rest and therefore the accessory muscles of respiration are required early (Montes de Oca *et al.*, 1996). Lung hyperinflation reduces the strength of the respiratory muscles and is one of the pathophysiological mechanisms of dyspnoea in these patients.

In patients with respiratory disease physical deconditioning occurs due to disease progression. The result of dyspnoea associated with many respiratory diseases is such that the patient restricts their activity in order to avoid becoming breathless and this adds to the rapid deconditioning, low confidence and further reduced functioning. Exercise training encourages the patient with respiratory disease to acknowledge that breathlessness can be controlled through breathing techniques and thus helps to break the vicious cycle of increasing dyspnoea with time and progression of lung disease.

Comprehensive pulmonary rehabilitation programmes aim to restore the patient to the highest degree of physical functioning by means of exercise therapy and education. The American Thoracic Society and European Respiratory Society have adopted the following definition of pulmonary rehabilitation in a position paper in 2006: 'Pulmonary rehabilitation is an evidence-based, multidisciplinary, and comprehensive intervention for patients with chronic respiratory diseases who are symptomatic and often have decreased daily life activities'. Integrated into the individualized treatment of the patient, pulmonary rehabilitation is designed to reduce symptoms, optimise functional status, increase participation, and reduce health care costs through stabilising or reversing systemic manifestations of the disease. The benefits of pulmonary rehabilitation have been demonstrated both in patients with mild and severe disease (BTS, 2001). Pulmonary rehabilitation includes practical exercise classes and education of exercise training, secretion clearance techniques, nutritional support, smoking cessation and advice on breathing control. Musculoskeletal assessment in these patients should include observation of posture, measurements of joint range of motion, muscle activity and strength. It should also include documentation of any pain on rest or movement. Questioning about the use of long-term steroids is required in patients with chronic respiratory disease, as this treatment may lead to reduced bone density. Chapters 5 and 7–9, which discuss exercise in the management of the thoracic spine and upper limb conditions, should be consulted for practical examples of appropriate exercises.

Range of movement and respiratory disease

The range of movement in the spine and shoulder girdle needs to be evaluated prior to specific exercise prescription in the patient with respiratory disease. Posture in sitting needs to be examined; typical abnormalities in patients with cystic fibrosis include forward head posture, tight suboccipital and cervical extensors, scapulae the abducted and protracted, an increase thoracic kyphosis and a reduced lumbar lordosis. The range of movement in the thoracic region is dependent on the movement at the apophyseal, costovertebral, costotransverse joints and ribs, and the length of the intercostals, pectoralis and latissimus dorsi. A thoracic kyphosis may be the result of limited range in the upper thoracic spine. Thoracic rotation and lateral flexion occur in the mid-thoracic spine and any restriction here or shortening of the latissimus dorsi or teres major will limit the range of shoulder elevation. The range of rotation in the glenohumeral joint may also be affected by the tightness in the anterior and posterior shoulder capsule and related muscles. Shoulder movements and scapulohumeral rhythm need to be observed.

Muscle function and respiratory disease

Both peripheral muscle strength and respiratory muscle strength are affected in patients with respiratory disorders. Respiratory muscle function may be affected by a number of factors including hypoxia, hypercapnia, acidaemia and malnutrition (Tobin, 1988). The combination of steroids, decreased exercise tolerance and chronic inflammation may lead to respiratory muscle weakness. Function may also be affected by biomechanical changes associated with hyperinflation of the lungs, which leads to flattening of the diaphragm so it is at a disadvantageous position in terms of the length tension curve.

In addition to the respiratory muscles, the peripheral muscles are also affected with generally a greater decrease in the strength of the lower limb muscles (a decrease of 20–30% in quadriceps strength has been reported) and relative preservation of upper limb strength (Decramer *et al.*, 1994; Gosselink *et al.*, 1996). Within the upper limbs, proximal muscle strength has been found to be more impaired than distal strength in patients with stable COPD (Gosselink *et al.*, 2000). Structural and biochemical abnormalities have been found along with a reduction in the percentage of type 1 muscle fibres. Metabolic abnormalities are probably due to hypoxaemia and inactivity. Lactic acidosis occurs at lower work rates in COPD patients when compared with controls and this is associated with impaired exercise tolerance.

Muscle function in patients with respiratory disease may also be limited by disuse, malnutrition, inflammatory markers, low levels of sex hormones, or prolonged use of systemic corticosteroids. Malnutrition may contribute to the muscle wasting and the patient with COPD may experience weight loss and an associated decrease in fat-free mass. Nutritional supplementation for 3 months was found to have a positive effect on maximal skeletal muscle strength (respiratory muscles and handgrip) in addition to body weight, mid-arm circumference and triceps skinfold thickness (Efthimiou *et al.*, 1988) in patients with COPD who received supplemental oral nutrition compared with controls. Respiratory muscle strength and hand grip strength improved alongside nutritional status.

Many respiratory conditions are associated with systemic inflammation (Gan *et al.*, 2004). Yende *et al.* (2006) examined the association between inflammatory markers and ventilatory limitation, muscle strength and exercise capacity in elderly patients, both with and without obstructive lung disease. Those with obstructive lung disease had lower quadriceps strength, lower maximum inspira-

tory pressure, higher systemic interleukin-6 levels and higher C-reactive protein levels than those who had normal lung function measures. Higher systemic levels of interleukin-6 were found to be associated with reduced forced expiratory volume in 1 second (FEV_1), quadriceps strength and exercise capacity.

Reduced levels of growth hormone and testosterone may contribute to muscle wasting. Van Vliet *et al.* (2005) compared circulating levels of hormones of the pituitary-gonadotrophic axis of men with COPD and age matched controls. The relationship between muscle force, exercise tolerance, inflammatory markers and hypogonadism was also explored. The hormonal differences were significantly higher for follicle-stimulating hormone and luteinising hormone, and lower testosterone in subjects with COPD. Low testosterone was significantly related to quadriceps weakness (r = 0.48) and C-reactive protein (r − 0.39) but not to exercise tolerance as measured by the 6-minute walk test.

Many patients with chronic respiratory disease will have a combination of these factors, all of which contribute to the decrease in muscle strength and have to be considered in exercise management.

Bone health and respiratory disease

Patients with obstructive lung disease have many risk factors that can predispose them to low bone density. In those with severe disease, the risk of osteoporosis increases as patients become more immobile, malnourished and more dependent on drug therapy. Sin *et al.* (2003) analysed data from the Third National Health and Nutrition Examination Survey and found that airflow obstruction was associated with increased odds of osteoporosis compared with those without airflow obstruction (odds ratio (OR) 1.9; 95% CI 1.4 to 2.5). Those with severe airflow obstruction were at an increased risk (OR 2.4; 95% CI 1.3 to 4.4). The authors concluded by highlighting the need for bone mineral density (BMD) evaluation in these patients to inform related management. Treatment of emphysema by lung volume reduction surgery has been found to result in an improvement in BMD (Mineo *et al.*, 2005). The increase in BMD correlated with residual volume, diffusing capacity of the lung for carbon monoxide and fat-free mass, suggesting that the improvement was related to improved respiration and nutritional status.

Oral glucocorticoids are frequently used in asthma. Inhaled glucocorticosteroids are used in asthma to reduce symptoms and theoretically should have low systemic effects but even in those on low-dose inhaled corticosteroids, BMD has been found to be lower than controls (El *et al.*, 2005). In this latter study on 45 female subjects, no correlation was found between disease duration, inhaled steroid treatment duration, cumulative inhaled dose and BMD measurements.

In subjects with cystic fibrosis, osteopenia and osteoporosis are seen and may be related to factors such as malnutrition and chronic use of corticosteroids (Hardin *et al.*, 2001). Total body bone mineral content in children with cystic fibrosis has been found to be significantly less than in age- and gender-matched controls (Hardin *et al.*, 2001). In children with non-cystic fibrosis bronchiectasis, osteopenia has been found to be more common compared with controls (Guran *et al.*, 2008). The risk increased with age but BMD was not related to the severity of lung disease, calcium intake or steroid use.

Exercise management of patients with respiratory disease

The exercise component of the pulmonary rehabilitation programme generally comprises aerobic, strength and flexibility exercises. Either continuous or interval aerobic training in the form of walking or cycling is a key component and is carried into the home programme. Extremity conditioning exercises are used to improve maximum oxygen uptake, strength, endurance and co-ordination (Ries, 1994; Siebens 1996). The type of exercise indicated is of low resistance and high repetition which can be tolerated by the patient.

Patients are assessed prior to commencing rehabilitation and an individual training programme is devised. Patients may need postural correction with the goal of obtaining a position so that the spine, pelvis and shoulder girdle are in a neutral position to permit optimal muscle function. The management of joint restriction includes the use of passive mobilisations followed by exercises. Upper limb flexion and spinal extension may be performed with breathing exercises. In sitting the patient can

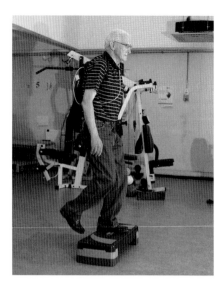

Figure 14.1 Patient performing step-ups.

perform extension and rotation with assistance if required to gain an increase in range. Home exercises need to be explained and the use of a mirror may help provide visual feedback to the patient.

Typical exercises to increase range of movement in the cervical and thoracic spine and shoulder joint include active-assisted rotation for the cervical and thoracic spine with the patient sitting on a chair, active thoracic spine lateral flexion with the patient in standing, and passive stretch of the anterior shoulder muscles. Figures 14.1–14.4 show examples of exercises that are performed in pulmonary rehabilitation and which benefit the musculoskeletal system. Exercises to maintain range of movement, in particular, in the shoulder and thoracic regions are included as part of the warm-up and exercise session. Examples of these are shoulder circles in each direction, trunk rotation and flexion and push-ups with hands against the wall at shoulder height.

Muscle strengthening as part of rehabilitation for patients with COPD is recommended. In addition to lower limb exercises, upper extremity training is also recommended to help performance in daily activities. Subjects with reduced exercise capacity who experience less ventilatory limitation to exercise and more reduced respiratory and peripheral muscle strength have been found to be more likely to respond well to exercise training (Troosters *et al.*, 2001). At this stage there is insufficient evidence to advocate high-intensity exercise and there is a

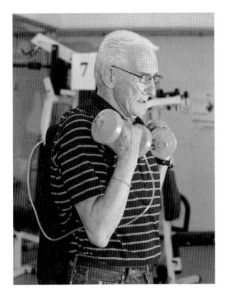

Figure 14.2 Patient using hand weights.

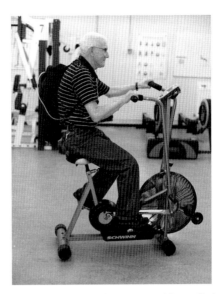

Figure 14.4 Patient exercising upper and lower limbs.

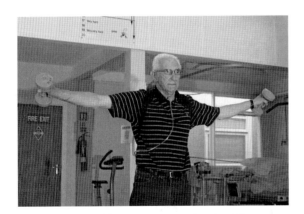

Figure 14.3 Shoulder exercises using hand weights.

need for studies to investigate the results of varying intensities of exercise. Low-intensity peripheral muscle conditioning, in the form of 10 different exercises, each performed for 30 seconds, has been shown to be well tolerated and led to improved muscle performance in patients with COPD (Clark *et al.*, 1996).

The effects of inspiratory muscle training have been extensively studied with varying results. However, an 8-week programme of high-intensity inspiratory muscle training resulted in a significant increase in inspiratory muscle function, increased thickness of the diaphragm, improved lung volumes and work capacity in subjects with cystic fibrosis

(Enright *et al.*, 2004) and healthy subjects, at 80% of maximal effort (Enright *et al.*, 2006). A Cochrane systematic review by Ram *et al.* (2008) identified five randomised controlled trials in which respiratory muscle training was investigated. The pooled results showed a significant effect of inspiratory muscle training.

Cardiac disease and musculoskeletal dysfunction

Limitations in physical functioning in patients after cardiac surgery and in those with cardiac disease

The causes of musculoskeletal problems post cardiac surgery may be the result of sternal retraction, positioning of the patient during the surgery (which lasts a number of hours), cannulation of the internal jugular vein and the relative devascularisation of the sternum due to harvesting of the internal mammary artery (El-Ansary *et al.*, 2000). Retracting the sternum involves the eversion of the upper ribs and this may be one explanation for pain in the anterior chest wall and thoracic joint dysfunction. The results of the alterations in the chest wall can be seen for at least 3 months post operatively, with pulmonary function demonstrating a restrictive pattern (Kristjansdottir *et al.*, 2004). After cardiac surgery involving a median sternotomy there may be limitation of movement in the shoulder girdle and upper back as well as pain over wound sites (LaPier and Schenk, 2002). The pain may be due to direct surgical trauma, and swollen and inflamed areas may lead to mid or lower cervical root irritation causing referred pain to the scapula or upper limb. Posture may also be affected and a flexed posture with forward head position may lead to shortening of some muscles and lengthening of others.

In post-thoracotomy or -sternotomy patients, passive movements of the shoulder joint may be limited as the patient may hold the upper limb immobile due to fear of pain. In the weeks following surgery the patient may be limited in forward bending or backward extension due to approximation of the incisional area or stretching of the area. Exercises prescribed need to considered in light of overall activity recommendations for patients and gradually increased. Despite current management aimed at regaining range of movement in the immediate post-operative period, a number of patients (approximately 30%) will develop musculoskeletal complications that affect comfort and/or function after cardiac surgery (Stiller *et al.*, 1997). Complications after harvesting the radial artery are rare other than persistent cutaneous paraesthesia in a small percentage of patients (Budillon *et al.*, 2003). In patients on long-term ventilation, restrictions in joint range may occur, and where possible, passive or assisted movements of the upper and lower limbs should be performed.

Cardiac rehabilitation is part of the overall management of patients post surgery and/or stenting, and in more recent years is prescribed for those with heart failure. In patients with heart failure there appear to be peripheral muscle changes with exercise training. Muscle mass and endurance are decreased in patients with heart failure, and on biopsy a decrease in type 1 fibres with an increase in type 11b fibres is seen (Sullivan *et al.*, 1988). Patients with heart failure have been found to have lower BMD than age-matched controls (Kenny *et al.*, 2006) and therefore interventions to increase physical activity are important in their management. Heart failure in elderly patients is often accompanied by other co-morbidities such as mus-

culoskeletal problems, cerebrovascular disease and respiratory disease, and such may influence function and activity (Lien *et al.*, 2002). The presence of osteoarthritis needs to be taken into account when rehabilitating these patients as heart failure may be exacerbated by the use of over-the-counter non-steroidal anti-inflammatory drugs (Page and Henry, 2000; Van der Wel *et al.*, 2007).

Heart failure is associated with changes in muscle mass, cellular structure, energy metabolism and blood flow. These are associated with decreased exercise capacity and are improved with exercise training (Warburton *et al.*, 2007).

Exercise management of musculoskeletal conditions in patients with cardiac disease

Cardiac rehabilitation has been defined as 'the sum of activity required to ensure cardiac patients the best possible physical, mental and social conditions so that they may by their own efforts regain as normal as possible a place in the community and lead a normal life' (WHO, 1993). Exercise is a major component of all phases of cardiac rehabilitation. It commences with walking in phase 1 and 2 and is increased to circuits in phase 3 in outpatient, exercise-based cardiac rehabilitation generally for 8–12 weeks. Patients are then expected to continue incorporating exercise into daily life (phase 4). The exercise components are aerobic-type activities and resistance training is generally reserved for low- to moderate-risk cardiac patients. Patients with cardiac disease may have other co-morbidities that may affect their ability to exercise.

In patients early post cardiac surgery, exercises need to be performed to prevent the risk of the patient developing a frozen shoulder (Tucker *et al.*, 1996). The scapula can be moved with the patient in side lying and active upper limb exercises encouraged. While Stiller *et al.* (1997) found that routine range of movement exercises did not lead to a change in the incidence of musculoskeletal problems at 8–10 weeks post operatively, upper limb and trunk exercises are advised to help anterior chest wall discomfort (El-Ansary *et al.*, 2000) and stretching exercises when the sternum is stable.

If a patient has osteoarthritis in any of the lower limb joints this will interfere with exercise performance. Therefore, the physiotherapist needs to address the limitations to movement including pain and may need to prescribe more non-weight-bearing exercise so that the patient may experience the benefits associated with exercise rehabilitation. Weight loss may also help in symptoms of osteoarthritis and facilitate exercise uptake.

Patients with heart failure have also been found to benefit from exercise rehabilitation and specifically muscle strengthening. A 12-week quadriceps resistance training programme in New York Heart Association (NYHA) class III patients led to improvements in muscle strength ($P < 0.01$), exercise capacity ($P < 0.01$), clinical status ($P < 0.01$) and quality of life ($P < 0.05$) (Jankowska *et al.*, 2008). The training programme was performed three times per week and consisted of resistance exercises of several exercise circuits of 10 repeated quadriceps resistance exercises. The weight lifted commenced at 35% of maximal weight. Bartlo (2007) analysed data from a number of trials on aerobic and strength training in subjects with congestive heart failure. Aerobic exercise was found to have a significant beneficial effect on dyspnoea, work capacity and ventricular function ($P < 0.01$) and strength training increased muscle strength ($P < 0.05$) and endurance ($P < 0.001$) and left ventricular function ($P < 0.01$).

In conclusion, while the exercise management of patients with cardiac or pulmonary disease focuses on increasing aerobic capacity it is important for the physiotherapist to recognise the limitations to exercise and pain, and limitation of movement that may result from musculoskeletal concerns.

References

Bartlo, P. (2007) Evidence-based application of aerobic and resistance training in patients with congestive heart failure. *Journal of Cardiopulmonary Rehabilitation and Prevention*, 27, 368–375.

British Thoracic Society Statement (2001) Pulmonary rehabilitation. *Thorax*, 56, 827–834.

Budillon, A.M., Nicolini, F., Agostinelli, A., Beghi, C., Pavesi, G., Fragnito, C., Busi, M. and Gherli, T. (2003) Complications after radial artery harvesting for coronary artery bypass grafting: our experience. *Surgery*, 133, 283–287.

Clark, C.J., Cochrane, L. and Mackay, E. (1996) Low intensity peripheral muscle conditioning improves exercise tolerance and breathlessness in COPD. *Respiratory Journal*, 9, 2590–2596.

Decramer, M., Lacquet, L.M., Fagard, R. and Rogiers, P. (1994) Corticosteroids contribute to muscle weakness in chronic airflow obstruction. *American Journal of Respiratory and Critical Care Medicine*, 150, 11–16.

Dillard, T.A., Piantadosi, S. and Rajagopal, K.R. (1989) Determinant of maximum exercise capacity inpatients with chronic airflow obstruction. *Chest*, 96, 267–271.

El-Ansary, D., Adams, R. and Ghandi, A. (2000) Musculoskeletal and neurological complications following coronary artery bypass graft surgery: A comparison between saphenous vein and internal mammary artery grafting. *Australian Journal of Physiotherapy*, 46, 19–25.

El, O., Gulbahar, S., Ceylan, E., Ergor, G., Sahin, E., Senocak, O., Oncel, S. and Cimrin, A. (2005) Bone mineral density in asthmatic patients using low dose inhaled glucocorticosteroids. *Journal of Investigational Allergology and Clinical Immunology*, 15, 57–62.

Enright, S., Chatham, K., Ionescu, A.A., Unnithan, V.B. and Shale, D.J. (2004) Inspiratory muscle training improves lung function and exercise capacity in adults with cystic fibrosis. *Chest*, 126, 405–411.

Enright, S., Unnithan, V.B., Heward, C., Withnall, L. and Davies, D.H. (2006) Effect of high-intensity inspiratory muscle training on lung volumes, diaphragm thickness, and exercise capacity in subjects who are healthy. *Physical Therapy*, 86, 345–354.

Efthimiou, J., Fleming, J., Gomes, C. and Spiro, S.G. (1988) The effect of supplementary oral nutrition in poorly nourished patients with chronic obstructive pulmonary disease. *American Review of Respiratory Diseases*, 137, 1075–1082.

Gan, W.Q., Man, S.F., Senthilselvan, A. and Sin, D.D. (2004) Association between chronic obstructive pulmonary disease and systemic inflammation: a systematic review and a meta-analysis. *Thorax*, 59, 574–580.

Global Strategy for the Diagnosis, Management and Prevention of COPD, Global Initiative for Chronic Obstructive Lung Disease (GOLD). (2007) Available at: www.goldcopd.org (accessed 2009).

Gormley, J. and Hussey, J. (2005) *Exercise Therapy: In Prevention and Treatment of Disease*. Blackwell, Oxford.

Gosselink, R., Troosters, T. and Decramer, M. (1996) Peripheral muscle weakness contributes to exercise limitation in COPD. *American Journal of Respiratory and Critical Care Medicine*, 153, 976–980.

Gosselink, R., Troosters, T. and Decramer, M. (2000) Distribution of muscle weakness in patients with stable chronic obstructive pulmonary disease. *Journal of Cardiopulmonary Rehabilitation*, 20, 353–360.

Guran, T., Turan, S., Karadag, B., Ersu, R., Karakoc, F., Bereket, A. and Dagli, E. (2008) Bone mineral density in children with non-cystic fibrosis bronchiectasis. *Respiration*, 75, 432–436.

Hardin, D.S., Arumugam, R., Seilheimer, D.K., LeBlanc, A. and Ellis, K.J. (2001) Normal bone mineral density in cystic fibrosis. *Archives of Disease in Childhood*, 84, 363–368.

Jankowska, E.A., Wegrzynowska, K., Superlak, M., Nowakowska, K., Lazorczyk, M., Biel, B., Kustrzycka-Kratochwil, D., Piotrowska, K., Banasiak, W., Wozniewski, M. and Ponikowski, P. (2008) The 12-week progressive quadriceps resistance training improves muscle strength, exercise capacity and quality of life in patients with stable chronic heart failure. *International Journal of Cardiology*, 130, 36–43.

Kenny, A.M., Boxer, R., Walsh, S., Hager, W.D. and Raisz, L.G. (2006) Femoral bone mineral density in patients with heart failure. *Osteoporosis International*, 17, 1420–1427.

Kristjansdottir, A., Ragnarsdottir, M., Hannesson, P., Beck, H.J. and Torfason, B. (2004) Respiratory movements are altered three months and one year following cardiac surgery. *Scandinavian Cardiovascular Journal*, 38, 98–103.

LaPier, T. and Schenk, R. (2002) Thoracic musculoskeletal considerations following open heart surgery. *Cardiopulmonary Physical Therapy*, 13, 16–20.

Lien, C.T.C., Gillespie, N.D., Struthers, A.D. and McMurdo, M.E.T. (2002) Heart failure in frail elderly patients: diagnostic difficulties, co-morbidities, polypharmacy and treatment dilemmas. *European Journal of Heart Failure*, 4, 91–98.

Mineo, T.C., Ambrogi, V., Mineo, D., Fabbri, A., Fabbrini, E., Massoud, R. (2005) Bone mineral density improvement after lung volume reduction surgery for severe emphysema. *Chest*, 127, 1960–1966.

Montes de Oca, M., Rassulo, J. and Celli, B.R. (1996) Respiratory muscle and cardiopulmonary function during exercise in very severe COPD. *American Journal of Respiratory and Critical Medicine*, 154, 1284–1289.

Page, J. and Henry, D. (2000) Consumption of NSAIDs and the development of congestive heart failure in elderly patients. *Archives of Internal Medicine*, 160, 777–784.

Ram, F.S.F., Wellington, S.R. and Barnes, N.C. (2008) Inspiratory muscle training for asthma. *Cochrane Database of Systematic Reviews*, 3, CD003792.

Ries, A.L. (1994) The importance of exercise in pulmonary rehabilitation. *Clinics in Chest Medicine* 15, 327–337.

Roussos, C.S., Fixley, M.S., Gross, D. and Macklem, P.T. (1976) Respiratory muscle fatigue in man at FRC and higher lung volumes. *Physiologist*, 19, 345–349.

Siebens, H. (1996). The role of exercise in the rehabilitation of patients with chronic obstructive pulmonary disease. *Physical Medicine and Rehabilitation Clinics of North America*, 7, 299–314.

Sin, D.D., Man, J.P. and Man, S.F. (2003) The risk of osteoporosis in Caucasian men and women with obstructive airways disease. *American Journal of Medicine*, 114, 10–14.

Stiller, K., McInnes, M., Huff, N. and Hall, B. (1997) Do exercises prevent musculoskeletal complications after cardiac surgery? *Physiotherapy Theory and Practice*, 13, 117–126.

Sullivan, M.J., Higginbotham, M.B. and Cobb, F.R. (1988) Exercise training in patients with severe left ventricular dysfunction. Hemodynamic and metabolic effects. *Circulation*, 78, 506–515.

Tobin, M.J. (1988) Respiratory muscles in disease. *Clinics in Chest Medicine*, 9, 263–286.

Troosters, T., Gosselink, R. and Decramer, M. (2001) Exercise training in COPD: how to distinguish responders from nonresponders. *Journal of Cardiopulmonary Rehabilitation*, 21, 10–17.

Tucker, B., Jenkins, S., Davies, K., McGann, R., Waddell, J., King, R., Kirby, V. and Lloyd, C. (1996) The physiotherapy management of patients undergoing coronary artery surgery: A questionnaire survey. *Australian Journal of Physiotherapy*, 42, 129–137.

Van der Wel, M.C., Jansen, R.W., Bakx, J.C., Bor, H.H., Olderikkert, M.G. and van Weel, C. (2007) Non-cardiovascular co-morbidity in elderly patients with heart failure outnumbers cardiovascular co-morbidity. *European Journal of Heart Failure*, 9, 709–715.

Van Vliet, M., Spruit, M.A., Verleden, G., Kasran, A., Van Herck, E., Pitta, F., Bouillon, R. and Decramer, M. (2005) Hypogonadism, quadriceps weakness, and exercise intolerance in chronic obstructive pulmonary disease. *American Journal of Respiratory and Critical Care Medicine*, 172, 1105–1111.

Warburton, D.E., Taylor, A., Bredin, S.S., Esch, B.T., Scott, J.M. and Haykowsky, M.J. (2007) Central haemodynamics and peripheral muscle function during exercise in patients with chronic heart failure. *Applied Physiology, Nutrition and Metabolism*, 32, 318–331.

World Health Organization. (1993) Rehabilitation after cardiovascular diseases, with special emphasis on developing countries. Report of a WHO Expert Committee. *World Health Organization Technical Report Series*, 831, 1–122.

Yende, S., Waterer, G.W., Tolley, E.A., Newman, A.B., Bauer, D.C., Taaffe, D.R., Jensen, R., Crapo, R., Rubin, S., Nevitt, M., Simonsick, E.M., Satterfield, S., Harris, T. and Kritchevsky, S.B. (2006) Inflammatory markers are associated with ventilatory limitation and muscle dysfunction in obstructive lung disease in well functioning elderly subjects. *Thorax*, 61, 10–16.

Musculoskeletal Disorders in Obesity

15

Grace O'Malley

Introduction

A positive relationship exists between musculoskeletal fitness and general health status. Previous research has demonstrated impairments of the musculoskeletal system in individuals who are overweight, and to date, it is unknown whether these impairments occur as a consequence of obesity or whether they independently impart an increased risk of weight gain. In the USA between 1988 and 2004 the level of functional impairment associated with obesity increased and a greater burden of disability may be seen in the obese population of the future (Alley and Chang, 2007). In adults, osteoarthritis is the condition best documented to be associated with obesity; however recent research describes other musculoskeletal disorders. Common disorders that may present to physiotherapists working with overweight and obese individuals include: disorders of the lower limb such as foot pain; osteoarthritis of the knee (Felson *et al.*, 1988); recurrent ankle injury (Timm *et al.*, 2005); low back pain (Leboeuf-Yde *et al.*, 2005) and slipped upper femoral epiphyses (Loder, 1996). Musculoskeletal disorders in the upper body of overweight individuals include: neck pain, headaches, rotator cuff ten-

donitis (Werner *et al.*, 2005), frozen shoulder, peripheral nerve entrapment (Descatha *et al.*, 2004) and diabetes-related disorders.

Pain and discomfort can act as barriers to physical activity, and physiotherapists and other health clinicians can help improve the health and functional independence of obese individuals by reducing pain and discomfort. The positive relationship between musculoskeletal fitness (MSF) and weight status is mediated by physical activity, as those individuals with high levels of physical activity are seen to have better musculoskeletal health (Huang and Malina, 2002). Physiotherapists have vast experience in the rehabilitation of individuals with multiple pathologies and are very often the key professionals to motivate change, improve attitude and build self-efficacy. As such, when an individual who is obese presents to a therapist with musculoskeletal complaints, efforts to improve the global health of the client should be made, and might furthermore, be considered not only ethical but also part of the duty of care.

In an effort to individualize the management of overweight and obesity, the physiotherapist must first be able to assess the degree of overweight, second examine the general physical condition of the individual and third, in agreement with the

Exercise Therapy in the Management of Musculoskeletal Disorders, First Edition. Edited by Fiona Wilson, John Gormley and Juliette Hussey.
© 2011 Blackwell Publishing Ltd

patient, define goal-oriented methods of improving the functional independence and quality of life of the client.

Musculoskeletal assessment

In assessing the general health of an overweight client, the physiotherapist should complete a global examination of musculoskeletal fitness. This examination should include measures for joint range of movement and muscle flexibility, muscle strength and endurance, standing balance, pain, posture and gait. Collecting accurate measures for joint range of movement can be a challenge due to the difficulty in identifying bony landmarks and as such, the use of functional measures may be more appropriate.

In addition to assessment of the musculoskeletal system, the physiotherapist should detail the client's medical history, the level of overweight with which the client presents and the level of both physical activity and sedentary pursuits in which the patient engages. Body composition can be assessed by measuring height, weight, waist circumference and by calculating the body mass index (BMI; weight (cm)/ height (kg)^2). Subjective measures of physical activity such as the Baeke Questionnaire, the International Physical Activity Questionnaire or a 7-day activity recall can be useful in clinical practice. Similarly, time spent in sedentary activity can be calculated by summing the number of hours spent using a computer, playing video games and watching television.

Furthermore, assessing cardio-respiratory fitness is useful to gain a greater understanding of the general fitness of the patient and can provide a reliable client-specific outcome measure. In many cases medical clearance may be required prior to testing cardio-respiratory fitness, however, measures such as a 10-m walk test, the 6-minute walk test or a shuttle test can used in appropriate clients. Regardless of the age of the client, a holistic assessment will enhance the therapist's understanding of the impairments associated with the client's health status, which will in turn, guide him/her on how best to reduce limitations to activity and enhance participation.

During a musculoskeletal examination, the therapist should be aware that palpation and provocative testing can be difficult to complete due to excess subcutaneous tissue and the inertia of the client's body segments. As such, the manual handling risk associated with certain tests should be considered.

Physical effects associated with obesity

Clinically, limitations of the physical system are easily observed in the overweight population and recently, research has begun to describe these. In addition, many overweight individuals will present with diabetes mellitus as a co-morbidity and this condition is independently associated with musculoskeletal symptoms.

Impaired joint range of movement and flexibility

Bony structure determines the primary degree of joint freedom of movement and is influenced by the extensibility of soft tissue structures. Range of movement parameters are commonly used in clinical practice and have been utilised as indicators and predictors of physical function (Koman *et al.*, 2000). Overweight and obese individuals may present with a reduction in joint range of motion (ROM). This may be due to increased subcutaneous adipose tissue blocking joint excursion, localised oedema, abnormal bony torsion or decreased muscle length. Regardless of the underlying cause, it can be assumed that limited joint ROM may lead to subsequent reductions in flexibility and suboptimal postural alignment. Reduced muscle flexibility is commonly associated with musculoskeletal conditions (Hertling and Kessler, 1996) and may predict the presence of musculoskeletal symptoms in adulthood (Mikkelsson *et al.*, 2006). Research suggests that those who are physically active have better muscle flexibility than those who are not (Huang and Malina, 2002).

Increased body weight has been shown to be inversely associated with lower limb range of motion and impaired hip ROM is described as a risk factor in recurrent non-specific low back pain (LBP) (Jones *et al.*, 2005). In a cyclical process, it is hypothesised that poor hip mobility increases spinal strain leading to LBP which, in turn can lead to reduced levels of physical activity, thus possibly increasing the BMI and subsequently increasing the strain on spinal structures.

Reduced ankle dorsiflexion ROM and the resultant equinus gait pattern has been observed to cause abnormal pronation of the subtalar joint, which may increase stress on the plantar fascia (Hill, 1995). Furthermore, both obesity and excessive subtalar pronation have been highlighted as risk factors for the development of chronic plantar heel pain and repetitive strain injuries (Irving *et al.*, 2007).

Tight quadriceps and hamstrings may increase compression of the patellofemoral joint, causing pain (Hertling and Kessler, 1996), and reduced hamstring and quadriceps length has been described in obese persons. Impaired hamstring length can affect pelvic tilt, drawing the pelvis posteriorly (Józwiak *et al.*, 1997). Thus, hamstring tightness may affect posture, gait and low back discomfort, and evidence suggests that impaired hamstring flexibility is a risk factor for LBP in both adults (Esola *et al.*, 1996) and adolescents (Salminen *et al.*, 1992; Sjolie, 2004).

Oedema

Many obese clients have underlying conditions that may induce joint and soft-tissue swelling. The therapist should be aware of conditions such as lymphoedema and lipidaemia (a disorder of abnormal fat deposition) to ensure appropriate management for affected patients. Lymph drainage requires intermittent changes in local pressure from exercise and movement and as such, sedentary overweight individuals may develop dermatological symptoms (Garcia, 2002). Lymphoedema results from accumulation of protein-rich lymph in tissues and is caused by inadequate lymph drainage. Conservative management is initially recommended, such as lymphatic massage therapy, limb mobility exercises, use of compression garments and limb elevation (Weston and Clay, 2007). The clinician should bear in mind that local tissue swelling post injury may be difficult to appreciate secondary to the large bulk of adipose tissue surrounding the joints.

Impaired balance and postural stability

Balance is described as the ability of the body to maintain a centre of gravity over its base of support with minimal sway and maximal steadiness. Factors that have been shown to influence balance include:

age (Colledge *et al.*, 1994), physical activity level (Hahn *et al.*, 1999), previous lower limb injury (Emery *et al.*, 2005) and height and weight (Odenrick and Sandstedt, 1984). Balance may be reduced in overweight clients due to muscle weakness, limited range of movement and low levels of physical activity. Research has shown that increased body weight is correlated with an anterior displacement of the centre of mass, which places obese individuals closer to their boundaries of stability and at greater risk of falling when exposed to daily postural stress (Hue *et al.*, 2007). Weight loss in the obese cohort has proven to incur significant improvements in balance capabilities (Teasdale *et al.*, 2007).

Furthermore, limited joint range influences standing balance (Lowes *et al.*, 2004). Reduced knee and ankle range of movement can increase postural sway (Potter *et al.*, 1990) and also impede the implementation of the ankle strategy for postural adjustment (Mecagni *et al.*, 2000). Reductions in joint range of movement can also affect standing balance through the alteration of muscle length/tension curves, leading to inefficient gait and stance (Damiano *et al.*, 2001).

Appropriate measures of balance should be chosen depending on the patient's age and general physical condition. Standardised tests such as the Berg balance scale, the timed up and go and timed single leg stance tests are useful; however, at all times the clinician should use the tests with caution, particularly if the client is morbidly obese or has a significant fear of falling.

Reduced muscle and bone strength

Muscle strength is an integral part of physical fitness and relates to the ability of a muscle to generate force at a given speed. Inadequate muscular strength can predispose individuals to an increased risk of musculoskeletal fatigue and injury (Riddiford-Harland *et al.*, 2006). Impaired muscle strength is commonly due to advanced ageing, systemic illness, degenerative disease, injury and obesity (Miyatake *et al.*, 2000). A positive relationship exists between muscle strength and physical activity (Neder *et al.*, 1999) and a negative relationship has been observed between strength and obesity (Riddiford-Harland *et al.*, 2006).

It is thought that in overweight individuals, the dampening and decelerating capability of lower limb musculature is impaired secondary to muscle weakness and the resistance offered by the body's weight, thus increasing the rate of joint loading (Mikesky *et al.*, 2000). Functional tasks such as rising from a chair have been shown to be adversely affected by obesity (Riddiford-Harland *et al.*, 2006). In addition, weakness of muscles such as the gluteals and posterior tibialis (which eccentrically control loading during the stance phase of gait) may also lead to hyperpronation and associated injury (Cornwall and McPoil, 2000). In order to improve postural muscle co-ordination and enhance balance capacity, strengthening of ankle dorsiflexors, ankle plantar flexors and both hip and knee extensors should be encouraged (Lowes *et al.*, 2004).

It is uncertain to date as to what role reduced muscle strength plays in the development of musculoskeletal impairments. It is clear, however, that reduced muscle strength in children impairs the development of bone strength, and that inadequate bone strength at the peak growth stage may increase the risk of sustaining fractures (Goulding *et al.*, 2000b). Strong developing muscle has a positive effect on the accrual of bone mass both in puberty and in adolescence (Gustavsson *et al.*, 2003). Engaging in physical exercise incurs loading forces upon bone by exercising muscle, which in turn, increases bone mineral content and density.

In the physically active obese child, greater body mass requires larger muscle force to move the body in space and as such will lead to greater bone strength (Slemenda *et al.*, 1997). However, inactive obese children with weaker muscles can have a reduction in bone strength and thus may become osteopenic, increasing the risk of fracture. In addition, studies of inactive overweight children have suggested that high BMI, adiposity and associated low bone density increase the risk of fracture when members of this group sustain a traumatic fall (Goulding *et al.*, 1998, 2000a; Molgaard *et al.*, 1998).

In the morbidly obese, it is evident that there is bone loss and increased skeletal fragility following weight loss. More significant increases in bone fragility are seen where weight is lost during a relatively short period of time, such as 3–4 months (Van Loan *et al.*, 1998; Fogelholm *et al.*, 2001), whereas moderate weight loss over a longer period (6 months) results in little or no bone loss (Ramsdale and Bassey, 1994; Shapses *et al.*, 2001). Similarly,

dramatic weight loss such as that induced by the roux-en-Y gastric bypass and gastric banding is also associated with significant bone resorption and loss (Berarducci, 2007; Carrasco *et al.*, 2009). Efforts should be made to ensure that weight loss interventions aim to minimise bone loss by including aerobic and resistance-training protocols.

Finally, particular attention should be given to weight loss initiatives targeting elderly people, as the health benefits of weight loss in this cohort are uncertain. Weight loss in this cohort may accelerate the loss of muscle mass which, correlates negatively with functional capacity for independent living. The co-existence of reduced lean mass and increased fat mass is defined by 'sarcopenic obesity', and characterises a group of individuals with high risk of functional impairment (Miller and Wolfe, 2008).

Altered biomechanics and gait

In adults, links have been made between obesity and musculoskeletal conditions such as osteoarthritis and chronic back pain (Visscher and Seidell, 2001). Knee osteoarthritis is more common in overweight individuals, especially women, with external knee adduction moments cited as the most important load factors in generating articular injury (Hurwitz *et al.*, 1998; Sharma *et al.*, 1998). A recent study investigating risk factors for lumbar disc degeneration found that there was a strong association (95% CI 1.3 to 14.3) between disc degeneration at follow-up and persistent overweight, classified as BMI ≥25 kg/m² at age 25 and 40–45 years (Liuke *et al.*, 2005). A causal link between obesity and low back pain is yet to be described, as epidemiological studies report contradictory results (Leboeuf-Yde *et al.*, 2005; Lee *et al.*, 2005).

Recent work has described greater ground reaction forces and knee-joint loading in those who are obese compared with those who are not (Browning and Kram, 2007). Furthermore, Messier *et al.* (2005) reported that for every pound of weight lost, there is resultant four-fold reduction in the load exerted on the knee for each step taking during daily activities.

Regarding gait, individuals who are obese may present with a shorter stride length and slower cadence, and spend more time in stance phase and double support in walking (Lai *et al.*, 2008). It is possible that individuals who are obese may adjust the characteristics of their gait (such as walking speed) in order to reduce ground reaction forces and moments about the knee joint. This point should be considered when prescribing walking to clients, as the cardiovascular benefits derived from walking at brisk speeds may be attenuated by the slower speeds required to avoid musculoskeletal discomfort. As such, if a cardiovascular benefit is not anticipated from the self-selected natural walking speed of the client, non-weight-bearing activities may be more appropriate, particularly in the management of severely obese clients. Few authors have investigated the effect of obesity on gait but preliminary results (Gushue *et al.*, 2005) propose that overweight children have altered knee joint kinematics during walking due to higher peak knee adduction moments (73–100% higher than normal weight children). The authors propose that gait adaptation may increase medial compartment loading of the lower limbs, and contribute to the development of varus/valgus deformities and osteoarthritic wear and tear.

Musculoskeletal pain

Cross-sectional investigation reports that those who are obese are more likely to report musculoskeletal pain and that the severity of pain reported increases with the level of obesity (Hitt *et al.*, 2007). The most commonly reported sites of pain include the back, the feet and the knees (Shiri *et al.*, 2008; Stovitz *et al.*, 2008) and individuals with a BMI >35 have been shown to be at a greater risk of pain (Rohrer *et al.*, 2008). Tukker *et al.* (2008) reported a dose response relationship between the degree of overweight and the presence of osteoarthritis, pain and disability. These authors also reported that approximately 25% of health problems of the lower limb were attributable to overweight and obesity. It would be prudent for therapists working with those who are obese, to investigate the presence of pain and discomfort and to determine where possible, the underlying cause for these complaints in order to establish an optimal treatment plan. In addition, it is recommended that pain be addressed as it is cited as a barrier to the physical activity required for health enhancement (Mauro *et al.*, 2008).

Diabetes mellitus

Diabetes mellitus is a chronic metabolic condition with associated microvascular and macrovascular complications. Physical activity is recommended as a cornerstone in the management of diabetes mellitus and can both aid glycaemic control and decrease the risk of diabetic complications. Diabetic individuals have a greater incidence of musculoskeletal conditions such as reflex sympathetic dystrophy/chronic regional pain syndrome type 1, frozen shoulder, limited small-joint (hands and feet) mobility, Dupuytren's contractures, carpal tunnel syndrome, flexor tenosynovitis, neuropathic joints (Charcot's), diabetic amyotrophy and diffuse idiopathic skeletal hyperostosis (Smith *et al.*, 2003). When treating this cohort the therapist should advise and educate on correct footwear and appropriate management of blisters. In some cases, the use of silica gel or air mid-soles may be indicated in an effort to protect feet and prevent blisters. During the rehabilitative phase of musculoskeletal conditions, the patient should be advised to avoid Valsalva-like manoeuvres due to the risk of vitreous haemorrhage. Similarly, the therapist should work closely with patients in whom physical activity is prescribed to avoid hypoglycaemic episodes and to ensure that any exercise undertaken is well planned and safe.

Limitations in rehabilitation of the obese patient

The main aim of intervention should be to improve the general function of the client. However, the obese client may present with factors that may limit the effectiveness of a therapeutic approach. The client may be restricted by a plethora of both intrinsic and extrinsic barriers depending on his/her age and such barriers should be considered prior to and throughout treatment. Adequate attention should be given to the importance of goal setting and motivational techniques to optimise treatment.

Extrinsic barriers to the rehabilitation of musculoskeletal complaints in individuals who are obese include: a lack of time; a lack of information; a lack of support by employers and or family members (particularly parents, where paediatric clients are concerned); lower socio-economic status; previously failed attempts to manage musculoskeletal and general health, and a lack of safe access to recreational areas to increase physical activity. In addition to these, therapists should also be aware of 'weight bias', which many individuals are subjected to both in the community at large and in their interaction with health professionals (Schwartz *et al.*, 2003). In order to engage with the client positively, gain his or her trust and work towards agreed goals for treatment, it may be necessary for the therapist to reflect on their own view of the obese client and to consider any prejudices that may negatively affect the client–therapist interaction.

Intrinsic barriers to effective holistic management of clients who are obese may include additional physical and psychological co-morbidities. Patients with cardiovascular complications may be fearful of exercises that challenge their cardiorespiratory capacity. Individuals with low levels of physical activity may be physically deconditioned and may have poor motor control and co-ordination. Such clients may require a gradual increase in the intensity and frequency of therapeutic exercise. Clients may have a fear of falling or may be embarrassed to participate in tests or treatment procedures, which induce perspiration and breathlessness. Clients may have physical impairments such as those described above and as such, therapeutic exercise should address these. Of great importance is the consideration that should be given to choosing between weight-bearing and non-weight-bearing therapeutic activities. Severely obese patients may benefit from first working in non-weight-bearing positions in order to minimise discomfort and anxiety. Following orthopaedic procedures, a risk-benefit analysis should be made regarding the advantages and disadvantages of various assistive devices. The safety of the client should always be paramount but where possible the use of wheelchairs should be avoided in an effort to maintain energy expenditure during the rehabilitation period. Similarly, the therapist must ensure that all assistive equipment prescribed is safe to use for bariatric clients with high body weights. In the case of elective orthopaedic procedures, the benefit of prehabilitation should not be underestimated as clients may find the post operative period easier to cope with, having been well prepared in advance of surgery.

Finally, certain manual therapy techniques may not be appropriate, given the inertia of the client's body segments and may pose a manual handling risk. In such cases, alternative treatment procedures may need to be considered such as the use of belts or hydrotherapy for manual therapy treatments.

Rehabilitation exercises for the overweight client

In order to rehabilitate a client who is overweight, certain modifications to therapeutic exercises may be necessary. Modifications may prove to be safer to the client and may reduce the manual handling risk to the therapist. The therapist should be aware of any assistance the client may require in getting down to the floor and may need to recommend the use of a chair/bench to aid a safe transition. Such transitions should be practised with therapist supervision until the client is confident and safe.

Figure 15.1a illustrates a modified quadriceps stretch whereby the client gets into a kneeling position (using a chair for assistance if needed) and then with ankles and knees together begins to gradually sit back on the heels with the ankles in plantar flexion (Fig. 15.1b). The client may use his or her upper limbs to ease into this position and should be encouraged to press the knees into the floor.

Figure 15.2a depicts the starting position for a seated hamstring stretch whereby the client sits with his or her back flat against a wall, the knees extended, the upper limbs outstretched with the scapulae set against the rib cage and the toes pointing to the ceiling. The client is instructed to bend forward at the pelvis to the point that he or she feels the hamstrings stretch and should keep the back and knees straight at all times (Fig. 15.2b).

Figure 15.3 illustrates a modified calf stretch whereby the client leans into a wall with the toes pointing forward and flexing forward on the front leg. The forefoot is prevented from rolling in by placing the edge of a book under the first metatarsal and the calf of the back leg is stretched by keeping the knee straight throughout the stretch.

Figure 15.4 illustrates a modified adductor stretch whereby the client sits with his or her back against the wall with the hips in 90° flexion. The client then flexes the knee and externally rotates the hip by placing the foot against the inner aspect of

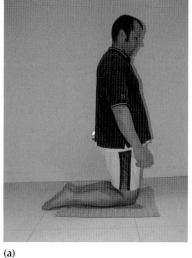
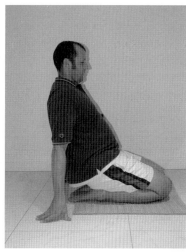

Figure 15.1 (**a**) A modified quadriceps stretch whereby the client gets into a kneeling position. (**b**) With ankles and knees together begins to gradually sit back on the heels with the ankles in plantar flexion.

(a)

(b)

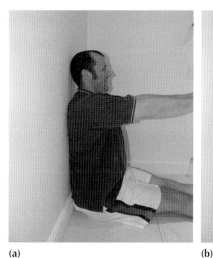
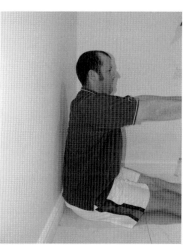

Figure 15.2 (**a**) The starting position for a seated hamstring stretch. (**b**) The client is instructed to bend forward at the pelvis to the point that he or she feels the hamstrings stretch and should keep the back and knees straight at all times.

(a)

(b)

the opposite thigh. The adductors are stretched by gently leaning and pushing the knee down to the floor.

Core stability work can aid in the management of back pain in this client cohort. Core stability training should commence with effective contractions of the abdominal wall and the therapist should be aware that excess abdominal tissue may make palpating the contractions difficult. The therapist might choose to use easy to understand instructions in order to stimulate contractions. Such instructions might include asking the client to concentrate on

preventing him or herself from going to the toilet by contracting the pelvic floor musculature. These exercises can then be progressed by contracting the abdominals while maintaining a balanced posture sitting on a ball (Fig. 15.5), while kneeling on a pillow (Fig. 15.6) and by getting into a modified four-point position (Fig. 15.7) and slowly extending one of the hips (Fig. 15.8).

Balance exercises can be used to improve postural stability and might include: toe walking; heel walking; single leg standing with the eyes open and closed; double leg standing; and single leg standing

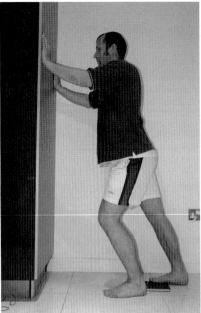

Figure 15.3   A modified calf stretch.

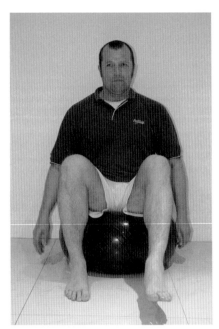

Figure 15.5   Contracting abdominals while maintaining a balanced posture sitting on a ball.

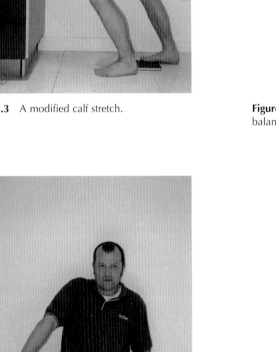

Figure 15.4   A modified adductor stretch.

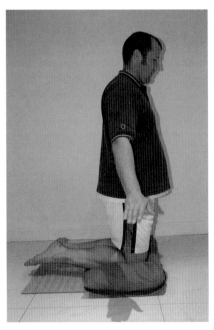

Figure 15.6   Contracting abdominals while maintaining a balanced posture while kneeling on a pillow.

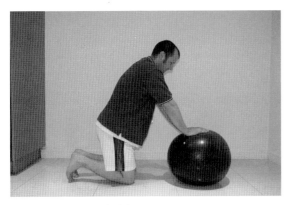

Figure 15.7 A modified four-point position.

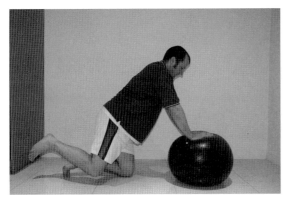

Figure 15.8 A modified four-point position and slowly extending one of the hips.

on a cushion or pillow with the eyes open and closed (Fig. 15.9).

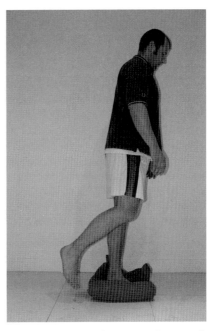

Figure 15.9 Single leg standing on a cushion or pillow with the eyes open and closed.

References

Alley, D.E. and Chang, V.W. (2007) The changing relationship of obesity and disability, 1988–2004. *Journal of the American Medical Association*, 298, 2020–2027.

Berarducci, A. (2007) Bone loss. An emerging problem following obesity surgery. *Orthopaedic Nursing*, 26, 281–286; quiz 287–288.

Browning, R.C. and Kram, R. (2007) Effects of obesity on the biomechanics of walking at different speeds. *Medicine and Science in Sports and Exercise*, 39, 1632–1641.

Carrasco, F., Ruz, M., Rojas, P., Csendes, A., Rebolledo, A., Codoceo, J., Inostroza, J., Basfi-fer, K., Papapietro, K., Rojas, J., Pizzaro, F. and Olivares, M. (2009) Changes in bone mineral density, body composition and adiponectin levels in morbidly obese patients after bariatric surgery. *Obesity Surgery*, 19, 41–46.

Colledge, N.R., Cantley, P., Peaston, I., Brash, H., Lewis, S. and Wilson, J.A. (1994) Ageing and balance: the measurement of spontaneous sway by posturography. *Gerontology*, 40, 273–278.

Cornwall, M.W. and McPoil, T.G. (2000) Velocity of centre of pressure during walking. *Journal of the American Podiatric Medical Association*, 90, 334–338.

Damiano, D.L., Quinlivan, J., Owen, B.F., Shaffery, M. and Abel, M.F. (2001) Spasticity versus strength in cerebral palsy: relationships among involuntary resistance, voluntary torque, and motor function. *European Journal of Neurology*, 8 (Suppl. 5), S40–S49.

Descatha, A., Leclerc, A., Chastang, J.F. and Roquelaure, Y. (2004) Incidence of ulnar nerve entrapment at the elbow in repetitive work. *Scandinavian Journal of Work, Environment and Health*, 30, 234–240.

Emery, C.A., Cassidy, J.D., Klassen, T.P., Rosychuck, R.J. and Rowe, B.B. (2005) Development of a clinical static and dynamic standing balance measurement tool appropriate for use in adolescents. *Physical Therapy*, 85, 502–514.

Esola, M.A., McClure, P.W., Fitzgerald, G.K. and Siegler, S. (1996) Analysis of lumbar spine and hip motion during forward bending in subjects with and without a history of low back pain. *Spine*, 21, 71–78.

Felson, D.T., Anderson, J.J., Naimark, A., Walker, A.M. and Meenan, R.F. (1988) Obesity and knee osteoarthritis. The Framingham Study. *Annals of Internal Medicine*, 109, 18–24

Fogelholm, G.M., Sievanen, H.T., Kukkonen-Harjula, T.K. and Pasanen, M.E. (2001) Bone mineral density during reduction, maintenance and regain of body weight in premenopausal, obese women. *Osteoporosis International*, 12, 199–206.

Garcia, H.L. (2002) Dermatological complications of obesity. *American Journal of Clinical Dermatology*, 3, 497–506.

Goulding, A., Cannan, R., Williams, S.M., Gold, E.J., Taylor, R.W. and Lewis-Barned, N.J. (1998) Bone mineral density in girls with forearm fractures. *Journal of Bone and Mineral Research*, 13, 143–148.

Goulding, A., Jones, I.E., Taylor, R.W., Manning, P.J. and Williams, S.M. (2000a) More broken bones: a 4-year double cohort study of young girls with and without distal forearm fractures. *Journal of Bone and Mineral Research*, 15, 2011–2018.

Goulding, A., Taylor, R.W., Jones, I.E., McCauley, K.A., Manning, P.J. and Williams, S.M. (2000b) Overweight and obese children have low bone mass and area for their weight. *International Journal of Obesity and Related Metabolic Disorders*, 24, 627–632.

Gushue, D.L., Houck, J. and Lerner, A.L. (2005) Effects of childhood obesity on three-dimensional knee joint biomechanics during walking. *Journal of Pediatric Orthopedics*, 25, 763–768.

Gustavsson, A., Thornsen, K. and Nordstrom, P. (2003) A 3-year longitudinal study of the effect of physical activity on the accrual of bone mineral density in healthy adolescent males. *Calcified Tissue International*, 73, 108–114.

Hahn, T., Foldspang, A., Vestergaard, E. and Ingmann-Hansen, T. (1999) One leg standing balance and sports activity. *Scandinavian Journal of Medicine and Science in Sports*, 9, 15–18.

Hertling, D. and Kessler, R.M. (1996) *Management of Common Musculoskeletal Disorders: Physical Therapy Principles and Methods*. Lippincott-Raven, Philadelphia, Pennsylvania.

Hill, R.S. (1995) Ankle equinus. Prevalence and linkage to common foot pathology. *Journal of the American Podiatric Medical Association*, 85, 295–300.

Hitt, H.C., McMillen, R.C., Thonthon-Neaves, T., Koch, K. and Cosby, A. G. (2007) Comorbidity of obesity and pain in a general population: results from the Southern Pain Prevalence Study. *Journal of Pain*, 8, 430–436.

Huang, Y.C. and Malina, R.M. (2002) Physical activity and health-related physical fitness in Taiwanese adolescents. *Journal of Physiological Anthropology and Applied Human Science*, 21, 11–19.

Hue, O., Simoneau, M., Marcotte, J., Berrigan, F., Dore, J., Marceau, P., Marceau, S., Tremblay, A. and Teasdale, N. (2007) Body weight is a strong predictor of postural stability. *Gait Posture*, 26, 32–38.

Hurwitz, D.E., Sumner, D.R., Andriacchi, T.P. and Sugar, D.A. (1998) Dynamic knee loads during gait predict proximal tibial bone distribution. *Journal of Biomechanics*, 31, 423–430.

Irving, D.B., Cook, J.L., Young, M.A. and Menz, H.B. (2007) Obesity and pronated foot type may increase the risk of chronic plantar heel pain: a matched case-control study. *BMC Musculoskeletal Disorders*, 8, 41.

Jones, M.A., Stratton, G., Reilly, T. and Unnithan, V.B. (2005) Biological risk indicators for recurrent non-specific low back pain in adolescents. *British Journal of Sports Medicine*, 39, 137–140.

Józwiak, M., Pietrzak, S. and Tobjasz, F. (1997) The epidemiology and clinical manifestations of hamstring muscle and plantar foot flexor shortening. *Developmental Medicine and Child Neurology*, 39, 481–483.

Koman, L.A., Mooney, J.F., Smith, B.P., Walker, F. and Leon, J.M. (2000) Botulinum toxin type A neuromuscular blockade in the treatment of lower extremity spasticity in cerebral palsy: a randomized, double-blind, placebo-controlled trial. BOTOX Study Group. *Journal of Pediatric Orthopedics*, 20, 108–115.

Lai, P.P., Leung, A.K., Li, A.N. and Zhang, M. (2008) Three-dimensional gait analysis of obese adults. *Clinical Biomechanics*, 23 (Suppl. 1), S2–S6.

Leboeuf-Yde, C., Axen, I., Jones, J J., Rosenbaum, A., Lovgren, P.W., Halasz, L. and Larsen, K. (2005) The Nordic back pain subpopulation program: the long-term outcome pattern in patients with low back pain treated by chiropractors in Sweden. *Journal of Manipulative and Physiological Therapeutics*, 28, 472–478.

Lee, C.Y., Kratter, R., Duvoisin, N., Taskin, A. and Schilling, J. (2005) Cross-sectional view of factors associated with back pain. *International Archives of Occupational and Environmental Health*, 78, 319–324.

Liuke, M., Solovieva, S., Lamminen, A., Luoma, K., Leino-Arjas, P., Luukkonen, R. and Riihimaki, H. (2005) Disc degeneration of the lumbar spine in relation to overweight. *International Journal of Obesity*, 29, 903–908.

Loder, R.T. (1996) The demographics of slipped capital femoral epiphysis. An international multicenter study. *Clinical Orthopaedics and Related Research*, 322, 8–27.

Lowes, L.P., Westcott, S.L., Palisano, R.J., Effgen, S.K. and Orlin, M.N. (2004) Muscle force and range of motion as predictors of standing balance in children with cerebral palsy. *Physical and Occupational Therapy in Pediatrics*, 24, 57–77.

Mauro, M., Taylor, V., Wharton, S. and Sharma, A.M. (2008) Barriers to obesity treatment. *European Journal of Internal Medicine*, 19, 173–180.

Mecagni, C., Smith, J.P., Roberts, K.E. and O'Sullivan, S.B. (2000) Balance and ankle range of motion in community-dwelling women aged 64 to 87 years: a correlational study. *Physical Therapy*, 80, 1004–1011.

Messier, S.P., Gutekunst, D.J., Davis, C. and Devita, P. (2005) Weight loss reduces knee-joint loads in overweight and obese older adults with knee osteoarthritis. *Arthritis and Rheumatism*, 52, 2026–2032.

Mikesky, A.E., Meyer, A. and Thompson, K.L. (2000) Relationship between quadriceps strength and rate of loading during gait in women. *Journal of Orthopaedic Research*, 18, 171–175.

Mikkelsson, L.O., Nupponen, H., Kaprio, J., Kautiainen, H., Mikkelsson, M. and Kujala, U.M. (2006) Adolescent flexibility, endurance strength, and physical activity as predictors of adult tension neck, low back pain, and knee injury: a 25 year follow up study. *British Journal of Sports Medicine*, 40, 107–113.

Miller, S.L. and Wolfe, R.R. (2008) The danger of weight loss in the elderly. *Journal of Nutrition, Health and Aging*, 12, 487–491.

Miyatake, N., Fujii, M., Nishikawa, H., Wada, J., Shikata, K., Makino, H. and Kimura, I. (2000) Clinical evaluation of muscle strength in 20–79-years-old obese Japanese. *Diabetes Research and Clinical Practice*, 48, 15–21.

Molgaard, C., Thomsen, B.L. and Michaelsen, K.F. (1998) Influence of weight, age and puberty on bone size and bone mineral content in healthy children and adolescents. *Acta Paediatrica*, 87, 494–499.

Neder, J.A., Nery, L.E., Shinzato, G.T., Andrade, M.S., Peres, C. and Silva, A.C. (1999) Reference values for concentric knee isokinetic strength and power in nonathletic men and women from 20 to 80 years old. *Journal of Orthopaedic and Sports Physical Therapy*, 29, 116–126.

Odenrick, P. and Sandstedt, P. (1984) Development of postural sway in the normal child. *Human Neurobiology*, 3, 241–244.

Potter, P.J., Kirby, R.L. and Macleod, D.A. (1990) The effects of simulated knee-flexion contractures on standing balance. *American Journal of Physical Medicine and Rehabilitation*, 69, 144–147.

Ramsdale, S.J. and Bassey, E.J. (1994) Changes in bone mineral density associated with dietary-induced loss of body mass in young women. *Clinical Science (Lond)*, 87, 343–348.

Riddiford-Harland, D.L., Steele, J.R. and Baur, L.A. (2006) Upper and lower limb functionality: are these compromised in obese children? *International Journal of Pediatric Obesity*, 1, 42–49.

Rohrer, J.E., Adamson, S.C., Barnes, D. and Herman, R. (2008) Obesity and general pain in patients utilizing family medicine: should pain standards call for referral of obese patients to weight management programs? *Quality Management in Health Care*, 17, 204–209.

Salminen, J.J., Maki, P., Oksanen, A. and Pentti, J. (1992) Spinal mobility and trunk muscle strength in 15-year-old schoolchildren with and without low-back pain. *Spine*, 17, 405–411.

Schwartz, M.B., Chambliss, H.O., Brownell, K.D., Blair, S.N. and Billington, C. (2003) Weight bias among health professionals specializing in obesity. *Obesity Research*, 11, 1033–1039.

Shapses, S.A., Von Thun, N.L., Heymsfield, S.B., Ricci, T.A., Ospina, M., Pierson, R.N. and Stahl, T. (2001) Bone turnover and density in obese premenopausal women during moderate weight loss and calcium supplementation. *Journal of Bone and Mineral Research*, 16, 1329–1336.

Sharma, L., Hurwitz, D.E., Thunar, E.J., Sum, J.A., Lenz, M.E., Dunlop, D.D., Schnitzer, T.J., Kirwin-Mellis, G. and Andriacchi, T.P. (1998) Knee adduction moment, serum hyaluronan level, and disease severity in medial tibiofemoral osteoarthritis. *Arthritis and Rheumatism*, 41, 1233–1240.

Shiri, R., Soloviena, S., Husgafvel-Pursiainen, K., Taimela, S., Saarikoski, L.A., Huupponen, R., Viikari, J., Raitakari, O.T. and Viikari-Junutra, E. (2008) The association between obesity and the prevalence of low back pain in young adults: the Cardiovascular Risk in Young Finns Study. *American Journal of Epidemiology*, 167, 1110–1119.

Sjolie, A.N. (2004) Low-back pain in adolescents is associated with poor hip mobility and high body mass index. *Scandinavian Journal of Medicine and Science in Sports*, 14, 168–175.

Slemenda, C., Brandt, K.D., Heilman, D.K., Mazzuca, S., Braunstein, E.M., Katz, B.P. and Wolinsky, F.D. (1997) Quadriceps weakness and osteoarthritis of the knee. *Annals of Internal Medicine*, 127, 97–104.

Smith, L.L., Burnet, S.P. and McNeil, J.D. (2003) Musculoskeletal manifestations of diabetes mellitus. *British Journal of Sports Medicine*, 37, 30–35.

Stovitz, S.D., Pardee, P.E., Vazquez, G., Duval, S. and Schwimmer, J.B. (2008) Musculoskeletal pain in obese children and adolescents. *Acta Paediatrica*, 97, 489–493.

Teasdale, N., Hue, O., Marcotte, J., Berrigan, F., Simoneau, M., Dore, J., Marceau, P., Marceau, S. and Tremblay, A. (2007) Reducing weight increases postural stability in obese and morbid obese men. *International Journal of Obesity (Lond)*, 31, 153–160.

Timm, N.L., Grupp-Phelan, J. and Ho, M.L. (2005) Chronic ankle morbidity in obese children following an acute ankle injury. *Archives of Pediatric and Adolescent Medicine*, 159, 33–36.

Tukker, A., Visscher, T. and Picavet, H. (2008) Overweight and health problems of the lower extremities: osteoarthritis, pain and disability. *Public Health Nutrition*, 1–10.

Van Loan, M.D., Johnson, H.L. and Barbieri, T.F. (1998) Effect of weight loss on bone mineral content and bone density in obese women. *American Journal of Clinical Nutrition*, 67, 734–738.

Visscher, T.L. and Seidell, J.C. (2001) The public health impact of obesity. *Annual Review of Public Health*, 22, 355–375.

Werner, C.M., Steinmann, P.A., Gilbart, M. and Gerber, C. (2005) Treatment of painful pseudoparesis due to irreparable rotator cuff dysfunction with the Delta III reverse ball and socket total shoulder prosthesis. *Journal of Bone and Joint Surgery, American Volume*, 87, 1476–1486.

Weston, S. and Clay, C.D. (2007) Unusual case of lymphoedema in a morbidly obese patient. *Australasian Journal of Dermatology*, 48, 115–119.

16 Osteoporosis

Nicholas J. Mahony

Introduction

Evolution has optimised bone structure, shape and mass to reflects its various functions: mechanical support and leverage for the musculoskeletal system; protection of vital organ systems; mineral storage and homeostasis; and within the marrow, lipid storage and haematopoiesis (Currey, 2003). Osteoporosis is one of the most significant bone disorders the therapist will encounter in modern practice. Diagnosis of osteoporosis is based on the combination of clinical risk factor assessment and bone mineral density measurement by a special low-dose X-ray technique (dual energy X-ray absorptiometry (DXA)). Treatment of established osteoporosis is complex, and has three main aspects: adequate nutrition, appropriate drug therapy and mechanical loading through exercise.

Exercise plays a role in preventive strategies in childhood and adolescence, maintenance of bone mass through adult years and interventions to slow age-related bone loss in later life. In addition exercise programs can be used to correct posture, improve balance, increase strength and co-ordination, with an overall effect to reduce falls. The therapist should take note that exercise without attention to diet or without appropriate drug therapy may be ineffective, those who over-exercise can develop osteoporosis, and finally that in severe osteoporosis certain types of exercise are dangerous and cannot be recommended.

Bone structure

The skeleton comprises some 206 individual bones adapted in shape and size for functions of protection, weight-bearing and movement. Bones consist of a dense outer cortical shell and a more porous inner trabecular network of struts and plates. The ratio of cortical to trabecular bone varies in different parts of the skeleton. Long bones such as the humerus and femur are over 75% cortical bone whereas vertebrae consist of up to 75% trabecular bone; and external and internal structure can be adapted at different sites in the skeleton according to the local mechanical function and loading that has to be endured (Currey, 2003).

Trabecular bone is light, only 15–25% of volume is calcified tissue the remainder being occupied by bone marrow, blood vessels and connective tissue. The large trabecular bone surface area provides

Exercise Therapy in the Management of Musculoskeletal Disorders, First Edition. Edited by Fiona Wilson, John Gormley and Juliette Hussey.
© 2011 Blackwell Publishing Ltd

70–85% of the interface between the skeleton and soft tissues for cellular metabolic activities (Keaveny and Yeh, 2002). In the proximal and distal ends of long bones trabeculae effectively redistribute forces and bending moments to the cortical shell of the mid-shaft. In vertebral bodies, trabeculae distribute axial compressive forces throughout the entire network. The type of cellular structure formed, as well as thickness and connectivity of the struts and plates are key determinants of trabecular bone strength (Gibson and Ashby, 1997).

Cortical bone in contrast has a more solid form, making it highly resistant to bending and twisting forces and able to withstand very high loads (usually only in one predominant direction). Sudden loads applied in unusual directions can lead to fracture (Martin and Burr, 1989). The mass of bone making up the cortical shell and the distance of the cortical shell mass away from the neutral axis determine the cortical bone strength; or more simply, the strength of cortical bone is determined by both bone quantity, amount of mineralisation, and by geometrical properties of shape and structure (Frost, 1997). Osteoporosis affects both cortical and trabecular bone but trabecular bone is affected to a much greater degree due to its higher surface area for unbalanced remodelling. Sites in the skeleton with a high proportion of trabecular bone such as the distal radius, the proximal femur and the vertebrae are therefore more prone to the effects of osteoporosis.

Bone ultra-structure

At an ultra-structural level both cortical and trabecular bone are made up of layers or lamellae. Within lamellae, collagen fibres are aligned along the lines of the predominant stresses encountered during everyday activity, and this accounts for bone's anisotropic properties (Turner *et al.*, 1995). In trabecular bone, two to three lamellae form the interconnected rods and plates. In cortical bone, two to three sheets of circumferential lamellae make up outer smooth surfaces; deep to this are the osteons or 'Haversian' systems, three to five layers of concentrically arranged lamellae with central canals containing blood vessels and nerves. Interstitial lamellae, consisting of partially remodelled osteons, fill in gaps between the osteons and circumferential layers (Khan *et al.*, 2001).

Bone matrix

Bone matrix comprises an organic phase (20–25%), a mineral phase (70%), and a small amount (5%) of water (Sommerfeldt and Rubin, 2001). The organic phase conveys strength, flexibility and toughness and is mainly type I collagen fibres, non-collagenous proteins, proteoglycans, glycoprotein, osteocalcin and osteonectin. The mineral phase consists of crystals of calcium phosphate hydroxides, known as hydroxyapatite, which gives bone its hardness and stiffness. When formed *ex vivo*, the non-organic crystalline structure of these components is brittle but when combined with the organic phase the resultant composite material has a much greater hardness, strength and resilience to load (Khan *et al.*, 2001). Smaller breakdown products of collagen, osteocalcin and osteonectin, can be measured in the blood and thus are useful as clinical markers of bone turnover.

Bone surfaces

All bone surfaces, both inner and outer, are covered with bone-lining cells in a thin continuous layer (Currey, 2003). The outer lining membrane, the periosteum, also has fibrous and vascular layers. The inner lining layer on trabecular bone surfaces and lining channels for blood vessels is known as the endosteum. A single layer of osteoprogenitor cells is found here and it represents the primary source of cells for new bone formation during modelling, remodelling and repair.

Bone cells

Bone cells are derived from pluripotent stem cells of the bone marrow. Numerous factors influence differentiation, subsequent development and roles in bone modelling and remodelling. Bone cells are of three types, bone-resorbing cells (osteoclasts), bone-forming cells (osteoblasts) and the predominant cell type (osteocytes, >90%). The first two cell types are found on bone surfaces whereas osteocytes form a network within bone.

Osteoclasts

Osteoclasts are large, multinucleate cells derived from macrophage precursor cells in the blood, and

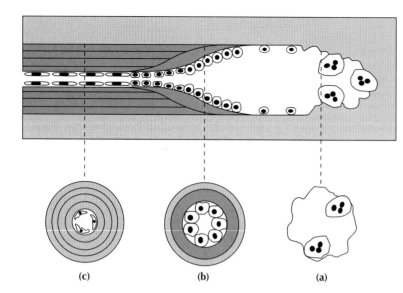

(c)   (b)   (a)

Figure 16.1 Cortical remodelling: (**a**) osteoclasts tunnelling a 'cutting cone' followed by smoothing in the reversal zone and (**b**) laying down of new concentric lamellae filling the cavity inwards to form (**c**) the Haversian canal and embedded osteocytes. (Adapted from Kanis, 1994, with permission from John Wiley & Sons Inc.)

have a resorptive function to remove bone matrix. Like macrophages, when signalled they have the capability to migrate into areas of damage for repair. Their ruffled borders attach to damaged bone surfaces in large lacunae on trabecular surfaces and in the cutting cones of basic remodelling units in cortical bone (Figs 16.1 and 16.2). They release enzymes, breaking down mineral and protein components of the matrix; acid secretions break collagen linkages with hydroxyapatite crystals, and collagenase and cathepsin further break down the protein elements. Activated osteoclasts can reabsorb bone at a rate of approximately $200\,000\,\mu m^3$ per day; which is far in excess of the maximum osteoid production and mineralisation rate of bone-forming osteoblasts.

Osteoblasts

Osteoblasts are mononuclear cells similar to fibroblasts, responsible for bone growth, repair and remodelling following osteoclastic resorption of damaged or older bone. They lie on inner trabecular bone surfaces and deep within osteons undergoing remodelling. Osteoblasts synthesise new bone matrix (osteoid) and then assist in mineralisation. They are activated by various growth factors, by micro-cracks in bone structure and by mechanical loading in a process called mechano-transduction. Their cell surfaces express many receptors; the predominant ones are parathyroid hormone (PTH),

oestrogen and 1,25-dihydroxy-vitamin D_3. However, glucocorticoid, growth and gonadal hormones also have effects on their function (Khan *et al.*, 2001). Osteoblasts lay down bone at the rate of approximately $0.5–1.5\,\mu m^3$ per day, and given their relatively short lifespan of several days it may take up to 10 generations of osteoblasts over several weeks to refill osteoclastic resorption cavities.

Osteocytes

Osteocytes are mature osteoblasts that have been enclosed within bone matrix during growth and remodelling. Embedded within bone, their fine cytoplasmic extensions form a communicating network via small channels (canaliculi) in the bone matrix with neighbouring osteocytes and cells lining surface layers (Khan *et al.*, 2001, Currey, 2003). Mechanical loading of bone has been shown to produce fluid shear stresses, which deform and in some cases damage this canalicular network. Damage and shear stress of the osteocyte network is purported to initiate and then modulate bone repair and remodelling mechanisms (Frost, 1987).

Bone development and ageing

The skeleton first appears as a cartilaginous template at 6 weeks of embryonic life; subsequent min-

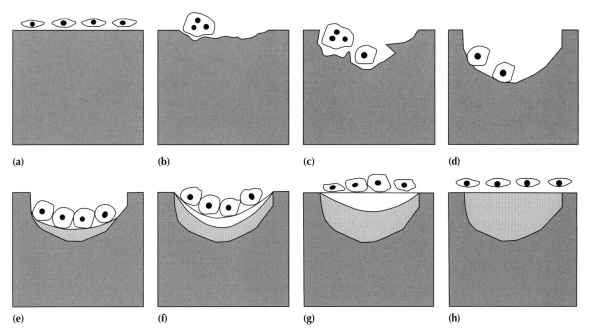

Figure 16.2 Trabecular remodelling: (**a**) resting phase; (**b**) osteoclast activation; (**c**) formation of resorption cavity; (**d**) smoothing by mono-nuclear cells (reversal); (**e**) differentiation of osteoblasts in erosion cavity (coupling); (**f**) matrix formation/mineralization; (**g**) complete matrix; and (**h**) lining progenitor cells cover new bone. (Adapted from Kanis, 1994, with permission from John Wiley & Sons Inc.)

eralisation and growth occurs for the next 25 years, and remodelling for the rest of adult life. Growth in width occurs through an appositional process of subperiosteal deposition and endosteal reabsorption, whereas longitudinal growth occurs at specialised cartilagenous growth centres – the epiphyses (Carter *et al.*, 1996). Bone mass as a whole increases at a rate of 7–8% during childhood and adolescence. Thereafter bone mass accrual occurs at a slower rate until late into the third decade. Then, after a period of mid life consolidation, in later years bone mass is lost due to age-related effects on remodelling (Forwood and Larson, 2000). The natural age-related loss of bone mass accelerates in females at the menopause due to declining oestrogen levels. In males there is a more gradual loss of bone with ageing in keeping with a slower decline in testosterone levels in the fifth decade. Figure 16.3 is a diagrammatic representation of age-related accrual, consolidation and loss of bone mass.

Achievement of peak bone mass at skeletal maturity is dependent on a variety of factors: genetics, levels of gonadal hormones, adequate nutrition, and exposure of the skeleton to mechanical stress.

Those genetically endowed with bones of greater width, thickness and of higher density due to accrual of greater bone mass during development have stronger bones and are less likely to have osteoporosis in later life.

Bone remodelling

Bone is a 'smart material' unlike inert materials such as concrete, because it possesses an adaptive mechanism which allows it to alter both its geometric (shape, length and width) and material properties (strength, stiffness and toughness) when exposed to varying mechanical stimuli. This process is called remodelling and is a dynamic biological balancing act of destruction and renewal, whereby approximately 10% of old bone is replaced by new bone each year. Normally remodelling activity is coupled so that no net bone loss occurs but with ageing the process becomes progressively unbalanced, ultimately leading to osteoporosis (Khan *et al.*, 2001).

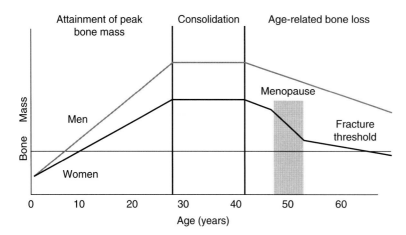

Figure 16.3 Age related changes in bone mass. (Adapted from Compston, 1990 with permission from John Wiley & Sons Inc.)

In cortical bone remodelling (Fig. 16.1), osteoclasts core out small tunnels or 'cutting cones' which move through bone at approximately 50 μm per day (Kanis, 1994). The space left by tunnelling osteoclasts, the resorption cavity, is then closed in layers by following osteoblasts, and as the layers of osteoid mineralise and new lamellae are formed, the osteoblasts become entrapped and become osteocytes. Successive lamellae are formed as osteoblasts add more and more layers in the 'closing cone' until the space is refilled, toward the central canal. The co-ordinated movement of the cutting and closing cones of the bone multicellular unit (BMU) through cortical bone has the effect to remove any small cracks within osteonal cortical structure which occur during normal everyday loading. In trabecular bone remodelling (Fig. 16.2) a similar process occurs on the surface of the struts and plates of trabecular bone. Firstly, osteoclasts gouge out old or damaged bone, and in reversal zones, the following osteoblasts fill in the grooves and indentations left behind.

In terms of localised structural adaptation, remodelling enables bone to adapt osteonal and trabecular structure to changes in directions and magnitude of predominating forces on the bone (Fig. 16.4). Resorption takes about 10 days and refilling with osteoid and mineralisation (reversal) can take 2–4 months (Currey, 2003). One of the short-term negative effects of remodelling is reduced bone mass, reduced trabecular thickness, reduced connectivity and ultimately decreased strength. In the normal healthy skeleton, however, this is soon

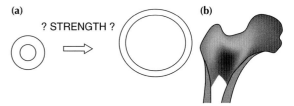

Figure 16.4 Bone adaptations to external stress through modelling/remodelling. (**a**) Change in distribution of bone material within the cortical collar results in increased cross-sectional moment of inertia and bone strength. Bone mass is the same in both cases but placing the mass further from the central axis increases resistance to bending in the larger diameter tube. (**b**) Laying down of trabecular bone in patterns according to the ambient compressive and tensile stress on the bone distributes load more effectively, increased loading leads to thicker, more inter-connected struts.

rebalanced by refilling but in osteoporosis this is a different matter.

Remodelling and osteoporosis

In osteoporosis the resorption in cortical and trabecular remodelling becomes unmatched by slower incomplete refilling. In trabecular bone, the struts and plates become thinner or disappear. Some trabecular bone may get thicker and thus stronger in one direction but lose strength in other directions due to loss of connectivity with loss of interconnecting struts. In cortical bone resorption cavities remain unfilled giving rise to areas of excess porosity known as stress concentrations. At a cellular level there is greater activation and overactivity of osteoclasts in the resorption phase, and underactivity in osteoblasts in the reversal phase, leading to a net excess of resorption. The overall effect is to weaken bone and make it more susceptible to fracture.

Recent advances in bone molecular biology have led to a greater understanding of the link between mechanical stress and cellular bone remodelling (Sommerfeldt and Rubin, 2001). The discovery of the RANK receptor (receptor activator of nuclear factor-kappa B) on osteoclasts, an activating binding-protein RANK ligand, and an inhibitory factor called osteoprotegerin (OPG) has led to new insights into the control of remodelling at the molecular level (Boyle *et al.*, 2003). Experimentally, in small animal models genetic alteration of these factors has been able to reproduce the bone morphology seen in osteoporosis and many other bone diseases. Currently, research is underway in North America into the molecular biology of bone remodelling in hibernating animals such as grizzly bears. These animals do not develop fragile bones despite no exercise or food and little exposure to sunlight for many months. An understanding of bone physiology at the molecular level using various animal models will hopefully lead to newer treatments for osteoporosis in the future, possibly without the need for exercise!

Osteoporosis

Osteoporosis is a systemic skeletal disease characterised by low bone mass and micro-architectural deterioration of bone tissue, with a consequent increase in bone fragility and susceptibility to fracture (World Health Organization (WHO) Study Group, 1994). In the European Union in 2000 there were an estimated 3.79 million osteoporotic fractures with an estimated cost of treatment of €32 billion. These figures are projected to double by 2050 (Reginster and Burlet, 2006). The causes of osteoporosis are multifactorial and include: genetic and environmental factors; hormonal, nutritional and ageing effects on bone material properties, as well as the effects of metabolic, bone and systemic diseases and their various drug regimens.

Aetiology

Genetic and environmental factors result in development of smaller bones, with fewer thinner trabeculae, thinner cortices and less accrual of bone mass during growth. Ageing leads to disordered remodelling; with advancing age over-dominance of resorptive activity leads to greater removal of older damaged bone unmatched by osteoblastic reversal. The result is a net loss of bone mass; thinner, less connected trabecular bone; and increased porosity in thinner cortical bone. Oestrogen withdrawal in females and hypogonadism in males will cause osteoporosis if it occurs at any age, but more usually gonadal insufficiency accelerates age-related remodelling failure in later life after the menopause in females. Hyperparathyroidism, secondary to calcium malabsorption, at any age in either sex, can also lead to decreased mineralisation (Kanis, 1994; Cummings and Melton III, 2002; Seeman, 2002).

In the elderly low trauma fractures must also be distinguished from 'pathological fracture' due to multiple myeloma or secondary metastatic deposits from tumours of the breast, thyroid and prostate. Many forget that osteoporosis can also affect younger patients. Patients with early gonadal failure, on high-dose steroid regimens for autoimmune or chronic inflammatory conditions, and post cancer chemotherapy are all at risk. Patients with nutritional deficiency due to anorexia nervosa, malabsorption syndromes due to coeliac disease or post abdominal surgery are also at risk of early osteoporosis (Seeman, 2002). In apparently healthy populations, lack of exercise, eating disorders, over-consumption of carbonated drinks and under-consumption of dairy produce are also implicated as major causes of poor bone health. Ultimately a combination of factors results in long-term failure of bone remodelling and repair, degradation of bone material properties and production of fragile bone of limited strength and stiffness that will fracture under normal loading conditions (Kanis, 1994).

Clinical presentation

Clinically osteoporosis should be suspected, when patients present with a low trauma fracture at a typical site: wrist, hip or spine, or if there are early signs of vertebral collapse on X-ray during the investigation of back pain. The clinical complications of osteoporosis depend on the site of the fracture although only vertebral and hip fractures result in an excess mortality (Cummings and Melton III, 2002). In the vertebral column pain, disability and spinal deformity are the main secondary problems. The most serious complications arise with hip fracture; up to 50% of patients will suffer permanent disability, and between 10–20% will die within 3 months to a year usually due to complications of prolonged immobility (Cummings and Melton III, 2002; Goldsby *et al.*, 2003; Kanis *et al.*, 2003).

Obviously the latter situation represents the clinical end point for osteoporosis, and it is far more preferable to detect those at risk earlier. Therefore, elderly patients with a strong family history of osteoporosis or early menopause, or younger patients with a history of steroid treatment, chemotherapy or any chronic disease and disability preventing normal biomechanical loading, should be investigated. Low bodyweight individuals, those with eating disorders and low body weight athletes, people on unusual diets, vegans and vegetarians, both male and female may be at risk and should also be investigated.

Investigation

In elderly patients presenting with bone pain or deformity, the medical practitioner must obtain a thorough history and perform an examination and investigations to rule out primary and secondary bone tumours; and, metabolic and endocrine disorders affecting bone. In the majority of patients this will entail, in addition to risk factor identification an estimate of bone quantity using DXA. The degree of attenuation of a dual beam of photons is correlated to bone mineral content and when divided by projected area of the site of interest an area density for the bone of in the scan area of interest is calculated. Thus DXA scans are two-dimensional images and it must be remembered that the density is not a true volumetric density but an area density. However, despite this and other errors introduced by non-uniformity of surrounding soft tissues, DXA-derived bone mineral density still remains the gold standard of clinical diagnosis in osteoporosis (Kanis, 2002).

The therapist should ensure that the patient has had a standard scan protocol in a centre specialising in osteoporosis. This usually assesses L1–L4 vertebrae, and both the left and right hip. However other regions such as the distal radius and even whole body scans can be done depending on the type of scanner device and protocols used. DXA scans report estimated area (EA, cm^2), bone mineral content (BMC, g), and area density (BMD, $g.cm^{-2}$) for regions of interest in a standard protocol of scans.

The measured BMD value is then compared with a database of mean values for the standard population. Due to racial variation in bone density these standard population databases may be different for people from different parts of the world. Scan results when compared with the same age and gender norms are referred to as 'Z scores'. However, it is more usual to compare measured values with a set of standard values typical of peak bone mass in young adults (age 20–30 years); this is known as the 'T score' (Cummings *et al.*, 2002).

In DXA terms normal bone density is then a T score of +1 to −1 SD around the mean, a difference of −1 to −2.5 SD from the mean is defined as osteopenia, and a T score of −2.5 SD or below is defined as osteoporosis (WHO Study Group, 1994; Kanis and Glüer, 2000). Severe osteoporosis is defined as the same 'T' score criteria as previously described plus an osteoporotic-related fracture (Kanis, 2002). The relevance of this is that longitudinal research has shown that fracture risk approximately doubles for every one standard deviation below mean T score. However it should be noted that any fragility fracture at any typical site also defines osteoporosis, even in the absence of low BMD from the DXA scan. It should also be noted that overall fracture risk in individual patients is determined only after a full evaluation of risk factors outlined above in conjunction with the DXA scan results. Ideally management should be prescribed by medical specialists working in osteoporosis clinics with experience in evaluation, diagnosis, investigation and treatment of the condition. Table 16.1 summarises the risk factors which may be implicated in early osteoporosis and DXA diagnostic criteria, and the associated diseases and their treatments.

Treatment and prevention of osteoporosis

The treatment and prevention of osteoporosis can been likened to the repair of a 'three-legged stool'.

Table 16.1 Summary of risk factors and diagnostic criteria for osteoporosis

Risk factors	Associated diseases	Drug therapies	Clinical criteria
FAMILY history	Cushing's syndrome	Corticosteroids	Low trauma fracture of wrist, hip, or spine
		Chemotherapy	
Smoking alcohol	Hyperparathyroidism	Immunosuppressants	**DEXA diagnostic criteria**
	Gonadal failure	Heparin	Osteopenia: T score −1 to −2.5
Low calcium intake	Acromegaly		Osteoporosis: T score ≤2.5
Low vitamin D	Insulin-dependent diabetes mellitus		Severe osteoporosis: low trauma fracture + any of above T scores
Acidic diet	Rheumatoid arthritis		
Female ageing	Renal failure		
Early menopause	Liver disease		
Asian and Caucasian	Anorexia nervosa		
Thin body type	Coeliac disease		
Immobility	Crohn's disease		
Low activity levels	Ulcerative colitis		

Over-attention to repair of one or even two legs of the stool can still result in failure, because if the third leg fails the stool will fall (Marcus, 1996). Treatment of osteopenia and osteoporosis has to consider all three main areas: adequate diet, appropriate drug therapy depending on grading and extent of osteoporosis, and appropriate skeletal mechanical loading by exercise.

The common drug therapies for osteoporosis include hormone replacement therapy, anti-resorptive medications, and recently developed bone-building medications. Nutritional advice should aim to promote adequate energy and protein intake, and according to age and gender adequate amounts of calcium and vitamin D should be present in the diet. Exercise prescription should be appropriate to age, level of mobility and bone status. In a younger fitter population with normal bone status high impact targeted bone loading exercises are recommended. At the opposite extreme in the frail elderly, exercise aims to maintain mobility and increase neuromuscular co-ordination to prevent falls. Targeted bone loading in this group can cause fractures.

Prevention is better than cure and strategies here aim for attainment of optimal peak bone mass by early adulthood by focusing on targeted bone loading exercise programmes and adequate nutrition in childhood and adolescence. Further prevention strategies through adult life can build bone and slow bone loss, however, they do not have the same magnitude of effect as that seen with bone-loading exercise programmes in childhood and adolescence.

Nutritional factors

Growth, development and maintenance of bone structure requires adequate protein intake to provide the necessary amino acid building blocks for collagen synthesis and adequate intake of calcium, and its co-factor in metabolism vitamin D_3, to form the mineral component hydroxyapatite. Growth, repair and remodelling also require energy, therefore adequate calorific intake is also required to maintain bone tissue integrity. Inadequate protein, mineral, vitamin D and low calorie intake for whatever reason will ultimately lead to poor bone quality; and no exercise programme can create strong healthy bones without proper nutrition. An example of poor nutritional practice associated with over-exercise occurs in the 'female athletic triad' – a clinical syndrome seen in gymnasts, ballet dancers and long-distance runners that is characterised by eating disorder, amenorrhoea and osteoporosis.

In the growing skeletons of children and adolescents, adequate amounts of calcium and vitamin D_3 are essential for the attainment of greater peak bone mass in early adulthood. Adolescent girls and boys require up to 1200 mg of calcium a day during the growth spurt. However, the need for calcium and vitamin D in adults and elderly populations is often underestimated. Recommended female daily allowances (RDA) for calcium and vitamin D_3, for use in conjunction with an exercise programme are shown in Table 16.2.

Practical guidelines

Most adults with normal bone density or mild osteopenia should take 500 ml of full fat milk or one of the newer milk products fortified with extra calcium and vitamin D once a day. In established osteoporosis milk intake would have to double to 1 litre of milk a day. For many this is impractical, therefore increasing intake of calcium-rich dairy produce plus a calcium and Vitamin D supplement once daily are usually required instead. Patients should be discouraged from following very strict vegetarian and vegan diets, or from fad diets with

Table 16.2　Age group and RDA for calcium and vitamin D_3

Age group (years)	Calcium (mg)	Vitamin D (IU)
Girls (9–11)	1000	200
Teenage girls (12–18)	1300	200
Women (19–50)	1000	200
Pregnancy	1000–1300	200
Women (51–70)	1300	400
Women (>70)	1300	800

Adapted from Exercise and Osteoporosis (www.sma.org.au).

excessive protein intake and the excessive intake of acidic carbonated drinks.

Drug therapies

It is important for the therapist to be aware of the common drug regimens for osteoporosis; although widely prescribed, many have side effects and if recognised must be reported to the prescribing doctor. Drug treatment should be tailored to the individual patient, taking into account other illnesses and possible interactions with other medications.

In early or pre-menopause, some women with osteoporosis may be prescribed hormone replacement therapy in the form of oestrogen. Oestrogen has been shown to prevent fractures, prevent bone loss and increase calcium absorption. However, due to a slightly increased risk of female cancers, newer selective oestrogen receptor modulator (SERM) medications have been developed. SERMs such as raloxifene have the same actions on bone as oestrogen without the increased risk of uterine and breast cancers. Calcitonin and the bisphosphonate group of drugs are the other commonly prescribed anti-resorptive medications for osteoporosis. Calcitonin is taken as a nasal spray and may be especially useful in the case of bone pain from vertebral collapse. The bisphosphonate group of drugs, alendronate, etidronate and risedronate, are very effective drugs but are particularly tricky to administer. They have to be taken in the morning on an empty stomach, and the patient must stand in the upright position and be well hydrated. Gastrointestinal upset is common and although these are very effective anti-resorptive drugs, many patients cannot tolerate their side effects. Newer injectable forms are now coming on the market with extremely long half-lives, which could potentially mean an injection once or twice a year rather than daily oral medication.

The last group of bone-building drugs, parathyroid hormone (PTH) and strontium ranelate, should only be prescribed in patients with severe osteoporosis. Timing and dosage especially of PTH therapy depends on initial serum PTH level and other factors in the patient history. PTH may actively stimulate new bone formation or bone resorption depending on timing and dosage and should therefore is only be prescribed in specialist osteoporosis clinics (Delmas, 2002).

Exercise and bone health

The evidence for the use of exercise in the management of osteoporosis comes from three areas: epidemiological studies on fracture rates from countries with different lifestyles; studies comparing bone density of athletes with inactive populations; and animal studies of bone remodelling. There is also an accumulating body of evidence from intervention studies looking at change in bone mass and fracture incidence with varying exercise programmes and in different age groups.

Comparative studies of fracture incidence in Europe, Africa and Asia have shown that even after adjustment for age-related decline in bone health, there was still an excess of osteoporosis-related fractures in those countries with more Western, urbanised sedentary lifestyles (Mosekilde, 1995). Studies on fracture incidence within Europe have suggested that effects of postmenopausal oestrogen insufficiency in females and decreasing testosterone levels with ageing in males may have been overemphasised and lifestyle and genetic factors may be more important in the development of osteoporosis (Kanis, 1993). Based on these findings Kanis has recommended habitual exercise as way of protecting the population from the effects of osteoporosis.

Studies on the bone density of athletes have shown significantly higher density in the impact loaded forearms of gymnasts when compared with runners, and higher bone density in the lumbar spine and hips of runners than that of non-impact loaded swimmers (Kannus *et al.*, 1996; Frost, 1997). Biological mechanostat theory suggests that prerequisite stresses and strain levels are required to activate bone modelling BMUs to maintain bone health (Frost, 1988). Essentially, strain levels of greater than 1500–3000 microstrain are purported to induce bone modelling processes and increase bone mass, cortical thickness and cross-sectional area; but much lower strain levels, 100–300 microstrain, are all that are required to decrease activation frequency of mechanically controlled bone remodelling and thus preserve bone. However, below this level, ~100 microstrain, there is increased activation of BMUs, loss of bone mass and thus any unloaded structures will disappear. At a cellular level, therefore, exercise could theoretically prevent bone loss in two ways: first, high strains could stimulate bone modelling, i.e. new bone formation, and, second, intermediate level strains could inhibit the mismatched remodelling processes causing osteoporosis.

General recommendations

Basic training theory suggests that, given the correct exercise mode, progressive overload in training by manipulation of FITT (*frequency/intensity/time/type*) with adequate time for repair or recovery will result in adaptation (Kannus *et al.*, 1996; Turner and Robling, 2005). It has also been shown that lack of force through the skeleton due to prolonged immobility due to enforced bed rest, or in zero gravity due to space flight will result in loss of bone mineral, the *disuse* principle of training.

Unfortunately many studies involving exercise and bone density do not consider basic physiological training principles. When evaluating training or exercise studies purporting to have an effect on BMD, one must also consider the basic principles of training listed below.

- *Specificity:* The major impact of the activity should be at the site where BMD is being measured as the response to loading appears to be a localized effect.
- *Overload:* To effect change in bone mass, the training stimulus must exceed the normal loading.

- *Reversibility:* The positive effect of a training programme on bone will be lost if the programme is discontinued.
- *Initial values:* Those with the lowest levels of BMD have a greater capacity for percentage improvement in training studies; those with average or above average bone mass have the least.
- *Diminishing returns:* Each person has an individual biological ceiling that determines the extent of a possible training effect. As this ceiling is approached, gains in bone mass will slow and eventually plateau.

Targeted bone loading

In terms of specificity, exercise can be divided into activity which is good for overall general health and that which is good for bone health. Swimming, cycling and may benefit general cardiovascular health but have little if any impact on bone mass accrual or prevention of bone loss and therefore bone strength. The concept of *targeted bone loading* is used to describe exercise which specifically stimulates bone modelling or inhibits bone remodelling processes and thus improves bone strength. For targeted bone loading, exercise must be weight-bearing and mechanical stress on the bone must be greater than those normally experienced by the skeleton during everyday activities (specificity and overload principles).

The way in which the force is applied to the skeleton also makes a difference. Jumps off a raised platform 0.3 m of the ground 20–30 times three times per day with total exercise duration less than 30 minutes/day, is more effective than a 2-hour walk or bike ride. Forces generated during the gait cycle of walking and running are attenuated as one moves up the skeleton and by the time forces reach the axial skeleton there is little substantive loading of the vertebral column (site specificity). In terms of practical exercise advice, walking and running will only benefit the bones of the lower limb, and other forms of loading need to be used to target the spine.

Exercise programmes to improve or maintain bone health should continue throughout life, and whenever clinically appropriate should involve targeted bone loading, that is, an exercise mode which

specifically exposes bone to loading at stresses and strains in excess to that encountered in everyday activities. Only in this situation will the training stimulus be great enough to produce adaptation. Exercise for osteoporosis can be thought of in three main areas according to chronological age:

(1) Optimum accrual of bone mass in childhood and adolescence
(2) Prevention of bone loss through adulthood
(3) Prevention of age-related bone loss and falls in older people.

Optimum bone accrual in childhood and adolescence

Childhood and adolescence is an especially important time to improve bone mass through exercise (Khan *et al.*, 2000; Janz *et al.*, 2004; Forwood *et al.*, 2006). Achievement of a higher peak bone mass by age 26–30 years means that later age-related decline in bone quantity starts from higher peak values and takes longer to reach fracture thresholds (Fig. 16.3).

In terms of training principles and targeted loading, regular short duration and high intensity physical exercise in childhood especially at or slightly before the pubescent growth spurt can significantly increase accrual of a greater bone mass by the third decade (Kannus *et al.*, 1996). It goes without saying that inactivity such as television, computer video games and vehicular transport for short journeys should be limited.

Exercise in young children should be weight-bearing, provided there are no contraindications to high impact, but most importantly the emphasis should be on fun. McKay and co-workers from Canada have developed simple exercise programmes, such as 'bounce the bell' and 'leaping lizards', to study effects of exercise on bone health in primary school children (McKay *et al.*, 2005). For example, the leaping lizards programme involves competitive team drills of running, jumps and turns performed over a short course marked by cones at 2.5 m intervals. The team that picks up all cones in the quickest time is the winner! Exercise duration is approximately 15 minutes (time) and the races can be performed on a daily basis (frequency). The therapist can adapt this simple routine and vary speed and length (intensity) of the course, and change running to hopping, galloping or bunny hops (type) etc. to ensure progressive overload.

In adolescents (<18 years) and younger adults (<28 years) the key to increasing bone mass accrual is again to encourage short duration, high-impact weight-bearing exercise. In this group, organised classes such as step aerobics and dance, or running, are more appropriate. In all younger age groups simply advocating any weight-bearing activity, such as fast walking and sporting activity of any type for at least 30 minutes per day, may be just as effective.

Prevention of bone loss through adulthood

In adults (30–50 years) small but significant differences in bone density have been shown between exercising groups and controls. Exercise modes in these studies include jogging, supervised and unsupervised weight-training, high-impact jumps or steps incorporated into an aerobics exercises. Results of these studies show only small gains, 1–2% increase or no change in bone density at the hip and spine in comparison with controls. The best results seem to be with high-impact jumping programmes (Bassey and Ramsdale, 1995).

Increasing bone mass over and above that seen in a healthy active population can probably only be achieved by resistance training. Several studies have shown that bone density at certain sites can be predicted by overall muscle strength in that general area of muscle attachment. Increases in BMD due to strength training programmes are site specific, and the magnitude of response is again governed by FITT principles in modulation of progressive overload. If resistance programmes are stopped, muscle strength and BMD will be lost, i.e. the disuse principle. A combination of a step-based aerobic programme, and gym exercises incorporating body resistance and weights, 12 exercises, 3 sets, 15 repetitions (weight depending on 1 or 3 RM (repetitions maximum)) has been shown to be effective programme in preventing decline and/or further developing bone mass in this group (Friedlander *et al.*, 1995). It should also be re-emphasised here that over-exercise in young adults can suppress levels of gonadal hormones, and result in low bone density.

Slowing age-related bone loss and prevention of falls in older people

Although weight-bearing exercises, such as aerobics and strengthening exercises are all useful for increasing BMD in the spine and walking can increase BMD in the hip (Bonauti *et al.*, 2002), it is important to determine bone status before exercise prescription. Exercise programmes for older people with normal density can focus on short duration, high-impact programmes. However, vigorous activity in those with established osteoporosis is potentially dangerous as it may cause further wedge fractures of the spine and as exercise in older people has not been shown to improve bone density, it cannot be recommended (Forwood and Larson, 2000). In particular exercise with sudden stop starts and or twisting movements, involving sudden abdominal flexion or impact loading should be avoided. In very frail elderly people with low bone density, exercise programmes should focus on improving muscle strength for mobility and balance, improving quality of life and preventing falls. Exercises that enhance posture, such as back extension exercises in a seated position or seated back and scapula extension against a wall can counteract anterior wedging in the spine.

Exercise programmes for osteoporosis: key information sources

There is now a vast resource of information with regard to exercise in individual patients with osteoporosis or for those who just want to improve their bone health. There are many fact sheets available giving general lifestyle advice on exercise and nutrition at all ages from reputable sources e.g. the Medicine and Science for Women in Sport Group of Sports Medicine Australia (2008; www.sma.org.au). The National Osteoporosis Society (2008) in the UK (www.nos.org.uk) has also produced two useful booklets, *Exercise and Bone Health* and *Exercise and Osteoporosis*, which contain exercise advice to prevent osteoporosis and exercise advice for those patients with established osteoporosis. For the therapist, Forwood and Larson (2000) have outlined safe exercise guidelines for those with established osteoporosis, in a series of postural exercises for frail elderly people. For a synopsis of the current research in the area of bone health and physical activity consult Khort *et al.* (2004). *Physical Activity and Bone Health* covers exercise and osteoporosis in its entirety with a variety of programmes to maximise bone mass accrual in childhood and adolescence, strengthen bone in adulthood and in the elderly, plus effective exercise programmes to slow age-related bone loss and prevent falls (Khan *et al.*, 2001).

It must be stressed that those in at risk groups for osteoporosis or osteopenia should always have an assessment of bone health in a specialist medical osteoporosis clinic prior to any exercise advice or programme. In addition it should be appreciated that the prescription of exercise alone in the absence of adequate nutrition and in certain cases without a pharmacological intervention will be largely ineffective and in certain cases may put the patient at serious risk of a fragility fracture.

Summary

In the treatment of osteoporosis, exercise can be employed as a primary prevention strategy in childhood and adolescence to maximise accrual of bone mineral by early adulthood. In the adult years, exercise is necessary to prevent or decelerate bone loss due to natural ageing processes, and, especially in urbanised societies, to counteract the negative aspects of a sedentary lifestyle. In the early adult years, targeted exercise programmes and resistance training are required to improve bone strength above normal levels. In later years, exercise may slow the rates of bone loss and additionally by maintaining mobility, balance, and muscle strength, and prevent the falls which can cause fracture of more fragile bones. In patients with established osteoporosis the therapist needs to work closely with allied health professionals in the provision of individually tailored, safe, and well-monitored exercise programmes. The therapist must also be mindful of the hazards of exercise prescription in patients with severe osteoporosis, as not all exercise is beneficial and some exercises are dangerous for fragile bones.

References

Bassey, E.J. and Ramsdale, S.J. (1995) Weight-bearing exercise and ground reaction forces: a 12-month randomized controlled trial of effects on bone mineral density in healthy postmenopausal women. *Bone*, 16, 469–476.

Bonauti, D., Shea, B., Iovine, R., Robinson, V., Kemper, H., Well, G., Tugwell, P. and Cranney, A. (2002) Exercise for preventing and treating osteoporosis in postmeopausal women. *Cochrane Database of Systematic Reviews*, Issue 2, CD000333.

Boyle, W.J., Simonet, W.S. and Lacey, D.L. (2003) Osteoclast differentiation and activation. *Nature*, 423, 337–342.

Carter, D.R., Van Der Meulen, M.C.H. and Beaupri, G.S. (1996) Mechanical factors in bone growth and development. *Bone*, 18 (Suppl. 1), 5S–10S.

Compston, J.E. (1990) Osteoporosis. *Journal of Clinical Endocrinology*, 33, 653–682.

Cummings, S.R. and Melton, L.J. (2002) Epidemiology and outcomes of osteoporotic fractures. *Lancet*, 359, 1761–1767.

Cummings, S., Cosman, F. and Jamal, S.A. (2002) *Osteoporosis: An Evidence-Based Guide to Prevention and Management*. American College of Physicians. Philadelphia, USA.

Currey, J.D. (2003) *The Mechanical Adaptations of Bones*. Princeton University Press, Princeton, New Jersey.

Delmas, P.D. (2002) Osteoporosis IV: Treatment of postmenopausal osteoporosis. *Lancet*, 359, 2018–2026.

Forwood, M. and Larson, M. (2000) Exercise recommendations for Osteoporosis. *Australian Family Physician*, 29, 761–764.

Forwood, M., Baxter-Jones, A. and Beck, T. (2006) Physical activity and strength of the femoral neck during the adolescent growth spurt: a longitudinal analysis. *Bone*, 38, 576.

Friedlander, A.L., Genant, H.K., Sadowsky, S., Byl, N.N. and Glüer, C.C. (1995) A two-year program of aerobics and weight training enhances bone mineral density of young women. *Journal of Bone and Mineral Research*, 10, 574–585.

Frost, H.M. (1987) The mechanostat: A proposed pathogenic mechanism of osteoporosis and the bone mass effects of mechanical and non mechanical agents. *Bone Mineral*, 2, 73–85.

Frost, H.M. (1988) Vital biomechanics: Proposed general concepts for skeletal adaptations to mechanical usage. *Calcified Tissue International*, 42, 145–156.

Frost, H.M. (1997) Why do marathon runners have less bone than weight lifters? A vital-biomechanical view and explanation. *Bone*, 20, 183–189.

Gibson, L. and Ashby, M. (1997) *Cellular Solids: Structure and Properties*, pp. 429–450. Cambridge University Press, Cambridge, UK.

Goldsby, R.A., Kindt, T.J., Osborne, B.A. and Kuby, J. (2003) *Immunology*, 5th edn. WH Freeman and Company, New York, New York.

Janz, K., Burns, T. and Levy, S. (2004) Everyday activity predicts bone geometry in children: the Iowa bone development study. *Medicine and Science in Sports and Exercise*, 36, 1124–1131.

Kanis, J.A. (1993) The incidence of hip fracture in Europe. *Osteoporosis International*, 19 (Suppl. 1), S10–S15.

Kanis, J.A. (1994) *Osteoporosis*. Blackwell, Oxford.

Kanis, J.A. (2002) Diagnosis of osteoporosis and assessment of fracture risk. *Lancet*, 359, 1929–1936.

Kanis, J.A. and Glüer, C.C. (2000) For the committee of scientific advisors, international osteoporosis foundation; An update on the diagnosis and assessment of osteoporosis with densitometry. *Osteoporosis International*, 11, 192–202.

Kanis, J., Oden, A. and Johnell, O. (2003) The components of excess mortality after hip fracture. *Bone*, 32, 468.

Kannus, P., Sievanen, H. and Vuori, I. (1996) Physical loading, exercise and bone. *Bone*, 18 (Suppl. 1), S1–S3.

Keaveny, T.M. and Yeh, O.C. (2002) Architecture and trabecular bone–toward an improved understanding of the biomechanical effects of age, sex and osteoporosis. *Journal of Musculoskeletal and Neuronal Interactions*, 2, 205–208.

Khan, K., McKay, H. and Haapasalo, H. (2000) Does childhood and adolescence provide a unique opportunity for exercise to strengthen the skeleton? *Journal of Science and Medicine in Sport*, 3, 150–164.

Khan, K., McKay, H., Kannus, P., Bailey, D., Wark, J. and Bennell, K. (2001) *Physical Activity and Bone Health*, 1st edn. Human Kinetics, Champaign, Illinois.

Kohrt, W.M., Bloomfield, S.A., Little, K.D., Nelson, M.E. and Yingling, V.R. (2004) Physical activity and bone health. *Medicine and Science in Sports and Exercise*, 36, 1985–1996.

Marcus, R. (1996) Endogenous and nutritional factors affecting bone. *Bone*, 18 (Suppl. 1), S11–S13.

Martin, R.B. and Burr, D.B. (1989) *Structure, function and adaptation of compact bone*. Raven, New York, New York.

McKay, H.A., MacLean, L., Petit, M., MacKelvie-O'Brien, K., Janssen, P., Beck, T. and Khan, K.M. (2005) Bounce at the bell: a novel program of short bouts of exercise improves proximal femur bone mass in early pubertal children. British. *Journal of Sports Medicine*, 39, 521–526.

Mosekilde, L. (1995) Osteoporosis and exercise. *Bone*, 17, 193–195.

National Osteoporosis Society. (2008) Camerton, Bath. Available at: www.nos.org.uk/NetCommunity/Page.aspx?pid=466&srcid=234> (accessed July 2008).

Reginster, J. and Burlet, N. (2006) Osteoporosis a still increasing prevalence. *Bone*, 38 (2 Suppl. 1), S4–S9.

Seeman, E. (2002) Osteoporosis II: Pathogenesis of osteoporosis in women and men. *Lancet*, 359, 1841–1850.

Sommerfeldt, D.W. and Rubin, C.T. (2001) Biology of bone and how it orchestrates the form and function of the skeleton. *European Spine Journal*, 10 (Suppl. 2), S86–S95.

Sports Medicine Australia. (2008) *Australian Sports Medicine Federation*. Available at: www.sma.org.au/information/women_in_sport.asp (accessed July 2008).

Turner, C.H. and Robling, A.G. (2005) Exercises for improving bone strength. *British Journal of Sports Medicine*, 39, 188–189.

Turner, C.H., Chandran, A. and Pidaparti, R.M. (1995) The anisotropy of osteonal bone and its ultrastructural implications. *Bone*, 17, 85–89.

WHO Study Group. (1994) *WHO Technical Report Series S43*. WHO, Geneva, Switzerland.

Index

Exercise Therapy in the Management of Musculoskeletal Disorders, First Edition. Edited by Fiona Wilson, John Gormley and Juliette Hussey.
© 2011 Blackwell Publishing Ltd